Roadmap to
The Correct
Prescription

Roadmap to
The Correct
Prescription

Aude Sapere

S.M. Gunavante

Fourth Edition
Revised & Enlarged

B. Jain Publishers (P) Ltd.
An ISO 9001 : 2000 Certified Company
USA — Europe — India

ROADMAP TO CORRECT PRESCRIPTION

5th Impression: 2010

All rights reserved. No part of this book may be reproduced, stored in a retrieval system or transmitted, in any form or by any means, mechanical, photocopying, recording or otherwise, without any prior written permission of the publisher.

© with the author

Published by Kuldeep Jain for
B. JAIN PUBLISHERS (P) LTD.
An ISO 9001 : 2000 Certified Company
1921/10, Chuna Mandi, Paharganj, New Delhi 110 055 (INDIA)
Tel.: +91-11-4567 1000 • *Fax:* +91-11-4567 1010
Email: info@bjain.com • *Website:* **www.bjain.com**

Printed in India by
J.J. Offset Printers

ISBN: 978-81-319-1159-4

DEDICATED

to

SHRI PRABODH M. MEHTA

who has silently but most

efficiently guided the progress of

Dr. SUBODH MEHTA MEDICAL CENTRE

from a small beginning

to its present status.

S. M. Gunavante

FOREWORD

This book is an example of how humanity benefits when a dedicated person like Mr. S.M. Gunavante comes in touch with a man of vision like Dr. S.K. Mankad, who occupies a decision-making position in a social service organisation like the Dr. Subodh Mehta Medical Centre. It speaks much for Dr. Mankad's vision that he was "dreaming" of conducting a course in homoeopathy for modern medical graduates, and still more so that, when he met Mr. Gunavante, he did not take much time to recognise that this man though a lay homoeopath, could help him in realising his dream. For my part, I am glad that when in the middle of November 1980, Dr. Mankad requested me to guide him in the effort, I readily agreed. Since then Mr. Gunavante used to hand over to me the course lessons prepared by him and I used to guide him with suitable points for writing the next lesson.

Little had I realised in the early stages of this effort that the ultimate result would be a nice, comprehensive book on all aspects of homoeopathy, except for Materia Medica, which naturally has to be read at source from the pen of masters. What is striking about this book is that it is simple, lucid and takes the reader step by step so imperceptibly into the deeper aspects of the science that even a novice hardly realises that he is already in the thick of it. The author has indeed taken great pains to consult various authoritative sources and present each aspect, be it the similimum, the provings, the evaluation of symptoms, the selection of the remedy, the potency question or the management of the case, with the mastery of detail that even veterans may find this to be a useful book of reference whenever needed.

I have no doubt that this book will help greatly in the further advancement of homoeopathy, and that whoever takes the trouble of studying it and follows the guidance given, will have little trouble in making his mark as a successful practitioner of homoeopathic medicine.

Bombay.

Date : 30th March, 1982.

Dr. Anil Bhatia
B. Sc., D.M.S. (Cal.)
DF. Hom. (London)

Principal
Smt. Chandanben Mohanbhai Patel
Homoeopathic Medical College,

Member
Central Council of Homoeopathy.

PREFACE TO FOURTH EDITION

Opportunity of this Edition has been taken by me to revise the book extensively with the object of presenting homoeopathic philosophy more comprehensively than before. The relative advantages and disadvantages of various repertories available today to the practitioners, especially those of Kent and Boger-Boenninghausen, have been more clearly defined. As practice makes a man perfect, twenty exercises for repertorisation have been added for the first time. The chapter on "How to Study the Materia Medica" has been entirely re-written presenting a novel and realistic method. This chapter also includes significant ideas on the practical application of Materia Medica on the basis of the "minimum syndrome of maximum value," and by using the most peculiar and indispensable symptom/feature as a pivot around which the similimum can be searched for. Further, the minimum essential characteristics of ten remedies have also been given, as a model.

All in all, I look forward to this edition providing all the philosophical and practical guidance one may need in the practice of this wonderful science of healing — homoeopathy — on the lines handed down to us by masters of the art.

20th July, 1990   **S. M. Gunavante**

Moraya Villa,
12th Road, Khar,
Bombay - 400052.

PREFACE TO THIRD EDITION

The call for a Second Edition of this work in less than two years is, indeed, very gratifying since it shows that it has met the needs and expectations of those interested in learning the fundamentals of homoeopathy. I have taken this opportunity to elaborate a number of points in order to enable students to easily grasp the new ideas. These include Dr. Sarabhai Kapadia's bold ideas on the repetition of high potencies. Practising homoeopathy as an art with the help of Kent's repertory is another important addition which it is hoped will be found useful and of much practical value by practitioners. Believing as I do strongly that Hahnemannian homoeopathy is the only law of truly scientific medical therapeutics, I offer this work to all those who are interested in alleviating human suffering, including the practitioners of modern medicine, who are bound to be struck by the marvellously curative powers of this science, if they only take some trouble to learn and practise it.

21st January, 1984.   **S. M. Gunavante**

Bombay - 400052.

PREFACE TO FIRST EDITION

Homoeopathy is marching ahead. It certainly will, so long as there are seekers after truth who are not afraid of investigating the claims made on behalf of any system of medicine and accepting them if found true. As Hahnemann said, "Homoeopathy demands nothing but to be put to the acid test of experience". It is a happy sign of the times that there are truth-seekers among practitioners of modern medicine who are open-minded and are eager to know what homoeopathy is and what it can do to help them in serving ailing humanity more efficiently. After all, the practice of medicine is one of the noblest of professions; and noblest is the man who takes it as a mission. Such nobility is twice blessed. It blesses the beneficiaries, with the cure of their ailments; and the beneficiaries, in turn, bless the practitioner not only materially, but also with honour, name and fame.

Dr. Subodh Mehta belonged to such a tribe of noble practitioners of homoeopathic medicine. From a professor of chemistry he rose to the position of a healer through homoeopathy. People with various ailments thronged to him in large numbers every day and he gave them relief and cure, free of charge, through the sweet little pills. Shortly before his death in 1970, a grateful populace contributed generously and presented him with a purse, with which he set up a trust charged with the tasks of continuing his mission of healing, and advancing the cause of homoeopathy.

It was my good fortune to come in touch with Dr. S.K. Mankad, Director of the Subodh Mehta Medical Centre, which is run by the Trust, a few months ago. Animated by a keen desire to launch some activity in fulfilment of the objects of the Trust, Dr. Mankad was at that time dreaming of organising a course of lectures on homoeopathy for allopathic practitioners who were asking him for enlightenment on this subject. I jumped at the idea and assured him of whatever assistance I could possibly render to realise his "dream." As we discussed the matter further, I felt encouraged by his confidence in me. In addition, fired as I was by enthusiasm at the magical cures effected by homoeopathy, I started writing out the course after consulting and studying whatever literature was available to me. This is how this book came to be written, and I have great pleasure in presenting it to those (not necessarily allopaths) who are desirous of learning how to master "without tears," the art of prescribing homoeopathic remedies.

An effort has been made in this course to give as much detailed information as possible and that logically and step by step so as to facilitate easy grasp of each subject dealt with herein. Selection of the homoeopathic remedy depends upon a mastery of the Materia Medica as well as the philosophy of this science. As this depends on the evaluation of several factors, any sure guidance given on this point can be an important contribution to the advancement and popularisation of homoeopathy. The author believes that such sure guidance, though known to homoeopaths, is not availed of by them for want of confidence in the method, which can only come through persistent practice. A brief description of classical literature on homoeopathy, to suit different stages of learning is also given, for the guidance of beginners.

When homoeopathy is a science, as it undoubtedly is, it stands to reason that the successful prescriptions of masters of this art should be capable of replication by any other prescriber, given the identical data. As a corollary, for a given case several doctors should be able independently, to return a verdict of the same remedy. How can we achieve this worthy objective? This can be done by taking care of two simple requirements, *viz.*, having an efficient *instrument* and mastering the *technique* of using it. An artist or craftsman who has one of these but not the other cannot deliver the goods. In homoeopathy, the instrument is represented by a complete and well-planned repertory (a complete Materia Medica with the Hahnemannian schema being the other side of the coin). Technique is represented by a mastery of the principles and philosophy as reflected in the ability to take the case (eliciting the characteristic symptoms) and evaluating the most important symptoms for repertorisation and if necessary, reference to the Materia Medica. The instrument should provide all the comparisons and differentiations between remedies with their grades of clinical confirmation, while the technique lies in our ability to use the instrument efficiently, i.e., speedily and accurately. When we master the technique through constant practise, our ability unconsciously rises to the level of an art or intuition. This logical process seems to explain how the master prescribers of olden days developed homoeopathic prescribing as an art, without such detailed repertories, but through enormous labour. When we look at the pinnacle of the skyscraper we feel dizzy; the artistry behind it seems mystifying; but when we analyse step by step the procedures followed by the artists till they reached the pinnacle, there unfolds before us a technique which any one with average intelligence and the will to "achieve" can master. It cannot be different with the process of selecting the similimum for a given case.

My plea, therefore, is to develop a perfect repertory which includes all symptoms known to have been reliably produced or repeatedly cured by the well-proved as well as the insufficiently proved drugs. The Boger-Boenninghausen's and Kent's repertories together, used as complementaries, provide us with much of the material required for this "perfect repertory." In my humble opinion, we should take the plan of Boger-Boenninghausen's repertory as a blue-print and, wherever it is found wanting, we should transfer rubrics and remedies from Kent into the former. An effort should also be made to incorporate additional rubrics on the basis of clinical confirmations of nosodes (including bowel nosodes) and ill-proved remedies. But this is a task for the future; for the time being, the two repertories together can solve most of our problems even in rare and difficult cases.

I have dilated on the usefulness of repertorisation and beg to be excused for it; but I did so only with a view to draw pointed attention to the fact that this is a very much neglected aspect of most of our homoeopathic practitioners. "Want of time" is a plea based on wrong notions of priority. In fact, careful case-taking, developing the skill in repertorisation by using "the minimum symptoms of maximum value" and administration of the correct remedy, in the appropriate potency from the outset is the best "time-saver" and "fame-builder."

Having personally experienced the difficulties of finding the remedy by reliance on a "knowledge of the Materia Medica", or reference to it alone without the aid of a complete repertory, and thereafter having experienced the ease with which one can find the remedy (or a group of two or three competing remedies) in the majority of cases with the help of a repertory, I felt that new students of this science should not have to go through the same mill of disappointment and discouragement from the outset and thus find an excuse to slide into "mixo-pathy" or even allopathy. Therefore, an "out of the beaten track" method of learning the Materia Medica through the repertory and "learning through treating" has been recommended and explained in this course. Readers and leaders of thought on this subject are requested to let us have their opinion as to how far this method really serves the intended purpose. We shall be only too glad to revise our opinion or introduce improvements in the method in the light of experience of a wide cross section of practitioners.

We have resisted the temptation to give, in this book, even an outline of the more important remedies in our Materia Medica, because even the best condensation would not do justice to the vast range of action of our polychrests. Such an effort is also not necessary in view of the fact that there are excellent books from masters of this art like Nash's *Leaders*, Allen's *Keynotes and Characteristics*, Tyler's *Drug Pictures* and Kent's *Lectures* which, if read in this order, will help the learner to grasp the genius of the remedies much better than through any other method. Yet, nothing can equal the confidence in the power, and facilitate acquisition of the comparative knowledge of the peculiarities, of each remedy which we can gain from the successful treatment of each case with the help of a repertory.

Apart from the good fortune of receiving encouragement from Dr. S.K. Mankad, I consider myself especially favoured by Dr. Anil Bhatia, Principal of the Govt. Homoeopathic Medical College, Bombay, who despite his busy schedule of work, went through the draft of this course and made valuable suggestions for its improvement. My thanks are also due to Dr. Bhanu D. Desai, who instilled faith in and guided me in the use of Boger-Boenninghausen's *Repertory*. I must especially acknowledge the guidance I have obtained from the writings of Drs. Dewan Harish Chand, Jugal Kishore, J.N. Kanjilal (and the *Hahnemannian Gleanings* of which he was the editor), S.P. Koppikar (and the *Homoeopthic Heritage* of which he is the editor) and the late Dr. P. Sankaran (and the *Indian Journal of Homoeopathic Medicine* edited by him), apart from other classical masters like

J.T. Kent, Gibson Miller, H.A. Roberts, Margaret Tyler, A. Pulford, F. Bellokossy, Elizabeth Hubbard, Sir John Weir, B.K. Sarkar, etc. Finally, I am grateful to Dr. H.L. Chitkara of New Delhi for having gone through the typescript critically and making a number of suggestions which have enhanced its utility.

While credit for all the good and proper ideas incorporated at appropriate places in this course belongs to the various authoritative sources which I have consulted, I hope to be excused for any deficiencies or inaccuracies in their presentation. Suggestions for improving the utility of this book (which may be sent to Dr. Subodh Mehta Medical Centre, 16th Road, Khar, Bombay) will be thankfully acknowledged and considered for incorporation in subsequent editions.

Finally, in consideration of the fact that, but for the inspiration provided by the Dr. Subodh Mehta Medical Relief Trust, this book would not have seen the light of day, and as this has been a labour of love for homoeopathy, I have relinquished all my rights in favour of the said Trust. I will consider myself amply rewarded if this work helps in the greater spread of Hahnemannian homoeopathy for the true cure of various ailments which humanity is heir to.

Bombay.

S. M. Gunavante

15th March, 1982.

DR. SUBODH MEHTA
MEDICAL RELIEF TRUST

Dr. Subodh Mehta Medical Relief Trust is a standing monument to the zeal of the man, whose name it bears, for the highest ideal of social service, namely, for healing the ailments of suffering humanity. The progress being made by the Centre, run by the Trust, from year to year is as impressive as the saga of Dr. Subodh Mehta's service to the ailing people who flocked to him for over thirty years at his residence, was inspiring.

Brilliant Career. Born in a lawyer family of Surat, Dr. Mehta passed his B.A., B.Sc. and M.Sc. with credit and took up his first assignment as an Assistant Lecturer in his alma-mater, the then Royal Institute of Science, Bombay. He rapidly climbed up the ladder of academic positions and rose to become Professor and Head of the Department of Chemistry, which post he held with distinction till his retirement in 1960. During this period he had prepared about 60 research papers on problems of organic and physical chemistry and his work received ungrudging recognition from scientific bodies in India and England. He had also the signal honour of presiding over the Chemistry Section of the Indian Science Congress, held in Calcutta in 1957.

Mission of Healing. The ways of providence are indeed unpredictable and young Subodh, who originally did not believe in the sweet little pills of homoeopathy, gradually came to see that they had cured him of his chronic indigestion. His scientific mind, therefore, would not rest until he found the secret of their power. He launched on an extensive study of this science which convinced him that homoeopathy is founded on an unalterable law of cure. Now, with his instinctive zeal for alleviating the sufferings of people, he launched on a mission of healing through homoeopathy using his newly acquired knowledge of the science to treat whosoever came to him for help. Very soon the trickle became a stream and as years rolled on, a time came when the number of patients who were all treated free of charge at his residence, became much too large, about 300 a day for a one-man mission. He then took on a few young qualified assistants for being trained to continue this mission of healing, some of whom are still working in the Medical Centre.

Establishment of the Trust. Dr. Mehta could not bear to see the helplessness of incurable patients and entertained fond ideas of research to discover cures for such problem cases. In order to give shape to his ideas and in recognition of his public services for over thirty years, his admirers and grateful beneficiaries founded a Trust in February 1968 wih Dr. Subodh Mehta as chairman, with the object of helping the advancement of learning in medical science in general and homoeopathy in particular. People's contributions poured in to swell the corpus of the Trust fund to Rs. 1,70,000.

A Sad Blow. At this promising juncture, a sad and shocking blow was dealt by fate as Dr. Mehta expired suddenly just about a month after the Trust was formed. The surviving Trustees did not allow this blow to daunt their spirits. They bent all their energies with even more determination to realise the objects of the Trust. They marched ahead step by step towards the establishment of a full-fledged Medical Centre. Following the growth of its activities steadily year by year, the Centre acquired in 1976 its own premises at 16th Road, Khar, Bombay - 52.

The Centre Today. The Centre today caters to a variety of needs of the Bombayman in respect of homoeopathic treatment, consultation in major branches of modern medicine as well as comprehensive diagnostic services — all at considerably concessional rates. The Centre is manned by eight homoeopathic doctors and forty honorary doctors of modern medicine belonging to various specialities.

The coming together of the homoeopathic system and the graduates of modern medicine under one roof has created interest about homoeopathy in the latter. To satisfy this interest, the Centre added one more wing to its activities, namely, in the field of education. A twelve weeks course of "Introduction to Homoeopathic Prescribing" for the benefit of graduates in modern medicine was launched on 12th April 1981. This book was specially written for the students of this course. The course has proved quite popular and the fourteenth batch was started on

22 January, 1984. To consolidate the training given in this introductory course, the Centre has also been running quarterly courses in homoeopathic Materia Medica and repertorisation. Further, in order to impart basic education in various aspects of health such as hygiene, nutrition, meaning of pathological tests and also to enable them to nip minor problems in the bud and render first aid before the doctor comes, two quarterly courses are being run for laymen and householders, *viz.* "Health through Homoeopathy" and "Homoeopathy for Beginners".

Acute shortage of space is very much felt by the Centre with the ever growing number of patients and its activities on the educational front. Expansion of accommodation has become imperative. And naturally, the Centre looks to the generosity of people to extend a helping hand liberally towards further expansion of its noble mission.

All donations to the Centre are exempted from Income Tax, vide Certificate No. B. C. No. Tech. 1/259 (2) 661-78-79, which has been extended to 31 December, 1988.

Current Trustees :

1. Shri Deepak S. Mehta (Chairman)
2. Shri Gulshan Lal Manaktala
3. Shri P.A. Sattawalla
4. Shri B.P. Baliga
5. Shri Naresh Kumar Jain.

ABOUT THE AUTHOR

A few words about the author of this book will be in order. Mr. Gunavante has described in his Preface how he came to write this book and it is a measure of the man that he has voluntarily relinquished his monetary interest in the book in favour of Dr. Subodh Mehta Medical Relief Trust.

Born in a middle class family in North Kanara in 1915, he had his schooling in Honavar. He used to top the class in school and in the matriculation examination held in 1933, in the then Bombay State, he was among the first 100. He could not pursue his studies owing to pecuniary difficulties and took up a job in the Oriental Life Insurance Co. in 1935. By dint of sincere devotion to duty he rose, from humble beginning to the position of Assistant Secretary (Development) in the L.I.C., before he retired in January 1975. During the last few years in service, as he held a responsible position in the Development Dept., concerned with the training of Life Insurance agents, Mr. Gunavante took active part in two training seminars, and wrote a number of booklets for training the agents in their sales and servicing work. He was also commissioned to write a textbook on "Marketing" for fellowship students of the Federation of Insurance Institutes.

Mr. Gunavante's *Introduction to Homoeopathy* came in 1950 when the Bombay Homoeopathic Association was holding a refresher course, and his friend Dr. G.L. Koppikar was its secretary. Under Koppikar's guidance he made extensive use of the Association's library, including old issues of the *Homoeopathic Recorder*. But the heavy work in his job allowed him no time to deepen his knowledge in this science and it was only after retirement that he could once again take up the pursuit of his beloved subject. Fortunately for him, at this stage he came in touch with Dr. Bhanu D. Desai, M.B.B.S., whose infectious enthusiasm and scientific method of case-taking and repertorisation not only impressed Mr. Gunavante, but were found to yield very fruitful results in practice. In his zeal to spread Dr. Bhanu Desai's methods, he assisted him in writing two articles for the *Hahnemannian Gleanings* on Boger-Boenninghausen's repertory. He also assisted Dr. Bhanu Desai in writing the book *How to Find the Similimum with Boger-Boenninghausen's Repertory*. Another book is *Bring up Healthy Children with Homoeopathy* by Dr. Desai, in the writing of which Mr. Gunavante has rendered much help.

It is not necessary for me to write more about this book than what the author himself says, and even more importantly, what Dr. Anil Bhatia, Principal of the C.M.P. Homoeopathic College, Bombay, who throughout displayed keen interest in the project, has said in his foreword. I can only say that it is a stroke of good luck for all of us that we came together inspired by the ideal of service to homoeopathy and the result is what the reader has in his hand just now.

Dr. S.K. MANKAD

Bombay.

30th March, 1982.

Director
Dr. Subodh Mehta Medical Centre
and *Hon. Director*
Sai Baba Medical Centre.

CONTENTS

	pages
Foreword--Dr. Anil Bhatia	vii
Preface to the Fourth Edition	ix
Preface to the Third Edition	xi
Preface to the First Edition	xiii
Dr. Subodh Mehta Medical Relief Trust	xix
About the Author – Dr. S.K. Mankad	xxiii

Lesson 1 : Basic Principles of Homoeopathy 1--17

Homoeopathic Philosophy—A Synopsis	2
The Law of Similars	4
Provings, the Basis of Materia Medica	6
Vital Force	7
How Do Homoeopathic Remedies Act :	8
Symptoms	8
Susceptibility	9
Treat the Patient as a Whole	9
Individualisation	10
Totality of Symptoms	10
Role of Diagnosis	10
Proper Diet Depends on Diagnosis	11
Treat the Basic, Underlying Cause, not the Result	11
Palliation and Suppression	12
Single Remedy	12
Minimum Dose - Potencies	13
Repetition of Dose	13
Signs of Curative Action	14
The Chronic Miasms	14
Removal of Exciting Causes	15
Selecting the Remedy	15
Self-Test	16

	Pages
Study in Depth	17

Lesson 2 : Homoeopathy and Modern Medicine — Search for the Curative Principle **18-32**
Discovery of the Law of Cure 20
Unrecognised Use of the Similia
  Principles in Modern Medicine 21
The Homoeopathic Trend in Modern Medical
  Thought 24
The Similia Principles in Ayurveda 25
Need for a Balanced View 26
Danger to Homoeopathy 28
Self Test 31
Study in Depth 32

Lesson 3 : Provings and Construction of Materia Medica **33-48**
Provings on Animals 35
Sources of Drugs 36
How to Know the Remedies Well 39
Books for Studying the Materia Medica 41
Books for Reference 41
A Novel Method of Studying the Materia
  Medica Useful for the Busy Neophyte 43
Self -Test 48

Lesson 4 : Evaluation of Symptoms **49-74**
Two Classes of Symptoms 49
Characteristic Symptoms 53
Totality of Symptoms 56
Kent's Approach to Evaluation of Symptoms 59
Key -notes 64
Peculiar Symptoms 66
Last Appearing Symptoms 69
Unmodified (Original) Symptoms 69
Only Phraseology Different 70

	Pages
Objective Symptoms	71
A Few Noteworthy Hints	72
Self-Test	74
Study in Depth	74

Lesson 5 : Taking the Case 75-88
Difference Between Homoeopathic Case-taking and that in Modern Medicine	75
How to Ask Questions	76
What to Record and How to Record the Symptoms	78
Case-taking Outline	79
Understanding Sensations	84
Acute Diseases	86
Self-Test	87
Study in Depth	88
Questionnaire	88

**Lesson 6 : Selection of the Remedy —
Repertorisation 89-123**
Repertorisation	89
Special Features of Different Repertories	89
More About Boger-Boenninghausen and Kent Repertories	94
Boenninghausen's Contribution	95
Genius of Kent	96
Scientific Method	96
Artistic Method	96
Secret of Artistic Work	98
Corroboration from other Prescribers	101
Two Repertories - One View	104
Step by Step Procedure for Repertorisation	104
Combining Two Eliminative Rubrics	106
Elimination Method - An Example	107
Two Eliminative Rubrics from Kent	107
Some Examples of Repertorial Study of Cases	109

	Pages
Bidwell's Comments	113
Learning from Repertorisation	121
Precautions in Using Particulars	121
Limitations of Repertories	122
More Exercises for Practice	122
Self-Test	123

Lesson 7 : Selection of Potency and Repetition of Dose 124-153

Advantages of Potentisation (Dynamisation)	125
Methods of Potentisation	126
Range of Centesimal Potencies	127
Fifty Millesimal Scale of Potencies	127
Scientific Basic for the Power Developed in Dynamisation	128
Dr. T.K. Bellokossy	129
Selection of Potency for Administration	131
High and Higher Potencies (1M and above)	133
Medium and High Potencies (30th, 200th and 1M)	135
Low Potencies and Crude-Drugs (Mother Tincture to 12c)	136
General Comments on Potencies	136
High to Low or Low to High	139
Curing by Lysis or Crisis	142
How Many Doses in the First Prescription?	143
Kent's General Guidelines	144
Kent's Specific Directions	145
Administering the Dose - How and When	148
Repetition of Dose	149
Self-Test	152
Study in Depth	153

Lesson 8 : Management of the Case 154-193

Criteria of Cure	155
Remedy Responses	156
Period Required for Positive Action	156

	Pages
What are the Types of Responses	161
Misconceptions about Aggravation	162
Why the Responses, and What to Do	165
Repeat same remedy in the same potency	172
Repeat same remedy in higher potency	172
Repeat same remedy in lower potency	172
Administer a complementary remedy	173
Administer a cognate of the last remedy	174
Administer an entirely new remedy	175
Zig-zagging (using a succession of remedies)	176
Alternating conditions	176
Change of remedy according to uppermost Miasm	177
Wait and watch	177
Advancing the Frontiers of Homoeopathy	178
Antidote	181
Intercurrent remedies	181
Relationship of remedies	181
Complementary relationship	182
Some examples of complementary action	182
Inimical or incompatible relationship	183
Antidotal relationship	184
Obstacles to cure	185
Surgical cases	186
Diet	186
Air pollution	189
Emotional environment	189
Drug effects - Tautopathy	190
Self-Test	192

Lesson 9 : The Chronic Miasms and Nosodes 194-211

Suppressions	196
Miasms and totality	197
Fragmentary presentation of diseases	198
Symptoms guiding us to the miasmatic background	198
Some characteristic differences between the three miasms	199

	Pages
Acute primary Infections	200
Nosodes - An Extention of Psora	201
The Duncan Method	203
Will Nosodes Complete the Cure?	203
Magical Cures with Nosodes	204
Tuberculinum	204
Psorinum	205
Variolinum	205
Pneumococcin	206
Medorrhinum	206
Pyrogen	207
Diphtherinum	207
Self-Test	210
Study in Depth	211

Lesson 10 : How to Study the Materia Medica...... 212-223
- Ability to differentiate between Remedies, A Must .. 212
- An effective method of studying Materia Medica 213
- Study Case Reports 214
- From Science to Art in Prescribing 215
- Take the Most Peculiar Symptoms First.................. 215
- The three legged stool 216
- Minimum Syndrome of Maximum Value 216
- Seek Confirmation from Materia Medica 219
- Referring cases to Materia Medica.......................... 219
- A System to Remain Abreast and Ever Ready 219
- Materia Medica to Repertory 220
- Repertory to Materia Medica 221
- Self-Test 222
- Arsenicum Album - A Study 222
- Physical Generals 223

Lesson 11 : Different Ways of Selecting the Remedy 224-233
- Key-note Prescribing 226
- Causation 229

	Pages
Organopathic remedies	232
Self-Test	232

Lesson 12 : Role of Therapeutic Hints 234-243
- Therapeutic Hints 234
- Clinical Therapeutics 235
- The Prescriber 235
- Homoeopathic Therapeutics 235
- Essentials of Homoeopathic Therapeutics 236
- Practical Homoeopathic Therapeutics 236
- Pointers to the Common Remedies 237
- Select Your Remedy 237
- Limitations of Therapeutics 238
- Taking advantage of Therapeutic Hints 239
- The Art of Selecting the Remedy 241
- Self-Test 243

Lesson 13 : Literature on Homoeopathy 244-257
- Elementary (Beginner's Stage) 245
- Principles and Philosophy (Four Books) 245
- Materia Medica (Four Books) 245
- Repertories (Two Books) 246
- Therapeutics (Thirteen Books) 246
- Middle (Graduate) Stage 248
- Principles and Philosophy (Two Books) 248
- Materia Medica (Five Books) 248
- Repertories (Four Books) 250
- Therapeutics (Five Books) 251
- Advanced (Post-Graduate) Stage 252
- Principles and Philosophy (One Book) 252
- Materia Medica (Eight Books) 252
- Repertories ((Four Books) 255
- Therapeutics (Seven Books) 256
- Journals (Three) 257

APPENDICES

Appendix

		Pages
'A' :	Questionnaire for Taking the Case	258
'B' :	Near-Specifics	267
'C' :	Prophylactics	278
'D' :	Causations	282
	"Never will since...."	284
	Suppressions - Bad Effects of	287
'E' :	Organopathic Remedies	289
'F' :	Some Important Differentiating Characteristics of Miasms	292
'G' :	Pseudo-Psora or Tubercular Miasm	297
'H' :	Miasms and the Children	298
'I' :	Exercises for Repertorisation	300
'J' :	Bryonia	307
	Belladonna	308
	Effects of Congestion	309
	Rhus-Tox	310
	Calcarea Carb	312
	Nux-Vomica	313
	Pulsatilla	314
	Sepia	316
	Lachesis	319
	Natrum Mur	320
	Nat Mur - Physical Generals	321
'K' :	Solutions of Repertorial Exercises	323
'L' :	Depth of Action of Remedies	328
'M' :	Anti Psoric Remedies	329
'N' :	Anti-Sycotic Remedies	329
'O' :	Anti-Syphilitic Remedies	330
'P' :	Anti-Pseudo-Psora (Tubercular)	330

References 331

Lesson 1

Basic Principles of Homoeopathy

> "When we have to do with an art whose aim is saving of human lives, any neglect to make ourselves thorough masters of it becomes a crime."
>
> — Hahnemann

1. Introduction. We have all come together with but one idea inspiring every one of us, *viz.* how to discharge our responsibilities to the ailing humanity by curing them of their various ailments gently, rapidly and permanently, and that, at as low a cost as possible. Our congratulations go out to those broadminded ladies and gentlemen who have set aside whatever prejudices and preconceived notions which they may have acquired about homoeopathy in the process of their academic life to listen to these lectures and find out the truth about homoeopathy. Truth ultimately triumphs and, as such, it need have no fear that by coming in touch with or listening to anything "different" it will lose itself.

2. Few things are more stimulating than to have one's pet prejudices attacked. For the allopathic physicians one of the most difficult obstacles in learning to prescribe according to the homoeopathic system, is to adopt the point of view that one must not use pathology as a sole basis for finding the remedy, but only as one of the important factors in the totality of symptoms; and that the same holds true about the need for diagnosis of the disease. The reason for this important difference will be apparent as we go deeper into this subject. It is hoped that by the time we come to the end of this course, we will have received ample guidance for finding the curative homoeopathic remedy easily and quickly.

3. It is appropriate at this stage to add that Hahnemann, the founder of this system, as well as all other pioneers of this system, were learned doctors of medicine in their own right. Though Boenninghausen was a sole exception to this, his learning and ability were so outstanding that King Wilhelm IV issued a cabinet order conferring upon him the right to practice as a physician. It would take a whole and absorbing book to tell how these doctors became so much attracted to homoeopathy that they even courted ridicule, penury and even risk to life in their zeal for the true art of healing. One or more events in their lives revealed to them in a flash the utter futility of the therapeutics they had learned in the colleges, as compared with the magical ability of homoeopathic remedies to cure baffling ailments gently, smoothly, rapidly and permanently. Boenninghausen himself was a patient of T.B. and he owed his life to homoeopathy. Constantine Hering, who was commissioned to write a thesis condemning homoeopathy, became its ardent exponent after studying its literature (which he had to do for writing the thesis), and even more so when his finger which became gangrenous after doing an autopsy, was saved from amputation by a homoeopathic remedy. Years later, at great risk to his life, he proved the deadly poison of a snake and introduced the valuable *Lachesis* to the Materia Medica. James Compton Burnett saw that the percentage of deaths in one section of his children's ward treated allopathically was high, whereas in the other section the children treated with homoeopathic *Aconite*, became convalescent and went home in a few days, and the ward was becoming empty. Nearer home, is the unique instance of Dr. Mahendralal Sirkar who, as Vice President of the British Medical Association (Bengal Branch), had denounced homoeopathy as quackery; but after repeatedly seeing the cases cured by Babu Rajendralal Dutta, a lay practitioner of homoeopathy, he was gradually convinced of the truth of the homoeopathic philosophy. He threw up his lucrative practice, and was unmoved by the boycott imposed by the British Medical Association because, he said, "Truth must be told, and truth must be acted upon". After passing through many tribulations he came to be recognised as a towering giant of homoeopathy in India.

HOMOEOPATHIC PHILOSOPHY — A SYNOPSIS

4. **Homoeopathy is a True Science of Healing.** It qualified to be called a science because it is based throughout on certain

fixed laws and principles. Announced to the world almost two hundred years ago, they are valid even today; in fact, their validity has been confirmed again and again through clinical experiences over this extended period of time wherever homoeopathy has been practised according to the principles. Some of the main principles are :

(1) The law of similars.

(2) Proving (or testing) of medicinal substances on healthy human beings, in order to ascertain the symptoms (of disordered functions) which the medicines produce on them. This record of symptoms constitutes the homoeopathic Materia Medica.

(3) The role of the vital force in health and disease. Vital force is nothing but what modern medicine calls the immune system, or the defence mechanism.

(4) Symptoms and signs are the sole expressions of the reaction of the vital force to the morbid inimical force which creates disorders of function and imbalance of health.

(5) Susceptibility of patients to morbid inimical forces on the one hand, and to the drugs on the other. This leads to the necessity of :

    (a) Treating the patient as a person, and not his parts (liver, lungs, digestion, etc.) alone and not the disease he is "diagnosed" to be suffering from.

    (b) Individualisation of the patient, to study his individual susceptibilities.

(6) "Totality of symptoms" of the patient.

(7) Role of diagnosis.

(8) Treat the cause, not the end-result.

(9) Palliation and suppression.

(10) Single remedy — no combination or alternations.

(11) Minimum dose — potentisation of remedies.

(12) Repetition of dose.

(13) Signs of curative action.

(14) The role of chronic *miasms* in the long-term and deep-seated disorders of health.

5. The following is a brief outline of these important tenets of homoeopathy. It will be seen that they are all based on sound logical reasoning as confirmed by the test of practical experience.

6. **The Law of Similars** *(similia similibus curentur)* : This principle or the law of cure was discovered by Hahnemann in 1790, almost two centuries ago. Hahnemann was a linguist, a master of sixteen languages, a master of chemistry and a doctor of medicine. He was yet a very sensitive soul whose heart grieved at the sufferings of others. He could not reconcile himself to the then prevailing cruel methods of bleeding, purgating and sweating the patients, nor to the thrashing of those considered insane or psychotic.

He, therefore, preferred to eke out his living by translating medical works. While translating Cullen's Materia Medica, the explanation given in it for the cure of intermittent fever by *Cinchona* led him to test the effect of the drug on the healthy human body, in order to see if it would not give him a clue to its remedial action in malaria. This experiment led him to the conclusion that "*Cinchona* cures intermittent fever by virtue of its power to produce in the healthy, a similar affection."

7. This experiment led Hahnemann to subject to the same test other medicines which experience had shown to be curative of certain well-defined diseases. He collected records of cases of poisoning with these medicines and also tested them on his own person and on members of his family. In every case he found that the positive effect of these remedies on the healthy human body corresponded with the morbid phenomena of disease they had been able to cure. After six years of labour on these lines, Hahnemann published his claim that medicines acted remedially by virtue of their power to cause derangements of health similar to those observed in the diseases they could cure. This

doctrine is expressed by the now well-known dictum, *similia similibus curentur*, i.e., let likes be treated by likes.

8. There cannot be two laws of Nature to govern the same phenomenon. It follows, therefore, and experience confirms this conclusion, that all other methods of treating illness which are not based on the Law of Similars, are palliative or suppressive, but not curative.

9. Let us listen to the words of Hahnemann who laboured up to the ripe old age of eighty-nine with full possession of his faculties, to perfect this science (he revised and improved six times his *Organon of Medicine*, which has been described as the 'high water-mark of medical philosophy'). Hahnemann gave "*Aude Sapere*" (Dare to be wise) as its motto, and thus gave a ringing call for boldness in upholding Truth, another name for Wisdom. Hahnemann said : "This doctrine appeals solely to the verdict of experience. Repeat the experiments, it cries aloud; repeat them carefully and accurately, and you will find the doctrine confirmed at every step; and it does what no medical doctrine, no system of physic, no so-called therapeutics ever did or could do — it insists upon being judged by results."

"Homoeopathy consists in the administration of a remedy for a disease which, if given to a person in health, is capable of producing symptoms similar (not identical) to disease — *similia similibus curentur* — likes by likes are cured :

You are palsied — you use *Strychnine*, which produces palsy.

You are gripped — you use *Colocynthis*, which gripes.

You are sick — you use *Antimony*, which produces sickness.

You have asthma — you use *Antimony*, which produces asthma.

You are relaxed in bowels — you use *Rhubarb*, which relaxes bowels.

"This is the law of likes curing likes. Refute these truths, if you can, by showing a still more efficacious, certain and agreeable method than mine; refute them not by words, of which we have already too many; but, if experience should prove to you, as it has done to me, that my method is the best, make use of it to save your fellow creatures and give the glory to God."

10. Hahnemann was an inveterate experimentalist; and in all his experiments he set his face sternly against *a priori* reasoning (i.e., drawing inferences from general to the particular). He based his conclusions on inductive logic, i.e., drawing general inferences only from repeated observations of particular events. "Prove all things and hold fast to that which is good" was the substance of his method and instruction. By his firmness in avoiding all "transcendental speculation into the hidden unknown processes going on in the body," and placing homoeopathy on the strong and unalterable foundation of observed symptomatology, Hahnemann provided mankind with a perennial law of therapeutics.

11. **Provings, the Basis of Materia Medica.** Once convinced that a drug can cure those disease symptoms which it produces when given to the healthy, Hahnemann's logical mind thought to itself that we must know the symptoms which the various drugs can produce, before we know what symptoms they can cure. He, therefore, set himself to the huge task of "proving" a large number of drugs, i.e. compiling the symptoms which they produced when given to healthy persons. Medical philosophers had, through the centuries, theorised about this law, mentioning it casually, in passing, but none had cared to take the next logical step of compiling the symptoms which drugs produced on the healthy. Unless these symptoms were known, there could be no question or opportunity of using them to treat and cure similar symptoms in the sick.

12. Hahnemann carefully and meticulously supervised the provings of a large number of medicines on healthy persons and had the symptoms experienced by the provers recorded in their own language, without any speculative guesses as to the physiological processes involved or the pathology which may have developed. This he did over a period of thirty years. These records were published in a number of volumes from time to time. The symptom records were then arranged by him in the form of schema (known as Hahnemannian Schema) under the headings of Mind, Throat, Stomach, Abdomen, Stool, Rectum, Urine, Genitalia, Respiration, Chest, Heart, Back, Extremities,

Sleep, Skin, Fever. This record constitutes the Materia Medica Pura, which guides the homoeopathic practitioners today and gives us a knowledge of medicinal power. It was only after many years of careful and laborious testing of medicines on himself and others, followed by deep reflection, that Hahnemann satisfied himself that the Law of Similars is a general rule of treatment which could be applied in practice.

Hahnemann's followers have added enormously to the nearly hundred medicines proved by Hahnemann, so that there is hardly a disease or natural morbific condition whose parallel or similia cannot be discovered among the nearly two thousand medicines whose symptomatology is found in the homoeopathic Materia Medica.

13. **Vital Force.** A truly curative medical science should have a well-proved and correct understanding of the relationship between health, disease and the therapeutic measures. The cornerstone of homoeopathy's understanding of this question lies in the importance it attaches to the vital force pervading the living organism, which governs all these three, *viz.* health, disease and therapeutics. Hahnemann asserted in Aphorism 10 of the *Organon* that the living body is incapable of any sensation or function of self-preservation without the vital force, the life force (or dynamis) as he called it. Without the vital force the organism is dead and resolves itself into its chemical constituents. It is the vital force which maintains all parts and functions of the body in admirable harmonious, vital operation as regards both sensations, functions and even self preservation. If the vital force is strong, no germs or bacteria can do any harm to it. The germs can thrive in the blood or tissues only if the vital force of the organism is primarily sick and affords a suitable soil for them. If it is weak and susceptible to the morbific agents (microbes) inimical to life, the fight between the vital force and the disease force (if the latter is stronger) manifests itself in the form of some disease. In acute diseases the vital force soon overwhelms the disease force, sometimes without even the help of any medicine. In chronic diseases, the vital force cannot conquer the disease unaided by the suitable remedies.

Vital force is nothing but the natural defence mechanism of the body comprising the Reticulo-Endothelial System (RES) and the Psycho-Neuro-Endocrine System (PsNES). It is well known that this mechanism, also called the immune system, rallies the forces to protect the body when it is threatened by harmful external forces. The reaction of the defence mechanism produces symptoms such as pain, fever, mucus, cough, etc. Fever inactivates many viruses; mucus in the respiratory tract envelopes and carries away the irritating material; a cough helps to throw it out as the mucus. The homoeopathic physician therefore regards these symptoms as a healthy reaction of the body's vital force, and as such seeks to support them instead of suppressing or opposing them. A strong vital force thus represents health, while a weak or disordered vital force is the cause of disease.

14. **How Do Homoeopathic Remedies Act?** When the balanced harmonious functioning of the body, over which the vital force presides, is disturbed by illness, the patient's susceptibility (a lowered state of resistance) to the similar remedy — a remedy which has proved its capacity to produce symptoms which are similar to those of the patient — is very much heightened; and thus, when the disease force is confronted by a similar drug force, the remedial force assists the vital force to overwhelm and cure the disease. This action of the similar remedy will be more clearly grasped from the analogy of how a runaway train can be overtaken and brought to a halt. This can be done only when another train runs in the same direction at a slightly greater speed till it overtakes it, and when the driver's cabins are closest, slows down to the same speed to allow the substitute driver to jump into it and bring it to a halt.

15. **Symptoms : the true representation of disease as well as unerring guide to therapeutics.** The deranged vital force (disease) manifests itself in the form of morbid signs and symptoms, which are perceived or felt by the patient and observed by the accurately observing physician. Symptoms are the only reliable external manifestation or expression of the internal disorder or turmoil in the body, and they constitute the only dependable guide to therapeutic action. They are divided into two classes : subjective and objective. Subjective symptoms are those which are felt by the patient alone, such as (1) **Mental** : *Pain, fear, delusions, suspiciousness, hatred, compassion, effects of grief or disappointed love,* etc. or (2) **Physical** : *Headache, colic, double vision, numbness, burning, itching, loss of smell, bitter taste* etc. They take the highest rank as expressions of the interior state of the organism. Nothing can supersede them. Objective symptoms are those expres-

sions of disease which are exposed to the senses of the physician and bystanders, such as different expressions of face, restlessness or torpor, ataxic gait, secretions (colour, consistency, odour), crying of the baby with hands on particular parts, signifying pain in that part, colic (in babies) indicated by flexion of the thighs over abdomen, etc.

16. **Susceptibility.** The deranged vital force is very sensitive and susceptible to certain morbific influences (call them allergic effects if you like), and thus suffers from a natural disease. Unless a person is susceptible (has weak resistance), he cannot be adversely affected either by pathogenic micro-organisms, infections, hot or cold weather, stressful situations, etc. No bacteria is the sole or absolute cause of disease. It will only be the exciting or proximate cause when there is a predisposing, antecedent cause, i.e. lower resistance, susceptibility. In other words, bacteria or viruses or other inimical forces in the environment can thrive only if the "soil" (vital force) offers favourable conditions for their growth. The nature of this susceptibility, and its extent, varies with individuals and it even varies in the same individual from time to time.

The deranged vital force is even more susceptible to the action of remedy which is capable of producing a "drug disease" (symptoms) similar to the symptoms of the natural disease it is suffering from. When the drug disease which is stronger meets the natural disease, the latter is over-powered (we are not yet able to explain exactly how this happens); and the disease loses all influences on the vital force. The natural disease as well as the drug disease (which is temporary) are thus both annihilated.

17. **Treat the Patient as a Whole.** The vital force has its sway over the whole body, all the organs and tissues of the patient. It is involved in resistance to disease wherever it may occur. Therefore, the aim of homoeopathic medicine is to restore the deranged vital force to its full power. It follows that there can be no 'local' diseases, or several 'local' diseases co-existing in the body. The patient does not suffer from more than one illness at a time, however many local manifestations this one illness may show. Each part of the body depends upon every other part, and all act together as one, in health and disease. No organ can become diseased without a preceding disturbance of the vital force. Therefore, it is a mistake to treat a part as if it stood alone. It is the individual patient as a whole who should be the object of treatment.

18. **Individualisation.** But since individual susceptibility varies (depending upon age, sex, environment, mental, emotional and physical stresses, habits and ways of life, heredity, congenital tendencies and pathological condition), it is necessary to study each patient as an individual. There may be five cases of headache or bronchitis (diagnostically), but each case will call for different homoeopathic remedy, based on his individual group of symptoms, as revealed by the totality of his symptoms. It is an axiom of homoeopathy that all aspects of treatment are governed by the principle of individualisation — examination of the patient, selection of the remedy, potency and repetition of dose, auxiliary treatment (diet etc.).

19. **Totality of Symptoms.** It is highly important to understand exactly what this peculiar expression used by homoeopaths means, because the totality of symptoms is the true and only basis for the truly curative homoeopathic prescription. Homoeopathy does not (really speaking, cannot) treat complaints pertaining to individual organs or functions to the exclusion of other parts nor, in finding out the curative remedy, does it go by the diagnostic label put on the ailment, as diagnosis only classifies diseases but does not take into account the patient's individuality. The exact meaning of the individual components of the totality, such as location, sensation, modality, concomitants, etc. will be explained in the next lesson. Suffice it to say that totality does not merely represent the numerical aggregate of all the symptoms, but their organic whole, in which all the elements are logically related and consistent, pointing to the pathogenesis of one remedy. The remedy emerging from a study of the totality has many facets (location, sensation, modality, mentals etc.) and together they represent the genius of a single remedy.

The next two points, diagnosis and treatment of the basic cause, are corollaries to the principle of individualisation.

20. **Role of Diagnosis.** In gaining a knowledge of the disease for purposes of homoeopathic therapeutics, the foregoing are very important considerations. But this does not preclude the physician from making a proper diagnosis of the case by taking the help of various diagnostic procedures such as palpation, auscultation, checking the reflexes; blood pressure, analysis of urine, stool, blood; X-ray of chest, stomach, kidneys, etc., manual examination of the cervix; E.C.G., E.E.G., etc.

Basic Principles of Homoeopathy

whenever necessary. Careful diagnosis helps prognosis; it prevents us from the risk of complacency in surgical conditions; it helps us in the way of auxiliary measures such as hygiene, diet, rest, etc. Even from the therapeutic viewpoint, diagnosis helps us to select the remedy of proper depth of action, as also to select suitable and effective potency so as to avoid aggravations on the one hand, and ineffectiveness on the other. Proper management of the case depends on diagnosis.

21. **Proper Diet Depends on Diagnosis.** For example, a tubercular patient with fever will require proteins and a nourishing diet, whereas in the case of jaundice fat-free diet will be compulsory. In acute peptic ulcer only milk diet will have to be advised. Then again, symptoms that may appear uncommon and peculiar may really be common to the disease from which the patient suffers. Unless we have a knowledge of diagnosis and the symptoms that go with it, we will not be able to identify the truly peculiar, uncommon, individualising symptoms which are of supreme importance in selecting the remedy. Further, without a knowledge of the significance of the diagnostic terms used in Materia Medica and Repertory, we will not be able to use them when necessary. The repertory section in Wm. Boericke's Materia Medica is full of such diagnostic terms, and there are also a few in Kent's as well as Boger-Boenninghausen's Repertory. Thus judicious medical practice calls for a knowledge of diagnosis.

22. **Treat the Basic, Underlying Cause, not the Result.** It is common nowadays to keep a watch on blood pressure, blood sugar (diabetes), and get pathological reports on urine, stool, complete blood count, E.S.R. (Erythrocyte Sedimentation Rate), Rheumatoid Arthritis Test, Montoux Test (Tuberculosis), etc. While all these pathological reports are useful to know the depth of the diseased condition, and are undoubtedly essential in treating a case, they are not of any direct help in selecting the remedy. Most of these conditions are the result of diseases, which in turn are caused by deranged vital force. Any treatment addressed to these resultant phenomena, and not to their underlying cause, will be but palliative. Removal of the result of morbid causes may alleviate suffering (like plugging a leaking ship), but does not constitute radical cure (stoppage of the leak). Functional changes always precede tissue changes and pathology. Good health follows only if we correct or remove the causes which have deranged the vital force leading to a state

of disease, and restore normal function of the organism. If this is done the pathology which has developed already will slowly regress and will be less and less troublesome. There are numerous cases treated homoeopathically which attest to this fact.

23. Palliation and Suppression. Fears of various kinds are driving patients now-a-days to seek quick relief by taking physiological dose of modern medicine (Aspirin, Paracetamol, sleeping pills for insomnia, Baralgan, colics, etc.,) or by applying local ointments on skin conditions, or by surgery of tonsils, and other growths. The result is first palliation and then suppression, followed by an actual aggravation of the first condition. It is not known, not even recognised, that physiological dosage always has biphasal action, *i.e.* primary action followed by secondary action, which latter is a reaction of the vital force (a reaction opposite to the primary action). Opium in physiological doses produces deep sleep, but it is followed by prolonged insomnia. Suppression of diarrhoea will often produce constipation. The use of salicylates and coal tar derivatives in rheumatic and allied complaints invariably sends the trouble to the central organs, especially to the heart.

As H.A. Roberts says in his *Principles and Art of Cure by Homoeopathy* : The one thing we should hold as our aim is to allow the vital force to express itself in its own chosen way when it is deranged. It is only when it shows itself clearly and without interruption in its natural development that we get a clear picture of the diseased state. Administration of the physiological medicine at such times changes the whole picture, suppressing one symptom after another until there is no expression of true condition of the patient. Without such clear expression of symptoms selection of the homoeopathic remedy is very difficult.

Similarly, by suppressing skin manifestations by local applications, or secretions like leucorrhoea by cautery, or removal of diseased sinuses or uterus by surgery, we are only cutting off the manifestation of disease through its chosen organs and are doing nothing to set in order the vital energy or to prevent further disease manifestations.

24. Single Remedy. Administering a single remedy at a time, which is another tenet laid down by Hahnemann, was a natural consequence of the fact that the Materia Medica contains the symptomatology of single remedies only. Since we do not know the effects which more than one remedy given at a time (in a combination or in alternation) can produce, it would be manifestly unscientific to administer remedies in mixture or in alternation. Is it possible to draw any lessons or conclusions about the effect of remedies for our future guidance, if instead of being used singly, they are used in combinations? Obviously not, and therefore this procedure is to be avoided. This injunction acquires greater validity when it is realised that the homoeopathic Materia Medica today comprise many remedies which have a broad range and depth of action and are alone capable of meeting all manner of symptom-complexes. Therefore, given proper selection of remedy according to principles, there is no warrant for mixing or using them in alternation.

25. **Minimum Dose — Potencies**. The question of dosage has long been the subject of controversy even among homoeopaths who have implicit confidence in the law of similars. The homoeopathic potencies with an infinitesimal content of the medicinal substance, have been as much derided and ridiculed by some, as they have been praised to the skies by others as magical in effect. Hahnemann, as a trained allopath, actually started with a massive dosage of the crude drugs in the allopathic fashion, and it is only the repeated aggravations that he experienced from such dosage that forced him to "dilute" the medicine, as he called it. Fortunately, being the most systematic and methodical chemist that he was, Hahnemann "diluted" drugs according to a definite scale and method (which will be explained later) and to his own surprise he found that the higher the dilution, the greater the power or potency it had; and hence they are now known as potencies. Yet, it must be said that the question of dose is still as open one, depending as it does on several factors such as the depth of action of the remedy, the acuteness or chronicity of the disease, the susceptibility of the patient, the plane of action expected of the remedy, etc. In the circumstances, while masters of the art have given us their own experiences, it is left to each physician to use the high, highest, medium or low potencies. The whole point which we wish to stress here is that, as in all other questions, the question of giving the smallest potentised dose was not decided *a priori*, but solely on the basis of clinical experience.

26. **Repetition of Dose**. The frequency of dosage is closely bound up with the potency, and the other factors involved in

determining the potency. Yet, Hahnemann has laid down one general rule, *viz.* that repetition should depend on the patient's reaction, and that the dose of the carefully selected remedy should be allowed to act as long as it is accomplishing its effect. So long as improvement is observed, repetition is contraindicated, as every new dose would disturb the process of recovery. Medicines do not cure; they merely stimulate the curative reaction of the patient. The call for repetition can only be the renewed call of symptoms.

27. **Signs of Curative Action.** The rational and scientific nature of the principles of homoeopathy is once again confirmed by its understanding of the progress of disease, and the progress of cure which should be its converse. It is well known that disease progresses from periphery to the centre. If peripheral symptoms of warning are suppressed by antipathic medicine, the disease strikes more and more vital organs (according to susceptibility). On the contrary, curative treatment should drive the disease from centre to periphery. Homoeopathic treatment conforms with this curative action, as laid down in Hering's laws of direction of cure. According to this law, when a medicine is acting curatively (i) the patient feels relieved from within outwards (more important organs like the brain, heart, etc. are first relieved), (ii) from above downward (first head, then chest, then abdomen, etc.), and (iii) his symptoms disappear in the reverse order of their appearance (the last one is the first to go).

28. **The Chronic Miasms.** Among the various obstacles to recovery which the physician has to contend with in the management of the case towards recovery, Hahnemann has elaborated on the three chronic miasms of Psora, Syphilis and Sycosis, as the most important. The Miasmatic theory was not a hair-brained idea he got one fine morning. Hahnemann found that many times even the best indicated remedy did not cure permanently as expected, and the cases came back again and again. Taking this as a challenge, he delved deep into the past histories of a large number of cases and came to the conclusion, after spending twelve years in investigating the sources of these chronic affections, that they are so inveterate that unless thoroughly cured by art, they continue to increase in intensity till death. They never disappear of themselves, nor can they be diminished by the most regular mode of life, etc. Dr. W. Younan, M.B., C.M. (Edin.) says : "The master's conception of chronic

Basic Principles of Homoeopathy

disease is so unique, and supplied such a want in the medical knowledge . . . that his earlier disciples and followers considered it as his masterpiece . . . It is due to his far-reaching genius that we possess such a wonderful therapeutics of chronic diseases." We dare say that even today there is no knowledgeable homoeopath who does not find daily confirmation of this doctrine of chronic miasms. More details on this subject will be discussed in the relevant lesson.

29. **Removal of Exciting Causes.** It goes without saying that Hahnemann was second to none in stressing the importance of hygiene, proper diet, congenial atmosphere (both physical and emotional) and in short, removal of all causes which excite the malady. He stopped the inhuman treatment (so much prevalent in his times) of insane people who came under his treatment. So long as the basic or exciting causes are not removed, medicines alone can do little, he emphasised.

30. In Aphorism 7 of the *Organon*, Hahnemann has given a few instances of the cause occasionally, after the removal of which the indisposition usually disappears on its own : Remove from the sickroom the strong-smelling flowers that have brought on faintness and hysterical manifestations; remove from the cornea the foreign body that is producing ophthalmia; remove the tight bandage that threatens to cause gangrene to a wounded limb; uncover and tie the severed artery that is causing shock; remove the foreign objects lodged in the nose, throat, etc. open the imperforate anus of the newborn infant.

31. **Selecting the Remedy.** In selecting the remedy, the physician ought to master the trinity, *viz*, the knowledge of the remedies in the Materia Medica (the drug pictures), knowledge of the diseased patient (*i.e.*, disease picture), and the art, or skill in matching the disease picture with the drug picture. This matching becomes easy if one knows on the one hand, the characteristic features of drugs so as to be able to differentiate one remedy from another, and on the other, if he develops the ability to elicit the characteristic symptoms of the individual patient. Both these are two sides of the same coin. The principles governing this aspect of skill in matching the disease and drug pathogenecy, as enunciated from their vast experience by masters of this art, will be discussed in detail in the appropriate lessons.

SELF-TEST

Please try to answer these questions first (at least orally to yourself) and refer back to the text later (para nos. given in brackets for confirmation).

(1) What were the circumstances under which Dr. Constantine Hering, a brilliant student in a Medical College, became a convert to homoeopathy? What were his contributions to the development of homoeopathy? (Para 3).

(2) Write a few lines about Dr. Mahendralal Sarkar. What did he say when he threw up his lucrative practice in allopathy and became a homoeopath? (Para 3).

(3) Why is homoeopathy a true science of healing? State a few of its basic laws. (Para 4).

(4) Describe how the basic law of similars is capable of universal application. (Para 4).

(5) What is the title of the book which is described as the 'high water mark of medical philosophy'? Who wrote it and how many times did the author revise and improve it in the light of his experience? (Para 9).

(6) What is the role of the vital force in maintaining good health? Is it capable of overcoming chronic diseases without the aid of appropriate remedies? (Para 13).

(7) How does any derangement of the vital force manifest itself to the observer? And why are these manifestations more dependable than diagnostic symptoms, as guides to the remedy? (Para 15).

(8) What is the role of diagnosis in homoeopathic therapeutics? (Para 20).

(9) What are the "two sides of the same coin" in selecting the homoeopathic remedy? Why do we call them so? (Para 31).

(10) Why was Hahnemann forced to use "dilutions" of remedies? Is there anything unique in these Hahnemannian dilutions? (Para 25).

(11) How can we know when a remedy is acting curatively? (Para 27).

STUDY IN DEPTH

For more detailed study, please read the following :

Ch. VI (pp. 56-64) on "Homoeopathy and the Fundamental Laws" from *Principles and Art of Cure by Homoeopathy* by H.A. Roberts.

Ch. IV (pp. 41-47) on "Vital Force as Expressed in Functions (in Health; in Disease; in Recovery; in Cure)" in the above said book by H.A. Roberts.

Ch. VII (pp. 76-86) on "Susceptibility, Reaction and Immunity" in *The Genius of Homoeopathy* by Stuart Close.

Ch. X (pp. 91-95) on "The Law of Cure" in the above said book by H.A. Roberts.

Books mentioned above are available with M/s. B. Jain Publishers (P) Ltd., Post Box - 5775 , New Delhi - 55.

Lesson 2

Homoeopathy and Modern Medicine — Search for the Curative Principle

1. Since the dawn of civilization the physicians of the day have naturally tended to adapt their practices to the prevailing dogmas. There was a time when affections of the liver and spleen were considered to be the source of all kinds of trouble. In the middle ages poisoned fluids of the body, or excess of blood in circulation were suspected to be the culprits and physicians felt that they failed in their duty if they did not resort to heroic measures like blood-letting and purging. Even notables did not escape the consequences of these cruel measures. Some of the victims of blood letting, among the great men of history are : Emperor Leopold II of Austria and his son Francis I (the latter in 1835); Goethe, Raphael, Mirabeau, Lord Byron (against his earnest protestations), Count Cavour the great Italian statesman (as late as in 1861), and in America, George Washington, known as the Father of that country.

2. This was followed by the dawn of morbid pathology and operative surgery in an endeavour to eliminate the diseased organs. Later still, came the discovery of microbic infection which is still holding the field, though the emphasis is slowly changing to a greater recognition of the susceptibility of the infected host. Side by side with the discovery of the role of vitamins, medical practice has tended to the removal of vitamin, mineral or nutritional deficiencies as curative measures. During a little earlier period, the internal secretions from the ductless glands, the hormones, impressed the physicians as being most responsible for many of the ills. One or more of these theories are still believed in and accepted as guides in the treatment of

diseases according to the inclination of the physicians, and the therapeutic indications given by the pharmacologists in their product information literature.

3. The result is that modern theory and practice of medicine prescribes Analgesics, Antacids, Anti-anaemia products (to remove deficiencies), Antibiotics (antimicrobial effects), Hypotensives, Diuretics, Antitussives, Corticosteriods (hormonal deficiencies), nutritional products (to remove deficiencies of vitamins and minerals) and tranquillisers or behaviour modifiers. There is thus specialisation (with specifics) for treating individual diseases and diseased organs as well as specialisation among practitioners, such as specialists in cardiology, gynaecology, E.N.T. diseases, pediatrics, etc. This specialisation carried to an extreme degree has become the hall-mark of contemporary theoretical and practical medicine, and the net result has been fragmentation of the patient, and fragmented approach of the practitioner to the diseased patient, though he is only one single (not fragmented) individual. The illogicality and unreality of this situation, which fails to give long term cures in the eyes of close observers, has been often commented on by even leaders of modern medicine who have glimpsed the need to see the man as a whole, but this realisation is yet a faint glimmer in the dark, and not the broad light of the day. It goes without saying that this situation is only a reflection of the mistaken approach to therapeutics which concerns itself with organs or systems but ignores the man himself, which believes in killing the microbes but ignores the "soil" which attracts them. If there are any principles of therapeutics behind all this they are obviously illogical. Is it possible that in this vast universe in which things happen like clock-work, the day following night, the seasons follow each other and the various laws govern physics and chemistry, etc. there is no logical, unchanging law which governs the curative action in the ailments of human beings? When theories change with every discovery of new facts and when practice endeavours to keep in step with these changes in theory, can we accept such theories as true and unalterable? The answer has to be a "No" if we care for truth and do not wish to delude ourselves.

4. One might say, I don't care for any principle or law of cure. Has not modern medicine given us its spectacular chemical, physiological and pathological data in regard to the etiology and progress of diseases and do we not get dramatic results

from the recently discovered drugs, the Sulphonamides, Penicillin, Streptomycin, Corticosteriods, etc.? We must agree that modern medicine has done all this, but can we forget the "side-effects," sometimes irreversible, which these powerful medicines have on the human system, the "iatrogenic" diseases they give rise to and above all, the fact that while they cure (read "suppress") the frank ailments, they insidiously attack other systems of the body and undermine their health, so that the patient goes from one ailment to a more and more serious ailment as time passes? On the other hand, in the words of Margery Blackie, M.D., a long-time colleague of Dr. Frank Bodman and a student of Dr. Douglass Borland, "Medicals find it difficult to believe that we (Hahnemannian homoeopaths) have a better method which gives equally dramatic and very often more lasting results. We have more entries for our post-graduate course than ever before, and more patients demanding homoeopathy."

DISCOVERY OF THE LAW OF CURE

5. Fortunately for the ailing humanity, the principles of application of the law of cure, "Let likes be cured by likes" was discovered by Hahnemann and he perfected its methods of practice till the last breath of his life, up ninety years of age. Learning from his critical observation and experiences he revised the *Organon of Medicine* six times, till it was near perfect. The passage of time has not dimmed the truth of the guidance he has laid down in this *magnum opus* for the practical application of homoeopathy in day to day practice. On the contrary, Hahnemann can be seen, through the *Organon*, by an unprejudiced observer as a seer who foresaw many of the conclusions which modern medicine is still groping its way to learn — to give only one example, the inseparable connection between the mind and the body, or the power of the micro-dose (hormones, vitamins).

Searle (*The Use of Colloids in Health and Disease*) found in 1920 that colloidal copper injected intravenously in large doses aggravates boils; injected intramuscularly in smaller doses it causes them to heal.

Wolf (*Endocrinology in Modern Practice*) stated in 1940 that glandular extracts in small doses stimulate an activity while larger doses act to depress that activity.

Alexander Fleming observed in 1946 (*Chemotherapy, Yesterday, Today and Tomorrow*) that in early work on sulfanilamide, complete bacteriostasis was achieved with a small *in vitro* inoculum, while the microbes grew freely if the inoculum was large.

UNRECOGNISED USE OF THE SIMILIA PRINCIPLE IN MODERN MEDICINE

6. Any principle or law to deserve that name should be of universal application. It can make no distinction as to whom it applies to. If the dictum that a medicine acts curatively in a given complex of symptoms (or disordered health) provided it has the power to produce similar symptoms when given to a healthy person, is true, we should be able to observe it even when an allopath or one practising any other system of medicine, prescribes remedies for conditions symptoms of which they have the power to produce in the healthy. In order to prove this fact Hahnemann has quoted a large number of such instances in his *Organon of Medicine* (the authoritative source book on the principles and practice of homoeopathy) quoting the names of the allopathic doctors who prescribed the medicines. A few of those cases are given in a bare outline below :

Veratrum alb. in cholera.
Agaricus in epilepsy.
Uva ursi in purulent urine.
Senna in colic.
Rose water in ophthalmia.
Turpentine in sciatica.
Wine in inflammatory fevers.
Nitric acid in salivation and ulceration of fauces.
Arsenic in cancer, buboes, ague.
Aloes in diarrhoea.
Millefolium in haemorrhage.
Nux moschata in fainting fits.
Scilla in pleurisy.
Cinchona in gastralgia and jaundice.
Cantharides in strangury and gonorrhoea.
Potash in tetanus.
Mercury in inflammation of mouth, salivation, and caries.

7. In the *Brittish Homoeopathic Journal* of April, 1980, Dr. R.H. Savage, B.Sc., M.B.B.S., M.F.HOM. writes, "It was quite a revelation to realise that homoeopathy is being used unwittingly by orthodox doctors in the midst of their allopathic prescribing." He has instanced the following examples :

Digitalis in heart failure. **Amphetamine** in hyper kinetic behaviour disturbances in children.

Silver nitrate (Argentum nit.) for purulent conjunctivitis or ophthalmia neonatorum.

Sulphur and sulphur containing drugs for itchy skin, skin rashes, eruptions, etc.

2% Sulphur ointment (British National Formulary, 1976-78) for acne, seborrhoeic dermatitis, pityriasis capitis.

Dapsone, Sulphapyridine : Dermatitis herpetiformis.

Magnesium sulphate paste : Localised pyogenic skin affections.

Ichthyol with wool fat and soft paraffin (rich in sulphur) : as a local anti-inflammatory agent.

Sulphasalazine. In ulcerative colitis without withdrawal bleeding. (Homoeopathic proving of sulphur has produced severe diarrhoea, with mucus and blood).

Selenium Sulphide. Scalp Seborrhoea; pityariasis versicolor. (Homoeopathic *Selenium* has itching eruptions in circumscribed areas, eczematous eruptions of scalp with falling of hair).

2.5% Suspension of Tellurium dioxide. As a shampoo in the treatment of Seborrhoeic dermatitis, (Homoeopathic *Tellurium* has itching eruptions of scalp).

Chrysarobinum. (Homoeopathic treatment of psoriasis, ringworm etc.) *Diathranol* or *Anthralin* topically for psoriasis (contains *Chrysarobin*). When *Chrysarobin* was used on one limb, the eruption disappeared from the other limb, indicating a systemic (homoeopathic) action.

Lugol's solution (5% Iodine and 7.5% Pot. iodide). Hyperthyroidism; but not all hyperthyroid patients benefited, because it is not the homoeopathic similimum in every case. Where it is homoeopathic, the effects are long lasting.

Sodium chloride. *Saline* washes in inflammatory conditions of eyes, mouth; *saline* irrigations for upper respiratory catarrh and sinusitis — (the *Natrum mur.* of homoeopaths).

Denol (provides protective layer of Bismuth on Peptic Ulcer). In the case of the select few with peptic ulcer who respond to Denol, Bismuth may be the homoeopathic remedy.

Colchicine. For acute gout.

Aurothiomatrate inj. increasing to 50 mg. monthly for arthritis. (Homoeopathic *Aurum met.* has swollen, painful, almost ankylosed joints).

Boric acid as a mouth wash. For aphthous ulcers. (Homoeopathic *Borax* is well-known for Aphthae of mouth, tongue, which bleed easily).

Ipecacuanha in small doses. As an expectorant when sputum is scanty (Martindale's *Extra Pharmacopoeia* for children, in croup and whooping cough) — Homoeopathic *Ipecac,* has violent cough, phlegm difficult to yield, suffocating cough, whooping cough, hoarseness).

Haloperidol. Mania, psychotic crises. (Homoeopathic proving has brought out catatonia, sensation of unreality, confusion, loquaciousness, excitability, disintegration of personality).

8. Dr. Savage points out that it is not the dosage of a remedy that makes it homoeopathic, but the similar nature of the symptoms in provings or toxicity of the substance, to the symptoms of the patient which make it so. He further points out that clinical trials as normally conducted do not cater for variations in individual responses, and yet the fact is that there are variations in individual responses to the same drug. There are many reasons for this, the homoeopathic effect being one of them.

9. There is thus considerable amount of data on which to base the hypothesis that many conventional drugs exert a curative effect on the patient by fulfilling the homoeopathic law of similars. Dr. Savage, therefore, urges that it should be possible for doctors in orthodox practice to test the hypothesis by observing which patients really seemed to be cured of their illness following administration of a drug and deciding critically as to why this patient did so well, when many others received only a partial cure. This observation could revolutionise drug therapy. Instead of "blasting" patients with increasing doses of drugs,

with consequent adverse reactions, it should be possible to individualise one's prescription to fit the patient, and one could expect a curative response with smaller material doses, or even the remedy in potency. . ."I do not say homoeopathy offers a cure for every illness, but the homoeopathic approach enables us to treat the patient as an individual and be selective in our choice of remedy without making him worse, and our prescribing costs can be reduced enormously."

10. **The Homoeopathic Trend in Modern Medical Thought.** We now give a few excerpts from an article by W.E. Young, M.D. published in the *Journal of American Institute of Homoeopathy*, Jan-Feb. 1966 — "Disease, be it natural or drug, manifests itself by symptoms and signs (pathogenesis), and in such wise only does it disclose itself to the physician or the scientific investigator. The question arises whether one should employ in the treatment of the sick an antigen of similar (homoeo) or opposite (contraria) pathogenesis. Experience, experiment and logic all conspire to instruct us that the *homoeo* principle is the one of choice. He then quotes a large number of authorities who support this view, and we give below the observations only of a couple of authorities on this subject :

"The similar antigen (toxoid, or toxin-like) is often to be preferred as a means of eliciting increased production of immune bodies, etc. than the toxin (idem, isopathic) antigen itself. Its advantages are many (Zinser, Enders and Fothergill, *Immunity*, 5th Edition, New York, 1939)."

"Lomhold (*British Journal of Dermatology*, 1920), Brown and Pierce (*Annals of Clinical Medicine*, 1924) concur on the following : The concentration of mercury in the blood of patients under full dosage is never more than 1-2 mgms. per litre. Spirochetes grow readily in horse serum containing as much as 20 mgms. per litre. Yet mercury increases antibody production in the humans and has a pathogenesis similar to the spirochete. Therefore, mercury must be considered as a homoeo specific antigen, and the beneficial effects, the result of increased immunological response.

11. In *The Art of Treatment* by Houston, W.R., edited by G. Minot, New York, 1936, we find the following : "This book will be unsatisfactory for those who wish to learn at a glance what is good for this or that. The emphasis is on approach, not dog-

matic solution. A very great difficulty is getting to know the man who has the disease. The presumption is likely to exist that if only the diagnosis is correct, correct treatment will inevitably follow from that. Nothing could be further from the truth. Treatment is not a mere corollary of diagnosis." If miliary tuberculosis is mistaken for typhoid fever and the patient adequately treated for typhoid, he will not be any the worse for the mistake. The diagnosis though bacteriologically wrong will be therapeutically correct."

12. Since the time of the earliest medical literature (*History of Medicine*), Vol. 1, pp. 114-115; E. Meryon, London, 1861), there has been the necessity to make a choice between the two principles, that of *contraria* and that of *similia*, in the rationale of drug therapy. The homoeopath does not hesitate to make a statement of general therapeutic principle and holds to the opinion that drugs, if used for their curative influence, must be employed on the basis of the *similia* principle, reserving at the same time the privilege of using drugs in accordance with other principles when that is the dictate of good medical judgement. But when he does so . . . he does it with the full realisation and hope that though at times effective, the body itself will remedy matters while the physician temporarily palliates aspect or aspects of the illness.

13. **The Similia Principle in Ayurveda.** Hahnemann has acknowledged that he is not the discoverer of this principle and that Hippocrates had propounded it long ago. In Ayurveda too there are mainly two modes of treatment. The first is called "Vipareeta" or "opposite" (that is *contraria contraris*), and the second is called "Vipareetarthakari" or "similar" (that is, the *similia*). In the former, the mode of treatment is opposite to the cause or manifestation of disease. In the latter, the mode of treatment is similar to the cause or manifestation of disease. The following aphorisms support the *similia* principle : "Samah Samam Shamayati" : or "Vishasya Vishamaushadam," or "Samam Samena Saanti," or "Ushnam Ushnena Shamayati." Another aphorism similar to the homoeopathic principle of *similia* is; "Kasya Aushadhasya Ayam Vyadhih Aaturo Va Yogyah" (*i.e.* the patient belongs to which medicine, or this symptom complex belongs to which medicine, is the point to be known thoroughly well — Vagbhat).

14. Charak (8/23) propounds the ideal mode of cure thus : "Prayogah Shamayet Vyadhim, Yo Anyam Anyam Udeerayet, Naasou Vishudhah, Shudhastu Shamayet Yo Na Kopayet."

That mode of treatment which annihilates an existing disease syndrome but gives rise to another new set of symptoms is not the method of ideal cure, whereas that method which removes a syndrome complex without exciting any other in its stead is the ideal cure. (Charak : 8/23)

15. In summing up this discussion, we find that the two principles of treatment, *viz. contraria contraris* and *similia similibus* have been known to and practised by medical thinkers in a way, since ages past. While modern medicine, with the aid of research projects, laboratories, guinea pigs and clinical trials, has gone far in developing and applying the principle of *contraria*, the *similia* principle had remained only a theory till Hahnemann's genius saw that if this theory is to be tested in practice, we should first ascertain what are the symptoms which each drug produces; it is only when we know them that we can see whether that same medicine can cure symptoms in the sick corresponding to those it has produced in the healthy. As stated earlier, he therefore began his "proving" of the medicines with a band of disciples who gathered round him in this noble task. Let us not forget that the provers had to undergo all types of sufferings patiently and record them for posterity. It is only when the theory was given a practical shape, that it became established as a practical science.

NEED FOR A BALANCED VIEW

16. The benefit of this discovery ought to have been taken advantage of by all medical men, but the narrow mindedness and selfishness of the leaders of thought in those years left no stone unturned to denigrate homoeopaths as quacks and hound them out of practice and even ostracise them socially. The tide seems to be turning now, as we find Kenneth Walker, M.B., F.R.C.S., a Harley Street specialist, writing in his book *Diagnosis of Man*, "An allopathic doctor can, if he retains an open mind, learn much from a homoeopathist. Homoeopathy has avoided some of the errors into which the allopathic school of medicine has fallen" (Dr. B.K. Sarkar's commentary on the *Organon* — p. 111). Had homoeopathy not been treated with such severe antagonism, mankind would have had the benefit of a more balanced view of both the systems, *viz. contraria* and *similia*. After all is said and done, it cannot be denied that both these systems have their respective roles to play in treating the

sick. In such a balanced view, the role which would properly belong to each school of thought would be somewhat as follows :

17. The homoeopathic remedy should be employed in all acute and chronic conditions, unless the signs, symptoms, physical examination (palpation, auscultation, etc.) and pathological reports where necessary (X-ray, ECG. Barium meal, sputum, etc.) reveal that the patient's condition is taking a serious turn and calls for urgent measures to afford him relief and save life. For this purpose, the physician should be guided by Aphorism 3 of the *Organon*, viz, he should know what is curable in the disease (or not curable), he should know what are the medicines which can cure the condition and thirdly he should know how to employ the medicine to effect a rapid and gentle cure.

18. Although the ruling principle is to cure by symptom-similarity circumstances arise occasinally when it becomes necessary to employ physiological doses for palliation. Hahnemann recognised this necessity in paragraph 67 of the *Organon*, in urgent cases where danger to life allows no time for the action of the homoeopathic remedy, e.g. in accidents, asphyxia, suffocation, freezing, drowning. This may reasonably be extended to cases of unendurable pain, when collapse is threatened during the passage of renal calculi, biliary concretions, etc. In exceptional cases it is permissible to use analgesics, in the same way as anaesthetics used in surgical and dental operations. As Stuart Close says : When all has been said and the scope of homoeopathy has been defined as clearly as possible, it is evident that there is a borderland between homoeopathy and its related sciences around which it is impossible to draw sharp lines of demarcation; and under such circumstances the physician must be governed by his own individual judgment.

Let it be pointed out that this is only a concession to the weakness of human nature, for, if the physician is skillful and enjoys the confidence of the patient, he may be able to afford relief even in renal or hepatic colic, with homoeopathic remedies alone. When possible this is the ideal way.

19. A warning, however, seems to be called for at this stage. The physician should not take what is stated here as an excuse for sliding into allopathic practice on all and sundry occasions,

for by doing so he will never be able to know the curative "power" of the homoeopathic medicines nor when and how to employ them. That homoeopathic remedies do have magically curative "power" even in the most serious conditions (except surgical), has been demonstrated by the masters of this art time and again. Therefore, this concession to use allopathic medicines should be taken advantage of only if, in spite of one's best effort (as it takes time and experience to become masters of this art), one is not sure of his choice of the homoeopathic remedy to achieve the urgent object. We recall here the confident assertion of Yingling (*Accoucher's Emergency Manual*) that the more threatening the condition, the more speedy and effective is the action of the indicated homoeopathic remedy. Therefore, one should master the art of homoeopathic prescribing by utilising every occasion and, if we may lay down a percentage, resort to allopathic therapy should not exceed 10% of the cases. We dare say that after just one year's practice on the above lines, the satisfaction which the physician gets in treating his patients successfully and also that of the patients in obtaining speedy cure of their ailments, will be very much more than if he were to do otherwise.

20. In this connection, it is significant that Dr. B.K. Sarkar after stating sixteen points of difference between homoeopathy and modern medicine, himself concludes with the statement : "The places of both are equally important. There is no conflict; there is complementary effort."

21. Long, long ago, in his preface to a text-book on homoeopathy Dr. Von Grauvogl wrote in 1845 : If homoeopathy should seek to treat all cases and every case simply and solely according to the law of similarity, it would fall into the same error as allopathy. Hence, these sciences are no contrasts in the sense of opposition, but rather complements of each other (*Hahnemannian Gleanings*, April, 1975, p. 153).

22. **Danger to Homoeopathy.** It would be appropriate at this juncture, to take note of what happened in the past when the clear lines of demarcation between homoeopathy and allopathy were allowed to be blurred, if not ignored. We shall give here a very brief gist of the documented book entitled *Divided Legacy — A History of the Schism in Medical Thought* by Dr. Harris L. Coulter Ph. D. (*Hahnemannian Gleanings*, October 1974). Homoeopathy entered the U.S.A. at a time when the people of

that country were more afraid of the treatment of the orthodox school (profuse bloodletting, leeches, blisters, huge doses of mineral drugs like *Calomel-Tartar emetic*, etc.) than of the disease. (George Washington was bled to death, for a fever which could have been cured overnight with *Aconite*). This gave rise to the Botanic and Eclectic schools of medicine. Meanwhile, popular publications like Hering's *Domestic Physician* and Humphry's *Guide Book with a Domestic Kit* carried homoeopathy to every household and practically the whole womenfolk — mothers, nurses, matrons, became enamoured of homoeopathy. The obvious cheapness of the homoeopathic medicines played a considerable role in its popularity. In consequence, many an honest and intelligent stalwart of the orthodox school, as well as people from elite circles like lawyers, legislators and literary men, became convinced of homoeopathy as a truly curative system of medicine and turned into strong fighters for the same. Many of President Lincoln's associates were strong patrons of homoeopathy.

Homoeopathy thus enjoyed its greatest influence and success in the two decades following the Civil War.

23. But this period of homoeopathy's triumph was equally the time of its greatest peril. With the relaxation of the external pressures from the allopathic and eclectic schools, whose stock was considerably low by this time, there arose a tragic conflict of opinion in the new school. "A small portion of them were willing to take the trouble and make the sacrifices implicit in the pursuit of Hahnemannian homoeopathy; the great majority rejected that course and attempted to "revise" Hahnemannism along lines which make it "easier to practice." The latter group became known as the "low potency men" and the former as "high potency group."

24. Helped by the widespread success of homoeopathy in the cholera epidemics of the 1830's and 1840's on the one hand and the craving of leaders of homoeopathy for quantitative strength of their organisation, there was a large influx of low-potency men in the American Institute of Homoeopathy. These "lows" played havoc on the doctrinal front :

(i) Inspired by Richard Hughes of Britian, the Materia Medica was re-oriented on pathological basis, subordinating the symptomatology to pathology, etiology and nosological diagnosis.

(ii) They launched an attack on the supposed super-abundance of drugs in the homoeopathic Materia Medica.

(iii) They even maintained that the "law of similars was only one possible rule for finding the remedy and that others existed which were equally valid." When the germ theory of disease came into vogue, many considered it an additional reason for abandoning the law of similars.

(iv) Finally, the "lows" rejected Hahnemann's rule that only one medicine was to be administered at a time, and by the 1880's literature was full of apologia for the mixing of medicines justified by the argument that "the homoeopathic Materia Medica was still incomplete."

(v) The 'lows' then went on to denounce the ultramolecular dilution and minimum dose as "a fanciful creation of Hahnemann . . . which is unsound in theory and very prejudicial to the interests of true homoeopathy." Using the medicines as palliatives, which were not homoeopathic to the patient's symptoms, the 'lows' were compelled to increase the size of their doses in order to obtain an effect (just as Hahnemann was compelled to reduce his doses, being completely homoeopathic to the patient, in order to avoid aggravation).

(vi) Rejecting the three basic rules of homoeopathy — Similar, Single and Minimum — the 'lows' could not but reject the theory of vital force as "unscientific . . . We object to making it the foundation of the homoeopathic healing art."

25. In consequence, on the educational and organisational fronts the 'lows' went on extending their influence by dint of their "democratic majority." Finding little ideological doctrinal and practical difference between themselves and allopaths, they became very eager to recruit the latter as members of the American Institute of Homoeopathy. Meanwhile, under pressure of circumstances, the orthodox school gradually abandoned harmful medications and took up many of the milder vegetable drugs used by homoeopaths and eclectics, and their intolerance against homoeopathy gradually became more polished. With industrialisation the people preferred quicker relief at any cost to the longer treatment based on homoeopathic principles, and they ran to pure allopaths. Thus has homoeopathy lost the attraction and sympathy of the people. The real death-knell for

the homoeopathic teaching institutions was rung as early as about 1910, when under the machinations of the American Medical Association (Allopathic), magnates like Rockfeller and Carnegie (who were the private benefactors of medical science and education) were led to allocate their funds to institutions which had the A.M.A.'s approval, and refuse them to others.

26. In recent years, faced by the flood of highly potent detrimental drugs of the modern medicine, people have started to think again of the really curative treatment of homoeopathy, as proved by the unmanageably increasing clientele of the few surviving homoeopaths with heavy fees. Yet, it is perhaps far too late to restore homoeopathy in U.S.A. to its old status, unless people take the initiative and turn the tide by recruitment of more truly homoeopathic practitioners to meet the demand.

27. The above history of homoeopathy in U.S.A., which had its golden period with stalwarts like J.T. Kent, H.N. Guernsey, Ad. Lippe, H.C. Allen, T.F. Allen, Constantine Hering, E.B. Nash, Caroll Dunham, S. Lilienthal, Raue and a host of others too numerous to mention, is given here so that the reader may have full knowledge of facts in order to judge for himself. It will also help us, in India, to avoid the pitfalls which may take us downhill.

28. During the course of the lesson so far we have dealt with the most important principle of *similia*. As we unfold more details of this science and its practice in future lessons, the readers will have a full understanding of what true homoeopathy is and what it can do as a curative system of therapeutics.

Self-Test

1. Which system of therapeutics has a better claim for our consideration — that which is based on everchanging "facts" or that which is based on a logical unchanging principle whose universality of application in practice, has stood the test of time? Where does homoeopathy stand in this respect? (Para 3).

2. It is said that the falling of the apple from a tree suggested the Law of Gravity to Newton. What is the corresponding incident that revealed the Law of Similars? (Para 5).

3. What is the Law of Similars? Explain in a few words what it means.

4. Mention a few remedies used by practitioners of modern medicine which to your knowledge are capable of producing similar symptoms in the healthy, to those which they can cure in the sick? (Para 6).

5. What are the practical aspects of treatment in which homoeopathy and allopathy can be taken as complementary to each other? (Para 18).

6. What were the six factors on the doctrinal front, by rejecting which one section of homoeopaths caused the downfall of homoeopathy in America in the 1880's? (Para 23).

STUDY IN DEPTH

Ch. II (pp. 8-22) — "General Interpretations." *Genius of Homoeopathy* by Stuart Close.

Ch. III (pp. 23-36) — "Schools of Philosophy," same book by Stuart Close.

Ch. IV (pp. 37-47) — "The Scope of Homoeopathy," same book by Stuart Close.

Ch. II (pp. 19-33) — "Introduction to the Study of Homoeopathy." *Principles and Art of Cure by Homoeopathy* by H.A. Roberts.

Books mentioned above are available with M/s. B. Jain Publishers (P) Ltd., Post Box - 5775 , New Delhi - 55.

Lesson 3

Provings and Construction of Materia Medica

Provings — How Made

1. Once Hahnemann was convinced that "in order to cure gently, quickly, unfailingly and permanently," we must select "for every case of disease a medicine capable of calling forth by itself an affection similar to that which it is intended to cure," he began "proving" drugs, *i.e.* testing their effects on "healthy but sensitive and susceptible human beings" and recording the symptoms they evoked, in order to use them, "with confidence" in the treatment of the sick. His list of fellow provers numbered fifty. Care was taken not only to elicit and record exact results, but to rule out errors. A prover would record his sensations when taking unmedicated powders and did not know when medicated powders were substituted, so that personal symptoms, unnoticed till his attention was focussed upon them, might be eliminated. All Hahnemann's work was thoughtful, painstaking to the last degree, and purely scientific. "A Materia Medica" he said, "should exclude every supposition, every mere assertion and fiction. Its entire contents should be the pure language of Nature, uttered in response to careful and faithful inquiry." Of such pure drug-provings the vast "Homoeopathic Materia Medica Pura," as he called it, is composed.

2. During some fifty years Hahnemann was poisoning himself, his pupils and his friends with remedies known and unknown, or known only to the ancients or the Arabians, in order to determine their exact, and especially their peculiar effects, physical, mental and moral (psychological). He proved nearly one hundred medicines upon himself. The provings have never proved detrimental to health (whatever the immediate sufferings may have been), but on the contrary, they tend, as Hahnemann

pointed out, to raise the resistance of the prover. And Hahnemann should know, who, having spent the greater part of his life in proving drugs, lived on, in full possession of health and senses, till only one year short of ninety.

3. Many remedies, since Hahnemann's day, have been added to our armoury against disease; but all subsequent work has been done on his lines. For the more exact purposes of homoeopathy, experiments in drug action on animals are useless, as Hahnemann pointed out; and that for two reasons. Substances poisonous to man are innocuous to many animals. Hedgehogs feed on *cantharides* and take no hurt. Rabbits eat *Belladonna* with impunity. *Morphia* makes dogs drowsy and to vomit, but excites cats. Horses are given large doses of *Arsenic* to improve their wind and to make their coats glossy. Rats are immune to diphtheria. Cats are said to be immune to tubercle, whereas guineapigs and monkeys are highly susceptible to that infection. All that experiments on animals may help us to find out is that certain drugs affect certain tissues of certain animals. That is all.

4. But more than this, homoeopathic provings were aimed at bringing out the very fine, very delicate and very definite and the subjective and mental symptoms (all important for our purpose), and these can be obtained only from humans. It is only men and women who, in provings, could have given us the mental symptoms which have led to so many brilliant cures — such as the depression to the verge of suicide of *Aurum*; the insane jealousy of *Lachesis*; the teror of insanity of *Mancinella*; the frantic irritability and intolerance of pain of *Chamomilla*; the suspicion and restlessness of *Arsenicum* : the terrors of anticipation of *Argentum nitricum*; the fear of death of Aconite and *Arsenicum*; the sensation of tallness and superiority of Platina; the sensation of unreality of *Medorrhinum;* the sensation of two wills of *Anacardium*; the indifference to loved ones of *Phosphorus* and *Sepia* — all straight cuts to the curative remedy — and these could only be got by provings on human beings. Even provings on the sick are not accepted, since sickness modifies the response of the organism to drugs, and from the sick no true drug-picture can be obtained.

Remedies also need to be proved on women as well as on men, in order to get their whole range of usefulness. The provings of *Lilium tigrinum*, for instance, entailed intense sufferings on the heroic women who undertook them, but they have given us a most useful remedy for the peculiar suffering of women in uterine displacements, after miscarriages, etc.

5. **Provings on Animals.** Provings on healthy human beings alone could give us the mental symptoms (such as irritability, aversion to company and even to loved ones, fear of darkness, sensitiveness to noise or music, anxieties of various sorts), or sensations of pain such as burning, throbbing, stitching, soreness; factors which modify symptoms (such as better or worse from heat or cold, pressure, lying on right or left side, before, during or after sleep or menstruation, etc.). Provings on animals would be incapable of giving us this detailed *subjective* symptomatology. Is not subjective symptomatology an essential part of disease, and is not homoeopathy, which lays much emphasis on it, a superior system of therapeutics than other systems of medicine which care little for these symptoms.

Determining the organs and tissues which are affected by different drugs (revealed post-mortem) through experiments on animals has led modern medicine to base its therapeutics on the treatment of organs and tissues to the total neglect of the man as a whole (including his subjective feelings). Consequently, it by-passes, even suppresses, the immune system (vital force) which governs the functioning of the whole organism. In the result while it undoubtedly scores local (organ based) victories, it loses in the final battle of curing the man.

6. Dr. Otto Leeser, M.D., Phil. D. in a highly learned article (*Hahnemannian Gleanings*, Sept. 1970) has shown that modern pharmacological methods throw intense light on the action of remedies on various bodily structures, and thus explain the mechanism of action of a remedy. But when it comes to practical application, such sporadic glimpses into intermediary processes are quite unfit to guide our therapeutic actions. For them, functional similarity remains the first principle. Compared to the complexity of biochemical processes in the organism, pharmacological experiments on partial systems are only pale imitators. As a guide to therapeutic action, the inhibition, or stimulation of this or that function is much too primitive. But the medicinal actions observed in provings on healthy persons, in the form of signs and symptoms are in no way affected or replaced by theoretical insights into how they arise. Structural comparison leads to applying antagonistic action (*contraria*

contraris) to individual processes (functions) taken out of context. On the other hand, comparison of signs of disturbed function (homoeopathic symptomatology) leads to accurate selection of a remedy which will support the reactivity of the sick organism in its totality. Modern pharmacology understands disease entirely in structural terms, molecular or larger, that is to say, eventually in mechanistic terms. Homoeopathy understands disease as a *dynamic disturbance* arising in a human being and manifested in the *experience of symptoms*. A mere structure, a mechanism, cannot experience symptoms. In view of this, the dependability of homoeopathic symptomatology derived from provings on healthy humans as a therapeutic guide, hardly needs reiteration.

7. **Sources of Drugs.** The drugs are drawn from six sources :

(1) Vegetable kingdom.

(2) Mineral kingdom.

(3) Animal kingdom.

(4) Nosodes, which are remedies derived from morbid tissues and secretions.

(5) Sarcodes, which are remedies prepared from healthy animal tissues and secretions.

(6) Imponderabilia, which include positive and negative magnetic forces, electricity, x-ray, sun-force, etc.

A few examples of remedies from each kingdom are given below :

(1) **Vegetable**
Aconitum Nepallus (Monkshood)
Aloes (Socotrine Aloes)
Arnica (Leopard's Bane)
Belladonna (Deadly Night Shade)
Bryonia (Wild Hops)
Chelidonium Majus (Calendine)
Cina (Worm Seed)
Chamomilla (German Chamomile)

China (Peruvian Bark)
Colchicum (Meadow Saffron)
Digitalis (Foxglove)
Gelsemium (Yellow Jasmine)
Hypericum (St. John's Wort)
Ignatia (St. Ignatius Bean)
Ledum (Marsh Tea)
Lycopodium (Club Moss)
Mezerium (Sparge Olive)
Nux Vomica (Poison Nut)
Phytolacca (Poke Root)
Podophyllum (May Apple)
Pulsatilla (Wind Flower)
Rhus Toxicodendron (Poison Ivy)
Sanguinaria (Blood Root)
Spigelia (Pink Root)
Secale Cornutum (Ergot)
Tabacum (Tobacco)
Thuja (Arbor Vitae)
Staphysagria (Stavesacre)
Terebinthina (Turpentine)
Veratrum Album (White Hellabore).

(2) **Mineral**
Acetic Acid (Glacial Acetic Acid)
Alumina (Oxide of Aluminium — Argilla)
Amyl Nitrosum (Amyl Nitrite)
Antimonium Crudum (Black Sulphide of Antimony)
Antimonium Tartaricum (Tartar Emetic)
Argentum Nitricum (Silver Nitrate)
Arsenicum Album (Arsenic Trioxide)
Aurum Metallicum (Metallic Gold)
Baryta Carb (Carbonate of Baryta)
Borax (Borate of Sodium)
Calcarea Carb (Carbonate of Lime)
Ferrum Met. (Iron)
Glonoine (Nitro-Glycerine)
Hekla Lava (Lava from Mt. Hecla)
Iodum (Iodine)
Kali Bichromicum (Bichromate of Potash)
Kali Carb. (Carbonate of Potash)
Kali Phos. (Phosphate of Potash)
Mercurius Solubilis (Quicksilver)
Mercurius Corrosivus (Corrosive Sublimate)

Magnesia Phosphorica (Phosphate of Magnesia)
Natrum Muriaticum (Sodium Chloride)
Natrum Sulph (Glauber's Salt)
Petroleum (Crude Rock Oil)
Phosphorus
Phosphoric Acid
Platina (Metal)
Silicea (Pure Flint)
Sulphur (Sublimated Sulphur)
Zincum Metallicum (Zinc).

(3) **Animal Poisons**
Agaricus Muscarius (Toad Stool — Bug Agaric)
Bufo (Poison of the Toad)
Apis (Honey Bee)
Bothrops (Yellow Viper)
Cimex (Bedbug)
Lachesis (Surukuku Snake)
Latrodectus Mactans (Spider)
Naja (Cobra Venom)
Tarentula Cubensis (Cuban Spider)
Tarentula Hispania (Spanish Spider)
Sepia (Inky Juice of Cuttlefish)
Cantharis (Spanish Fly)
Crotalus Horridus (Rattle Snake)
Vipera (The German Viper).

(4) **Nosodes**
Bacillinum (Maceration of a Typical Tuberculosis Lung)
Diphtherinum (Potentised Diphtheric Virus)
Medorrhinum (Gonorrhoea Virus)
Pyrogenium (Artificial Sepsin)
Psorinum (Scabies Vesicle)
Variolinum (Lymph from Small-pox Pustule)
Syphilinum (Syphilitic Virus)
Lyssin/Hydrophobinum (Saliva of Rabid Dog).

(5) **Sarcodes**
Adrenaline
Cholesterinum (Epithelial Lining of Gall Bladder)
Lac Caninum (Dog's Milk)
Pituitrin (Pituitary Gland)
Thyroidinum (Dried Thyroid Gland of Sheep)

(6) **Imponderabilia**
Electricity
Radium Brom.
Magnetis Poli Ambo.
Magnetis Polus Australis.
X-Ray.

8. **Sources of Symptomatology.** The symptomatology contained in the Materia Medica is mainly derived from the provings on relatively healthy individuals. Cases of poisoning, toxicology, has contributed the extreme symptoms and in part the pathology. There are also "clinical symptoms," that is, new symptoms appearing after administration of a remedy repeatedly verified), or symptoms cured during medication (also provided they are repeatedly verified), pathology which is cured such as open fontenelles, rickets, albuminuria, etc. has also been added to the Materia Medica. Nash called these clinical symptoms as symptoms "born of breach presentation," and thus justified their inclusion in the Materia Medica for, do we throw away a baby born of breach presentation?

HOW TO KNOW THE REMEDIES WELL

9. It must be said at once that it is no easy task to acquire and retain in one's memory a detailed knowledge of even fifty of the most important remedies, the polychrests, *i.e.*, remedies with a wide range of action. Yet it can become comparatively easy if we follow a method. The essence of homoeopathy is individualisation — the individuality of the patient has to be matched with the individuality of the remedy. We master the individuality of each remedy by studying its important *striking* features. Suppose you are asked by your father from Poona to meet his friend at the railway station in Bombay and give him some help. You have not met him before. Your father has given a brief description of his friend in his letter to you, *viz.* that he is six ft. two inches tall, is bald, wears thick glasses, is very thin, a black wart of his left forehead, has lost some incisors and has a scar above his right eyebrow. In trying to identify the gentleman from the fast moving crowd at the station, will you not first stop all *tall* men with *baldy* head (the most striking features which are uncommon), before checking up if they have the other identifying features? You will be satisfied that one of them is the man you want only when you find the *peculiar combination* of the clearly visible signs. Infact, one who answers

the description fully will not have to be examined for his lost teeth. In the same way, each remedy has several peculiar features, each of which may be common to some other remedies, but the combination (or totality) of features will belong to one remedy alone. Sometimes even two or three features of the friend (or remedy) may be so outstanding that with their help alone we may be able to recognise him even from a long distance. What are those distinguishing or individualising or differentiating features in the remedies corresponding to the facial features of the friend just described? If we understand these features, then we shall have gone a long way to an understanding of the personality of the remedies. These differentiating symptoms, according to the general experience of masters of this art, fall under the following broad heads:

(i) *Mental symptoms.* Such as fear, anxiety, irritability and anger, sadness, depression, tearfulness, aversion to company, loathing of life, etc.

(ii) *Modalities.* Conditions which modify, *viz.* aggravate or ameliorate the illness, pain, etc. such as the time of agg. Agg. from warm or cold air or draft, or wet or dry weather, Agg. from movement, position when lying (left or right side), agg. or amel. from touch or pressure, eating, drinking, stool, or before, during or after urination, menstruation, coition, sleep, etc. These modalities may be general, applying to the whole person, or particular, applying only to parts of the body.

(iii) *Sensations of pain.* Such as burning, cutting, soreness, throbbing, pulsating, cramping, bursting, etc. These again may be General or Particular as in the case of Modalities.

(iv) *Location of complaints.* Such as occiput, forehead, inner or outer canthi, zygomae, throat, stomach, abdomen, hypochondria (left or right), hypograstrium, genitalia, side of body (right or left), skin eruptions, glands, bones, etc.

(v) *Concomitant complaints associated with the chief complaint.* Such as dim vision before headache (*Kali bichromicum*); child cries before urinating (*Lycopodium*), pain in testicles while coughing (*Zincum*), involuntary urination while coughing or sneezing (*Causticum*), etc. Concomitants are those which seemingly have no relation to the leading symptoms from the standpoint of theoretical pathology. We might almost term them as "unreasonable attendants" of the case in hand.

Provings and Construction of Materia Medica

(vi) *Peculiar, rare, strange, uncommon, characteristic symptoms.* Such as head sweats profusely during sleep, wetting the pillow far around (*Calc. carb.*); stitching pains better by lying on the painful side (*Bryonia*); discharge of a tough stringy mucus, which can be drawn into long strings, and which adhere to the parts (*Kali bichromicum*); pain in small spots (*Kali bich.*); violent colic, sensation as if abdominal wall is drawn to the spine by a string (*Plumbum*), etc.

BOOKS FOR STUDYING THE MATERIA MEDICA

10. Meanwhile, we may recommend a few books for study, which will help the beginners to understand the personality of each remedy :

(1) The first book we recommend for all beginners is the *Leaders in Homoeopathic Therapeutics* by Dr. E.B. Nash. This book provides an excellent introduction to homoeopathy for beginners, covering philosophy, Materia Medica, therapeutics, potency, etc. with a "dose" of infectious enthusiasm as well. A dry subject is made very interesting as well as instructive. It repays repeated reading, and even veterans find it necessary to refer to it occasionally.

(2) *Key-notes and Characteristics* by H.C. Allen. It furnishes important key-notes of leading remedies (on the lines of Nash's *Leaders*) and within a short compass, provides us with a number of most dependable, characteristic key-notes and peculiar symptoms. Valued by many of the best prescribers.

(3) *Homoeopathic Drug Pictures* by Margaret Tyler. Fully justifies its title; presents drug-pictures as seen by various masters, garnished by therapeutic marvels & philosophical comments from the pen of an able prescriber. A must-be-read book.

(4) *Lectures on Materia Medica* by Dr. J.T. Kent. Unique for its detailed pictures of remedies, which leave a lasting impression on the mind about the true essence of remedies.

BOOKS FOR REFERENCE

11. The description of remedies given in these books informs us of the "genius," the red-thread, the guiding indications of remedies. But before prescribing on the genius of a remedy,

even if it comes out strong after repertorisation, it is advisable to make sure that the patient's characteristics match the remedy's as fully as possible. This can be done by referring to a complete Materia Medica and the regional symptoms (throat, chest, abdomen, etc. as the case may be) given therein. The following books are good for this purpose :

(1) *Materia Medica with Repertory* by Dr. William Boericke is both comprehensive and handy for day to day use and is as good for study as for reference. It also contains a useful repertorial section, with many pathological rubrics.

(2) *Materia Medica of Homoeopathic Medicines* by Dr. S.R. Phatak. Though not containing as many remedies as Boericke's, this book covers a wider spectrum of each remedy, especially the mental aspect, thus qualifying it as essential for reference before any other Materia Medica.

(3) *A Synoptic Key of the Materia Medica* by C.M. Boger reveals at a glance the regional affinities and modalities together with a useful synopsis of each remedy. There is also a repertorial section for bed-side use.

(4) *A Dictionary of Practical Materia Medica* (in three volumes) by Dr. John H. Clarke, M.D. is a comprehensive sourcebook which repays constant reference. In particular, the introductory essays at the beginning of each remedy are most enlightening, containing comparisons and "sensations as if."

(5) *The Guiding Symptoms of Our Materia Medica* (in ten volumes) by Dr. Constantine Hering, M.D. is a most valuable set, which may be taken as the final court of appeal. Dr. Jugal Kishore B.Sc., D.M.S. (Cal.) in his learned introduction to the Indian edition brings out the following salient points about these volumes :

(i) Hering admitted in these volumes only such symptoms as had not only appeared in a prover or provers, but had been verified at the bedside a number of times.

(ii) He laid down evaluation of symptoms in four grades : 1, 2, 3 and 4 for the first time in the Materia Medica, just as Boenninghausen had done with remedies for the first time in his *Therapeutic Pocket Book.*

(iii) Dr. H.C. Allen's Key-notes of leading remedies is based entirely on the *Guiding Symptoms.*

(iv) Dr. Kent based his *Lectures on the Materia Medica* mostly on Hering's *Guiding Symptoms,* using it as his "text."

(v) The greatest debt owed by Kent in the construction of his repertory was the evaluation or grading of the remedies for which he took Hering's evaluation.

(vi) Another useful feature is the mention of various pathological conditions or diseases in which a particular symptom was found to be cured by a particular drug — mentioned at the end of that symptom in brackets.

(6) *Hering's Condensed Materia Medica* (Condensed from the *Guiding Symptoms* and containing the leading remedies) is handy and useful for day-to-day reference, if one wants to avoid the much larger volume of the *Guiding Symptoms.*

(7) *Materia Medica of Graphic Drug Pictures and Clinical Comments* by Dr. A. Pulford, covers in just 318 pages, the kernel of the remedies together with uniquely useful clinical comments.

(8) *Hahnemann's Materia Medica Pura.* The original source of the subject is placed last on the list because of the mass of symtoms.

A NOVEL METHOD OF STUDYING THE MATERIA MEDICA USEFUL FOR THE BUSY NEOPHYTE

12. Allopathic physicians who may not have much time to devote to the intense study of the Materia Medica and are yet eager to learn to prescribe homoeopathic remedies may take heart. There is a method by which they can practise scientific homoeopathy, and take their own time — a year or two to acquire a fairly good understanding of the "drug pictures." This method is through finding the remedy for a case, first, with the help of the Repertory and then studying that remedy in the Materia Medica before administering it to the patient.

13. **What is a Repertory.** A Repertory is an alphabetical index of the various symptoms in the Materia Medica. The symptoms are classified under the various headings of the schema, such as Mind, Sensorium, Vertigo, Head, Eyes, Ears, etc. All the remedies which have produced a particular symptom in the provers (which has been verified as cured in disease), are shown against that symptom. The relative value of each remedy in respect of that symptom is shown in four grades in Boenninghausen's and three grades in Kent's Repertory. The remedies shown in capital letters in Boenninghausen's are the highest grade, and carry four marks. In Kent's the highest grade remedies are in bold letters and carry three marks. The next grade remedies carrying 3 or 2 marks respectively are in bold types and italics in the respective Repertories. The next lower grade remedies (with 2 or 1 mark) are in italics and ordinary types respectively. The lowest grade remedies in ordinary types in both repertories designate an occasionally confirmed symptom, while the higher grades are more frequently verified.

14. The following examples will make this clear :

"Love, unfortunate : *Aur.*, Calc.p., Caus., Cimi., COF., *Con.*, HYO., IGN., Kali-c., **Lach.**, **Nat-m.**, Pho., **Pho-ac.**, Sep., **Stap.** (Boger-Boenninghausen's repertory)

"Love, ailments, from disappointed : Ant-c., *Aur.*, *Calc-p.*, Caust, *Cimic.*, *Coff.*, *Hell.*, **Hyos.**, **Ign.**, Kali-c., *Lach.*, **Nat-m.**, Nux-v., **Ph-ac.**, Sep., *Staph.*, Tarent. (Kent's Repertory).

15. It will thus be seen that the Repertory not only shows at a glance all the remedies which are known to have produced and cured a symptom, but also shows the grade (or importance) they occupy as curative of that symptom. Even years of study of the Materia Medica will not give us such information so readily.

16. The method we advocate of treating a case by first referring to the Repertory and then consulting the Materia Medica being novel and unorthodox, may be criticised as "impractical" or even as "dangerous" by those who are accustomed to follow the beaten track and never venture away from it. We are aware that a good knowledge of the genius of remedies is helpful even in repertorising, but there are grades and degrees of knowledge, and where do we draw the line where one can say, "I know enough"? On the contrary, the need for a repertory was felt even

by Hahnemann who, through the provings, had lived and suffered from the symptoms of the remedies. It is admitted on all hands that remembering the detailed symptoms of remedies is almost impossible. It is also admitted that a high degree of differentiation between remedies is involved while selecting the remedy for a case. Is there any better and easier way of making these differentiations of remedies in respect of a number of symptoms comprising the totality than by reference to the repertory? Kent in the preface to his *Lectures on Materia Medica* has said that the trio — *Organon* (philosophy) the Materia Medica and the Repertory — must join in our hunt for the similimum. Dr. Glen I. Bidwell, M.D., in *How to Use the Repertory* says : "Constant use of the repertory leads us to the study of our remedies in a scientific, rational manner, from centre to circumference, from the mind to skin . . . thus learning to observe the disordered patient rather than pathological changes in the organs or parts." Dr. P.S. Krishnamurthy of Hyderabad, who studied Kent's Repertory and Materia Medica under Dr. Elizabeth Hubbard, says that the art (of selecting the correct remedy) comes from "constantly studying Materia Medica through Repertory and Repertory through Materia Medica. We must find out the symptoms of Materia Medica in the repertory; similarly, while studying repertory, we must search the Materia Medica for the rubric, as a symptom, . . . consulting the *Guiding Symptoms* as the appellate jurisdiction both for Materia Medica and Repertory."

17. Dr. P. Sankaran in his small but valuable booklet, *The Value of the Repertory*, says : "In fact, I believe that we may not comprehend even one drug thoroughly and completely even if we were to devote a life-time to its study. Under the circumstances, the use of a Repertory will considerably enlarge our vision, and help us to succeed in our work."

18. The advice of Dr. A. Pulford, M.D., in his article : "How Do You Approach the Materia Medica to Find the Similimum?" (*Homoeopathic Recorder*, 1930 — Reproduced in *Homoeopathic Heritage*, New Delhi, August, 1979) is even more specific. He says :

"There are various methods of approach to the Materia Medica used by various physicians. Our advice would be to procure a copy of either *Kent's Repertory* or Boger's revised *Boenninghausen's Repertory with Characteristics*, and using this as a basis.

"In our examination of the patient, if properly done, you will learn what is individualistically characteristic of your patient *i.e.*, rare, strange and peculiar, and his most important symptom or symptoms. You then pick out those and take them to the rubric or rubrics covering them, in the Repertory of your choice, and there you will find a list of remedies covering these symptoms, thus saving yourself the trouble of having to wade through the entire Materia Medica. Each additional symptom, or symptom qualifier, is apt to reduce the number of remedies which must be compared.

"For example : Mr. A comes to you with lumbago. You turn to your Repertory, to the section labelled "Back," then to pain in the lumbar region. There you will find the 600 or more remedies of the Materia Medica reduced to 200. Yet some maze ! Now, here comes the part that shows the importance of having your symptoms qualified. You find your patient is worse mornings in bed. This reduces your list to 26, which is some better. But your patient volunteers : "I must sit up before I can turn over in bed." Your Repertory says — *Nux*, and *Nux* only. Now you take the patient's symptoms and compare them with the provings of *Nux*, and the chances are 100 to 1 that *Nux* covers the entire case.

"Again, suppose Mr. B. comes in with a bad case of vesicular erysipelas. You turn to your Repertory to the section called "Skin," then to the rubric marked Erysipelas, then to the subrubric marked vesicular and there you will find instead of 600 remedies with which to compare, just 45. But you learned that your patient had a yellow stool, which cuts the list down to 17. You learned that the stool was watery which in turn cuts that list to 14. You further learned that the stool was forcibly expelled, coming out like a shot, which further cuts your list down to 10. Then the patient finally volunteered :

"My diarrhoea is always worse immediately after eating or drinking." That at once puts the characteristic mark or stamp of *Croton tiglium* on the case. By comparing your collected data of the patient with the proving of *Croton tig.* the chances are 100 to 1 that you will not have to change your prescription.

"So you see how this method makes your approach to the Materia-Medica more easy and a time saver. With all these advantages and labour-saving devices, there is no excuse for our not being able to do equally as good work as our masters before us did. They had none of these advantages. Try to learn to find the characteristics, the rare, strange and peculiar symptoms, the mark of stamp of each individual drug, not for prescribing purposes but for reference."

19. We hope it will be seen from the above that the Materia Medica and the Repertory are two sides of the same coin. A really good comparative study of remedies becomes possible when we study both together in the manner suggested by Dr. Krishnamurthy.

20. **Constant study of Materia Medica — a Must**. Let not the reader conclude from what we have said about studying the Materia Medica through the Repertory, that this procedure is sufficient. Far from it, constant study of the Materia Medica in order to grasp the essential characteristics of the remedies is a must. Dr. Clarke says in his *Prescriber*: It is impossible to carry all the symptoms of the Materia Medica in one's head but it is quite possible to remember a very large number of the characteristic symptoms and modalities (or conditions) of the chief remedies. And after all, the best Repertory any one can have is in his own memory. Only it must be possible to supplement it whenever required. Every remedy has a number of symptoms and modalities which are general in respect to it. That is to say, they qualify a very large proportion of its manifestations. So that when the practitioner meets with them in a patient, he will be able to select the remedy even if the particular symptoms are not in precise correspondence. Our advice would be to study two polychrests each week, reading each remedy together from Nash's *Leaders*, Allen's *Key-notes*, Tyler's *Drug Pictures* and Boericke's *Materia Medica*. The student will then get acquainted with the definite characteristics and range of action of the different remedies. This is like the "Rogues' gallery of portraits" in the crime branch of the police with a study of *modus operandi* of each criminal, helping the officer to identify the culprit in each case. The five of the rogues (who can cause as well as cure ill-health), *viz.* (i) Mentals, (ii) Physical Generals, (iii) Key-notes (strange, rare and peculiar symptoms), (iv) concomitants and, lastly (v) particulars with their qualifying modalities will be the main points for study, comparison and differentiation.

21. The reader will now be eager to learn the technique of repertorisation. However, before we take up this subject it is

essential to clearly grasp the comparative value of different symptoms which alone qualify for our attention while making a repertorial study of a case. Then again, we should also master the art of "taking the case," i.e. interrogating the patient for the purpose of eliciting all the symptoms which are of importance for repertorial study.

SELF-TEST

1. What care was taken by Hahnemann to see that the provers did not report personal symptoms induced by the knowledge that they were taking drugs which would produce symptoms? (Para 1).

2. What is the difference, in understanding the nature of disease, between modern pharmacology and homoeopathy? (Para 5 and 6).

3. What are the five classes of characteristic features which help us in differentiating one remedy from another? (Para 20).

4. What is a Repertory? What is the type of help it gives to the physicians? (Para 13-18).

Lesson 4

Evaluation of Symptoms

1. We have seen earlier that the disease makes itself known to the physician by signs and symptoms, and that the totality of the symptoms is the sole representation of the disease. The patient presents a large number and varied types of symptoms. Are all of them of the same value ? And how do we match them with an equally large and varied assortment of symptoms produced by each remedy in the Materia Medica?

2. The answer to these questions is provided when we remember that the susceptibility of each individual varies, which in turn calls for individualisation of his symptoms, *i.e.*, finding out what are his individual symptoms (no matter what diagnostic label we put on his disease), and compare them with similar individualising features of remedies. There may be three patients of pneumonia and each one of them may need different remedies according to the individual or characteristic symptoms presented by them.

3. **Two Classes of Symptoms**. To begin with, therefore, let us note that there are two classes of symptoms in every case of disease : *First*, those that pertain to the disease, that is, the *common* or *diagnostic* ones, and *second*, those that pertain to the *patient*. The advanced cases that present gross pathology, the ultimates of the disease, present but few symptoms as such. If we refer to the Materia Medica we shall find that almost every leading remedy has these common or diagnostic symptoms, such as headache, indigestion, sleeplessness, fever, etc. When the symptoms are so common to many remedies, how can we differentiate between them for applying them to the sick individual patient? We cannot differentiate them. That is why we say that we cannot base our prescription of these common or diagnostic symptoms. Dr. H.A. Roberts, M.D. says in *Principles and Art of Cure by Homoeopathy* :

"If we allow ourselves to become influenced by the diagnosis in making our remedy selection, we are very apt to become confused and fail to help our patient. We may be faced with a diagnosis of some grave condition such as some form of deep abscess, a grave pneumonic condition, an internal haemorrhage, or any one of a host of conditions. Selection of the remedy on the basis of the diagnosis may, and probably will, fail completely. However, the symptoms of the patient are an infallible guide, and the more serious the condition, the clearer cut are the indications for the remedy. If we allow ourselves to be guided by these symptoms, we shall probably save the patient, even though this remedy selected on the basis of the symptoms totality may never have been used under like diagnostic conditions before."

4. Does this mean that a knowledge of diagnosis and pathology is of no use in prescribing for a disease? Kent says : "It is necessary to know them, but he would put in a different way". He urged that "all become acquainted with diagnosis and pathology in order not to prescribe for the disease . . . If the physician does not know what the common symptoms are, *i.e.*, what symptoms represent the various diseases, he will make the mistake of trying to fit a remedy to such symptoms. The symptoms common to Bright's disease are dropsy, albumen in urine, weakness and the disturbed heart action. Any physician who would pretend to prescribe on these would show a great folly. The remedies that have produced such a complex of symptoms are very numerous. To prescribe on such a group must lead to failure. However, if there is no albumin in the urine and no signs of structural kidney change there, the symptoms mentioned become representative of the patient and become valuable features in the totality of the symptoms. It will at once be seen what a relative proposition each case of sickness becomes. Symptoms quite identical may be common or important . . . in accordance with the character of the sickness the patient suffers from."

5. Kent further clarifies that all the symptoms (general and particular), with the common left out, are always strange, rare and peculiar, and therefore, characteristic. To collect these is the only way to secure a firm basis for a homoeopathic prescription. In the highest sense, the general symptoms represent the patient; in a lesser sense the particulars (regional symptoms) represent the parts of the patient and hence in a lesser degree

the patient. The general symptoms that are mental are the very highest in importance. How did the master arrive at these classifications of symptoms? Kent says again, "It is truly by comparing our Materia Medica symptoms with disease symptoms that we have learned to classify them into symptoms that represent the patient as a whole, symptoms that represent his parts and symptoms that represent disease."

6. A few more examples to show how reliance on the common symptoms of disease alone does not help us in finding the remedy (but the symptoms peculiar to the patient do) will be in order. They are taken from Dr. Gibson Miller's classical monograph *On the Comparative Value of Symptoms in the Selection of the Remedy.*

"The common or pathognomonic symptoms of dysentery are bloody, mucous stools, pain and tenesmus. From these alone we can determine the group of remedies that corresponds in general to this disease, and in J.B. Bell's *Diarrhoea and Dysentery,* over fifty remedies are mentioned; yet from these alone it would be impossible to discover the individual remedy for the case under treatment. If, however, the patient has much thirst, and every time he drinks he shivers, and each drink is followed by a loose stool, then these symptoms, being unusual in the disease, would consequently be peculiar to the patient and guiding to *Capsicum* as the remedy.

"Dyspnoea, oedema and palpitation of the heart, albuminuria, are the common symptoms of many kidney troubles and from them alone we cannot determine the curative remedy; but if we find in addition there is a strong craving for fat, intensely strong-smelling urine, and a sensation as if the urine were cold when passed, then these would be peculiar to the patient, and point to *Nitric Acid* as the remedy.

In hysteria we have an illustration of the danger of the prescribing for the symptoms that are common to the disease, and hence not peculiar to the patient. It seems the most natural thing to be prescribed upon the peculiar and incongruous symptoms that characterise this disease; but when we realise that this incongruity is the very essence of the disease — in other words, is pathognomonic of it — we then perceive that we have been prescribing for the symptoms that represent the disease and not for those that characterise the patient. In such cases the true guides to cure, if discoverable, are to be found in the changes of desires, the aversions, the loves and hates, and these are particularly difficult to find, for the hysterical patient conceals her real hates and loves and relates what is not true."

7. Now let us see what Dr. J.H. Clarke, author of the *Dictonary of Materia Medica*, has to say on this point. He says in his *Prescriber* : "It often happens that those symptoms which are of the greatest value in correctly naming the disease, are of the smallest value in diagnosing the remedy. The times and conditions under which the various symptoms are better or worse are often of more consequence than the actual symptoms. And yet these characteristics would give little or no help in the diagnosis of the disease." For instance, Miss T., 60, consulted me about a pain which had troubled her more or less for twenty-five years. It affects the right side of the head and right cheek. In the temple are violent sharp shoots of pain. In the cheek it is a sudden pain, burning as if on fire. It is worse while eating : worse by touch, better after eating. It is worse if the patient is chilled; and is sometimes worse from 3 to 8 p.m. or at night.

8. In dealing with a case like this it does not assist us much whether we name the affection "neuralgia neuritis," or "Tic douloureux;" we must deal with it on the strength of its characteristic symptoms. The three important points of this case were : (i) the locality of the pain (one-sided, that is, right side); (ii) suddenness of pain — violent, sharp, shooting and burning; (iii) the conditions of aggravation, *i.e.*, aggravation by chewing, by the least movement or touch; and aggravation between 4 and 8 p.m. or night. On the basis of these characteristics of the patient, *Lycopodium* 200 was prescribed, and two months later the patient wrote to say, "the pain was relieved in a most wonderful way."

9. If this patient had applied to an old school practitioner, all these details would have been useless to him; all he would have needed to base his prescription would have been the word "neuralgia." It would have signified nothing, so far as his prescription went, whether it was right side, left side, or both sides. It would not have mattered what made it better or what made it worse, or at what time of the day it came on. To the homoeopath these are everything.

Evaluation of Symptoms

10. The above examples with comments, we hope, will sufficiently impress the reader that a sure way to invite failure in homoeopathy is to first label the disease and try to find a drug to match it.

11. **Characteristic Symptoms.** Now we come to the question, how do we identify the characteristic symptoms, characteristic in the patient as well as the drug? Hahnemann gives very clear instruction in Para 153 of the *Organon* : "In this search for a homoeopathic specific remedy . . . in the comparison of the collective symptoms of the disease with the symptoms of medicines, the more striking, singular, uncommon and peculiar (characteristic) signs and symptoms of the case are especially and almost solely to be kept in view; for it is more particularly these that must correspond to the very similar ones in the symptoms of the selected medicine, in order to cure." Hering in his preface to the *Guiding Symptoms* points out that Hahnemann in giving his practical advice uses the word "characteristic" in paragraph after relevant paragraph of the *Organon*, 95, 101, 102, 104, 153, 164, 165 and 178.

12. In the footnote to Para 153 of the *Organon*, quoted above, Hahnemann says that Dr. Von Boenninghausen "has lately increased our obligation to him by setting forth the characteristic symptoms." Therefore, let us see what Boenninghausen says in elaborating what we are to understand by the expression "more striking, singular, uncommon and peculiar (characteristic) signs and symptoms." He lists seven considerations for interpreting what constitutes a striking or singular symptom. (From the preface to *Boenninghausen's Repertory with Characteristics* by C.M. Boger).

(i) *Changes of personality and temperament* — Especially the striking alterations — *i.e.*, mental symptoms covering emotions, moods, disposition in dealings with others in day-to-day life.

(ii) *Peculiar sensations of the patient* — But not the diagnostic symptoms of the disease which can seldom or never suffice for the sure selection of the similar remedy.

(iii) *The seat of disease* — Almost every drug acts more definitely upon certain parts of the organism, the whole body being seldom affected equally, even in kind. For example, the specific curative powers of *Sepia* in those stubborn and sometimes fatal joint abscesses of the fingers and toes is extraordinarily conclusive evidence upon this point, for they differ from similar gathering in location only, while the remedies so suitable for abscess elsewhere remain ineffectual here.

(iv) *The cause* — Without it the choice of the homoeopathic remedy cannot be made with safety. Practice has shown the knowledge of the exciting cause (such as sprains, bruises, burns, or whether the symptoms localise themselves internally in the stomach, chest, abdomen etc.) or externally (head, feet, back, etc.) greatly restrict the list of remedies from which the selection is to be made. While these diseases are due principally to external impressions when there is already a natural predisposition thereto, there are another set of causes, *viz.* the natural disposition which is sometimes highly susceptible (idiosyncracy). This natural predisposing cause of disease, according to Hahnemann, depends upon the uneradicated miasms of psora, syphilis and sycosis, or drug diseases and poisonings, when these factors combine to undermine the health, they present a proportionately deeper rooted disease, just that much harder to combat. In such cases antipsoric remedies very much excel all others in efficacy.

(v) *The concomitants* above all, demand the most thorough examination in finding the similimum for the whole case. Commonplace accompaniments of a disease are unimportant unless they appear in a singular manner. They generally belong to another sphere of disease than that of the main one; and because of this they so decidedly lead us to the remedy, that they acquire an importance far out-ranking the symptoms of the main disease. They evidently belong to those which Hahnemann called striking, extraordinary and peculiar (characteristic) and hence lend their individuality to the totality. Dr. C.M. Boger says that the system of concomitants also makes homoeopathy distinctly safer, rendering it less dependent upon a previously constructed diagnosis which is often deceptive. Dr. H.A. Roberts has tersely stressed the role of concomitants by saying that "just as the single symptom is made complete by its qualifying condtion of aggravation or amelioration, in the same way as the concomitant symptom lends completeness to the totality."

(vi) *Modalities* — (*i.e.*, conditions of aggravation and amelioration) are the proper and most decisive modifiers of the characteristics, not one of which is utterly worthless, not even the

Evaluation of Symptoms 55

negative ones. They have developed in importance with the growth of homoeopathy. Roberts points out that "We must take into consideration that every symptom of note has these modifying conditions of aggravation and amelioration, as to time, the time of day or night, the time of season, the time of the moon; the aggravation or amelioration from thermic conditions; from motion or rest of the part affected or of the condition as a whole; from lying down or sitting or standing, and the position taken during such conditions, waking or sleeping, and the aggravation and amelioration from such positions and circumstances; the various positions in motion that aggravate or ameliorate; the desires or aversions to eating and drinking, especially in feverish conditions; aggravations from certain foods and drinks. These are all modifications that are of the utmost importance in evaluating the symptoms." Continuing, he says; "Conditions of aggravation or amelioration may in themselves become generals, if they appertain in the same way to several parts of the body; they then become conditions of the man as a whole, or general symptoms, even though they seemingly express themselves in local parts. For instance, if a headache is aggravated by motion; if the pain in the knee is aggravated by walking or stepping; if there is pain in the shoulder from raising the arm; then the agg. from motion becomes a general as of the whole man, although it seemingly appears in dissociated parts."

The importance of modalities in the selection of the remedy will be appreciated from Boenninghausen's note of caution: "When the symptoms seem to point to a particular remedy with which the modalities, however, do not agree the physician has most urgent reason to doubt its fitness . . . he should seek another remedy."

(vii) The time of the day (24 hours) when the symptoms occur, recur again and again, or aggravate or ameliorate is a special modality of much greater importance than even the other modalities in general, for hardly any disease lacks this feature and the provings also supply this peculiarity in respect of many remedies. To illustrate this we need only refer to influences which the time of day exerts upon cough, diarrhoea, etc. A few examples will be illustrative : 1 a.m. agg. of *Arsenicum-album*; 3 a.m. agg. *Kali-carb.*; 4 a.m. agg. of *Nux-vomica*; 7 a.m. agg. *Podophyllum*; 10 a.m. agg. *Gelsemium* and *Natrum-mur.*; 11 a.m. agg. *Nat-mur.* and *Sulphur*; 4 p.m. agg. of *Lycopodium*; 6 a.m. and 6 p.m. agg. of *Nux-vomica*; 9 p.m. agg of *Bryonia*; 12 midnight agg. of *Arsenicum-alb.* etc.

A complete list of these time aggravations is to be found in *A Concise Repertory of Homoeopathic Medicines* by Dr. S.R. Pathak, M.B.B.S. By the way, this time modality also called "periodicity" includes seasons, and periodic recurrences on alternate days, weekly, fortnightly, yearly, etc.

13. **Totality of Symptoms** : In selecting the remedy for a given case Hahnemann has laid stress on two essential aspects being taken into account, *viz*. the characteristic symptoms, about which we have already discussed in detail, and the "totality of symptoms." This totality pertains not only to characteristic symptoms which, of course, occupy a high rank in totality, but also other symptoms of location and sensation, so that a complete picture of the disease is represented. In Para 104, of the *Organon* he refers to the "Totality of symptoms that specially mark and distinguish the case of disease;" in Para 151 he states "The physician will find several other symptoms, besides the complaint of a few violent sufferings, which furnish a complete picture of the disease; in Para 152 : "Totality of symptoms;" in Para 153 he refers to "Collective symptoms;" Para 154 : If the antitype, constructed from the list of symptoms of the most suitable medicine, contain those peculiar, uncommon, singular and distinguishing (characteristic) symptoms, and if these are met with in the disease to be cured in the greatest number and in the greatest similarity, this medicine is most appropriate homoeopathic specific remedy for this morbid state." Lastly, Para 169 : "Totality of the symptoms of disease." It is obvious from these quotations that though "totality" must contain the characteristic symptoms, it does not exclude symptoms which may not be characteristic or peculiar if their omission leaves the disease picture incomplete.

14. We shall perhaps have a better appreciation of what "totality" signifies if we note what H.A. Roberts has to say. He says, and we have condensed what he has explained at length :

15. In disease one organ cannot suffer alone any more than one cell can suffer by itself. Therefore, in every disease we find groups of symptoms pertaining to different organs or systems. If one of those symptoms is the chief complaint, the others are its concomitants.

16. As regards remedies, it has been proved by years of experience that a medicine will remove a group of symptoms similar to the group which it is capable of producing . . . No

Evaluation of Symptoms

medicine can cure any disease unless it acts on all the disturbed parts, either directly or indirectly.

17. Now, since the medicinal character of the drug is represented not by a single effect but by a group of effects, and on the other hand, those same group of effects are found in disease states, these peculiar grouping of effects (which vary from one remedy to another and for the same remedy from one individual to another) are the best guides in establishing relationship between a drug and a disease. No medicine can effect a cure unless it has a curative action upon every diseased part, and in just the proportion that each part manifests disorder in the individual patient.

18. Therefore, it is only upon the totality (or group) of symptoms in the individual case that we can base our prescription; and to constitute the totality we require many individual symptoms showing the characteristics and personality of the patient.

19. There is a final over-riding consideration which makes it hazardous to ignore totality in selecting the remedy. As pointedly stressed by Boger in his *Synoptic Key* : "The prescriber has to keep in mind the fact that the actual differentiating factor may belong to any rubric whatsoever." In other words, the larger the characteristic symptoms base, of which concomitants (or group effects) are an important part, the greater the assurance of not missing the differentiating factor; and conversely, if we fail to pay due heed to totality, we are apt to omit or overlook the very differentiating factor of factors which would have led us to the curative remedy.

20. Finally, here is a gem from Gibson Miller's *Comparative Value of Symptoms*. After affirming at page 5, Hahnemann's directive that our main reliance should be placed almost exclusively on the peculiar or characteristic symptoms of the patient, and not on those that are common to the disease. Miller now gives (at page 7) an apparently contradictory advice that "it would be foolish to ignore the symptoms that signify the disease . . . for however helpful the peculiar symptoms may be, it is the totality of the symptoms that determines the choice." Let us see how he argues this point :

"In the foregoing, stress has been laid on the supreme importance of paying the greatest attention to the symptoms that are peculiar to the patient, but it would be foolish to ignore the symptoms that signify the disease. They must indeed be taken into consideration, but subsequent to, and of much less value than, those that are predicated of the patient. In a very large number of cases no one remedy corresponds to all the peculiar symptoms, but three or four seem to have equal numbers of them, and of approximately the same value. In such a state of affairs the remedy that has also the common symptoms best marked must prevail. It must ever be kept in mind that there must be a general correspondence between all the symptoms of the patient and those of the remedy, and that however helpful the peculiar symptoms may be in calling attention to certain remedies, yet they are not the sole guides; for, after all, it is the totality of the symptoms that determines the choice."

We trust that it will be clear from the above discussion that while characteristic symptoms are our best clues for calling our attention to certain remedies, and we must begin our repertorial work with them, and especially with the general modalities, it pays to seek confirmation of those remedies by taking the particular (regional) symptoms of the disease.

21. **Take Only Positively Existing Symptoms.** It is sometimes found that a remedy selected on the basis of totality is effective even though it is not indicated against some of the symptoms in the totality, so much so that we are apt to consider the remedy to be contra-indicated by the absence of these symptoms. For example, *Calc-c.* may work even if the patient is not obese, and in fact is "emaciated," (You will find *Calc-c.* against the rubric "Emaciation"). Or *Phosphorus* may work even when the patient has no craving for salt. Such examples may appear to contradict the principle of totality, but that is not so. Such erratic cases occur when we have failed to evaluate the symptoms into those of higher value and those others of lower value. We should select the remedy on the basis of symptoms of higher evaluation (outstanding) in the patient, and the absence of symptoms of lesser evaluation in the patient (though holding a high value in the remedy) should not be taken as a contra-indication.

This brings us to a very useful tip which Margaret Tyler has given after narrating a case of terrier suffering from cysts between toes for two years, very crippled at times, cured with three doses of *Calc-c.* 200. She says : The chilliness and desire

Evaluation of Symptoms

for sweets were so outstanding that they were used to throw out all remedies not common to both. Remedies in low types were ignored. The symptoms were so outstanding that all low grade remedies could be ignored. Now, she draws the important conclusion : "Note the value of Clarke's statement that only positive symptoms should be considered. *Calc.* has dread of bathing, but this dog liked to sit in the river on a cold day. *Calc.* is not affectionate, which the dog is; yet *Calc.* cured." Lesson : Only positively existing symptoms of high value in the patient should be considered for finding the remedy.

22. Match Patient's Symptoms with the Remedy — Not Vice Versa. It needs to be stressed that in each case we have to match the patient's characteristics with those of the remedy, and not the other way round. We cannot expect all the symptoms of a remedy (even its leading ones) to be found in the patient. For example, left-sidedness is characteristic of *Lachesis*, but we cannot reject this remedy in a case just because its complaints are not left-sided, if most of the patient's characteristic symptoms match the characteristics and the drug picture of *Lachesis*.

23. Accidental Symptoms. While repertorising it is often found that certain symptoms do not fit into the picture of a remedy presented by a majority of the characteristic symptoms. The beginner gets confused as omission of such a symptom detracts from "totality." In this connection it should be remembered that the true "totality" is more than the mere numerical sum or the whole of symptoms. It may even exclude some of the particular symptoms if they cannot at the same time be logically related to the case, because a prescription can only be made upon those symptoms which their counterpart are similar in the Materia Medica. Such symptoms which do not fit are known as "accidental symptoms."

Remember : "Nothing in the Particulars can contradict or contra-indicate strongly marked Generals; at the same time, strong Particulars must not be neglected on account of one or more weak Generals." The prescriber must weigh the importance of the "accidental symptoms" before deciding to ignore them as "accidental."

KENT'S APPROACH TO EVALUATION OF SYMPTOMS

24. The best description of Kent's approach to evaluation is to be found (apart from his *Lectures on Homoeopathic Philoso-*

phy), in Dr. Glen Bidwell's *How to Use the Repertory* and Dr. Margaret Tyler's *A Study of Kent's Repertory*. We shall first take a summary from Bidwell.

25. "In order to analyse our case with rapidity, we must go about it logically; we must have a starting place and a place to end. The start is made with the generals, and the particulars end it.

About the value of symptoms, looking to Kent we find that he uses three classes : Generals, Particulars and Common. The Generals and Particulars have the greatest importance in our prescription.

"As Generals, Kent includes all things that are predicated of the patient himself. Things that modify all parts of the organism are those that relate to the general state; and the internals that involve the whole man, the more they become generals.

"Things that relate to the ego are always general, *i.e.*, when he refers his complaints to "I" *e.g.*, when he says : "I am so thirsty," "I burn so," "I am so cold," "I cannot tolerate heat," etc. The things he says he feels are always general. His desires and aversions are general; menstruation is general, for when a woman says, "I feel so and so during menses" she has no reference to her uterus or ovaries; her state, as a whole is different when she is menstruating.

"On examining a series of particular organs, we find a certain modality or feature which runs so strongly through them that it may express the patient himself. Here we have a general composed of a series of particulars. (Modalities or sensations common to more than two particulars get their rank raised to Generals). This most often happens with sensations (characters of pain), such as cramping, burning, heaviness, numbness etc."

26. Kent's evaluation may be presented schematically as follows as given by Margaret Tyler (with additional comments from Bidwell) :

(1) **Mentals** :
 Will : with loves, hates, fears (emotions).
 Understanding : With delusions, delirium
 Memory.

Evaluation of Symptoms

(2) **Strange, Rare and Peculiar** :
These may occur among mentals, physical generals, or particulars and will therefore be of varying importance and rank.

(3) **Physical Needs** :
 (i) Sexual perversions (loves, hates).
 (ii) Cravings and aversion for foods and drinks.
 (iii) Appetite and thirst.

(4) **Physical Generals** :
Reaction to heat and cold;
 to wet, damp or dry; to time; electricity (storm, thunder); oxygen (air, hunger); to menstruation; to position, gravitation pressure, motion; with air or sea or car-sickness; food aggravations and ameliorations.

(5) **Particulars** :
(Relating to a part, and not to the whole; — always *qualified*).

(6) **Common Symptoms** (Generals, *i.e.* patient as a whole, or particular, pertaining to parts — All of which *not qualified*).

27. Bidwell has elaborated on these symptoms for our easy understanding :

Mentals : They form the first grade, and are again divided into three classes :

(i) *Will* : The group of symptoms referred to the *will* are of first importance in individualising the case for Repertory study. In sickness the patient's nature often becomes changed. He may become quarrelsome, angry, irritable, tearful, hating his loved ones, fearful, intolerant of sympathy, etc. These are often the most difficult of all symptoms to obtain as they are most often concealed from the world, from friends and the physician. Among the symptoms of this group we shall find "ailments from" anger, bad news, grief, love, joy, reproach, sexual excesses, contrariness, cursing, cowardice, hatred, irritability, jealousy, loquacity, quarrelsomeness, indifference, sadness, etc.

(ii) *Perversions of understanding* : These are manifested by delusions, hallucinations and illusions, etc. These take the second place in value for Repertory work. Other symptoms belonging to this group are : absorbed, clairvoyance, confusion, dullness, comprehension, both difficult and easy; ecstacy, excitement, imbecility, mental activity, ailments from mental exertion, etc.

(iii) *Perversions of memory* : Such as absent mindedness, errors in answers, mistakes in writing and speech, disorders of speech, etc. are symptoms with the lowest value of the mental symptoms.

Note : If mental symptoms are marked, especially if it is a change from normal, they are of the utmost importance to the case. Get these symptoms clear, then give them the highest standing in your Repertory analysis. The remedy which includes them will be curative.

Physical Loves and Hates : These are sub-divided into two groups :

(i) These include perversions of the sexual sphere, including menstrual generals. They will cover aggravations before, during and after menses; effect of coition, urination, etc. Undue desire or aversion to sex.

(ii) Loves and hates referred to the stomach, such as cravings and aversions for foods, for hot or cold foods and drinks; appetite; thirst — especially if they affect the body as a whole and not the stomach alone.

Physical Generals : These include things affecting the entire physical body, such as :

(i) Weather and climatic influences.
(ii) Extremes of temperature.
(iii) Foods that aggravate.
(iv) Positions, motion, etc., as they affect the body as a whole (as worse from standing, under *Sulphur* and *Valerian*)

Evaluation of Symptoms

(v) Pressure.
(vi) Bathing or wetting.
(vii) Touch.
(viii) Rubbing.
(xi) Jarring.
(x) Defecation.
(xi) Periodicity : Time, parts of day, seasons.
(xii) Moon phases.
(xiii) Sides of body such as left or right; exertion from left to right or right to left; alternating sides; or changing about in various parts of body.
(xiv) Congestions.
(xv) Contractions.
(xvi) Discolouration of parts.
(xvii) Atrophy, etc., are all classed in this group of generals.
(xviii) Special senses are often so closely related to whole man that a great many of their symptoms are general, as various odours that make one sick, the smell of cooking nauseates, the sight or smell of food sickens, over-sensitiveness to sounds, noise, light etc.
(xix) Sleep.
(xx) Dreams.
(xxi) Character of discharges: taking the normal as our guide, any change, a decrease or increase or perversion would constitute a symptom.

(1) **Particulars.** The symptoms that are predicated of a given organ are things in particular. The more they relate to the anatomy of a part, the more external they are, the more liable they are to be particular; but when they are qualified by peculiar modalities, their rank is raised from particular to general; such as thirst during the cold stage, or before it; thirst for large or small quantities (insatiable) of water; thirstlessness during period of high temperature raging thirst with no desire to drink — all these are peculiar to individual patients and to a few drugs. This is how a common useless symptom becomes transformed into a "strange, rare and peculiar" one, as it applies to the patient himself.

Note : The generals always rule our non-agreeing particular.

One strong general rules out one remedy and rules in another.

(2) **Common Symptoms** : That which is pathognomonic is always common. For instance, if we had a pleurisy it would be a common thing to want keep the chest wall quiet and you would get the symptom worse from motion, one of the keynotes of *Bryonia*, but if there were no other symptoms of *Bryonia* present, we could not make a prescription on that rubric alone. Common symptoms must be considered last in every case of repertory study, be they general or particular, mental or physical. Running through all symptoms from generals to particulars we have two divisions :

(a) Strange, rare and uncommon.
(b) Common.

But unless we become familiar with symptoms that are common, it will be difficult to know what are uncommon, strange, rare and peculiar. Knowledge of pathology and the character of diseases helps us to differentiate the common from the uncommon symptoms. However, when peculiar modalities qualify common symptoms, they become striking and peculiar and help to individualise the picture for Repertory work.

For example, diarrhoea is a common symptom which, by itself, does not help us to individualise. But if we get diarrhoea from milk, or diarrhoea after weaning, we are then able to select the drug for the patient more easily. Similarly, the number of remedies with headache are so numerous that unless we ascertain the qualifying conditions, such as aggravation from sun or noise, or from grief, individualising the remedy for the patient will be very difficult. You see how a common symptom with too many drugs against it, becomes transformed into a strange, rare and peculiar and therefore a general symptom pertaining to the patient himself, with very few remedies to choose from.

Many remedies are common to certain diseases. Many remedies are also to be found against a single symptom rubric. In both cases, the large list of remedies is of no help in selecting a single remedy. It is only when qualified by modalities (agg. or amel.) that the list gets reduced to a few remedies to select one from.

28. Key-notes. This word was coined by Dr. Guernsey to indicate that certain peculiar symptoms provide the key, and point straight to a remedy. Many of the old master prescribers like Drs. Ad. Lippe, H.N. Guernsey, P.P. Wells, C. Hering, H.C.

Allens and J.H. Allen, Farrington, Dunham, Swan and many others (men who made homoeopathy famous in America) were all users of the legitimate keynote. Key-notes were essential in those days before reliable Repertories were developed. The keynote led to the proper and easy study of remedies similiar to the case.

The Key-note is described as the guiding and controlling notes as in a piece of music, as without such a note there would be no harmony or music. When criticised that Key-notes ignore totality, Guernsey said that if correctly identified, they will be found to cover the totality as well. Stuart Close defines a Key-note as a minor generalisation based upon a study of many particulars. For example, aggravation from motion is a Key-note of *Bry.* since this modality applies to all complaints (mental or physical). That which is characteristic in a large way is rarely shown as a single symptom. "Worse in a warm or closed room" is a generalisation (Key-note) drawn from the observation of particular symptoms in numerous cases of *Pulsatilla*. The Key-note runs like a red thread through all the morbid symptoms of a given remedy.

The Key-note is apt to be abused by those who fail to distinguish its above features, and confuse it with Peculiar symptoms. As Elizabeth Hubbard points out, "strange, rare and peculiar symptoms often become Key-notes, although not all Key-notes are strange symptoms; for instance, "hunger at 11 a.m." is a key-note of *Sulphur*, but it is not a strange or peculiar symptom. The same is the case with 4-8 p.m. aggravation of *Lycopodium*. But a Key-note which is also peculiar is "the more you belch, the more you have to belch" of *Ignatia*, or the well known aggravation from downward motion of *Borax*.

In order to restrain the tendency of relying too much on a single symptom (Key-note or Peculiar), Hering recommended the formula of "three-legged stool," *i.e.* at least three (more are welcome) characteristic symptoms which together support a general likeness to the constitutional action — pathogenetic power — of the remedy, as a dependable guide in the choice of the remedy. Kent also supported the use of the Key-note provided it is not ruled out by contradicting general symptoms of the patient. He further pointed out that if Key-notes are taken as final, and if Generals do not confirm, then failures will come. If used only as pointers they are good short cuts to a small group of remedies from which one should select the most similar by further study.

We have explained the distinguishing features of Key-notes and Peculiar, uncommon symptoms, and the best way of using them safely. However, the most difficult part of our duty, if we are to use the Key-notes or Peculiar symptoms, is to discover them while taking the case.

29. Peculiar Symptoms. We shall now give some typically peculiar and uncommon symptoms which can render our task of finding the remedy easy.

Modalities, strange :
Burning pain, amel. by hot application : *Ars.*
Coryza amel. by cold bath : *Calc., Sulp.*
Pain, agg. by slight pressure, but amel. by hard pressure : *Chin., Lach.*
Vertigo, on closing eyes (K. 98) :
Pain in teeth, from getting wet (440) : *Lach.*
Epistaxis brought on by washing face (K. 338)
Pain in bladder, amel. by walking in open air (647): *Tereb.*

Peculiar Sensations :
Chilly, but agg. from warmth (1276) — "Laughs with pain" (62) "Sensation as if she were double" (24) — "Teeth feel long": (431) — "Empty sensation inside the head" (114) — "Numbness of forearm on grasping anything (1037) : *Cham.* — "Feels as if legs are not his own" (1043) : *Agar, Bapt.* "Lump in rectum, not amel. by stool" (623) : *Sep.*

Peculiar Concomitants :
"Thirst with chill" (528) — Thirstless during fever (530) — Thirst without desire to drink (528) — Headache during menses (142) — Lachrymation during coryza (245) — Vision dim during vertigo (277) — Urination involuntary, laughing when (660).

Side of Body : Right side (1400) : *Apis, Bell, Bry., Calc., Chel., Colo., Lyc., Nux-v., Puls.*
Left side : *Arg-nit., Graph., Lach., Phos., Sep.*
Right to left : *Lyc.* — Left to right : *Lach.*
Crosswise (Diagonal) — *Agar., Led., Rhus-tox.*
Alternating sides (1400) — *Lac-c., Cocc.*

Evaluation of Symptoms

Extension of Pain :
Chest, pain, heart, extending to nape of neck and shoulder (850) — *Naja*.
Uterus, pain extending upwards (734) : *Lach., Murex., Sep.*

Pain, wandering (1389) : *Kali bi., Ox-ac., Sabad.*

Pain, small spots : Nates, stitching pain in : (1145) : *Calc-p.*

Mode of onset of pain : Pain appears suddenly and disappears suddenly (1377) : *Bell., Kali-bi., Nit-ac.*
Pain appears gradually and disappears gradually (1377) : *Stann.*

Alternating states :
Constipation alternates with diarrhoea (607) : *Ant-c., Chel., Podo., Nit-ac., Nux-v., Op.*
Asthma alternates with eruptions (764) : *Hep., Kalm., Sulph.,*
Chest and rectal symptoms alternate (822) : *Sil.*
Chill alternating with sweat (1262) : *Phos.*

Periodicity of complaints : (1390); annually; at the same hour; seventh day; fourteenth day; twenty-first day; twenty-eighth day.

Aggravations in relation to Sleep :
Before sleep (1401); during sleep (1402); after sleep (1402).
Agg. or amel. in relation to menses : Before menses (1373); at the beginning of menses (1373); during menses (1373); after menses (1374) — Menses amel. (1374).

Absence of (normally) expected symptom :
Fever without thirst — K. 530
Vomiting without nausea : 400 (S.R. Phatak's Rep.)
Painless ulcers — K. 1337.
Painlessness (when pain would be normally expected) — K. 1390.

Other strange symptoms :
Asthma better lying down : *Psor.*
Asthma better in knee-elbow position : *Med.*
Headache amel. eating — (139) : *Anac., Kali-bi., Sep.*

Stool passes easier when standing — (608) : *Caust., Alum.*
Says he is well, though really ill — (95) : *Arn.*
Hates (averse to) loved ones — (9) : *Sep.*
Haemorrhoids, walking amel. — (621) : *Ign.*
Hearing impaired, amel. by noise (323) : *Graph.*

Discharges :
Coryza, Urine, Expectoration, Leucorrhoea, Menstrual blood (bright, dark, clotted), from eruptions and ulcers; sweat. (i) colour (ii) quantity (iii) odour, offensive or putrid, (iv) consistency, thin, thick, stringy, etc., (v) acridity, burning, excoriating. (vi) staining, difficult to wash off.

30. **Other Strategies.** While the above rules guide us in the evaluation of symptoms in all normal cases, occasions arise when it becomes difficult to put them in practice either for want of the guiding characteristic symptoms or because the case has become very much confused by the variety of medicines taken before the patient comes to us. On such occasions, the physician's skill and artistry in selecting the remedy are put to the severest test. There are fortunately a few other methods which if carefully applied, may help us in such cases. They are briefly following :

(i) The "last appearing symptoms."

(ii) The "unmodified (original) symptoms," irrespective of whether they are confirmed by the present symptoms or not.

(iii) The artistic method described in Lesson 5 by which the prescription is one where the given picture of the case is almost not the indication for it, and the selected remedy may not contain the present troubles of the patient prominently, so far as is known. The cure of impotence by Lippe with one dose of *Lac-can* (based on the history of diphtheria in which the symptoms alternated sides) and the cure of deafness by Dunham with Mezerium (taking suppression of eczema of the scalp as the basis) are examples of such art in prescribing.

(iv) The wall breaking (etiological) method of Rev. Cannon Upcher quoted in Lesson 5.

Evaluation of Symptoms

(v) The anti-miasmatic method as discussed in Lesson 7.

(vi) Using "cardinal" symptoms (or qualified particulars as Kent calls them) as explained at length in Lesson 6.

31. Last Appearing Symptoms. R.G. Miller draws attention to one more guideline in selecting the remedy, obviously applicable to intractable chronic cases. He says : "Ranking close behind, or even at times taking precedence of the peculiar and general symptoms, must be placed the last appearing symptoms of a case. These symptoms, to be of any real importance, must, of course, be outstanding and definite, and if so they are always of the first importance in the choice of the remedy. So much is this the case that where no remedy can be discovered that corresponds to the case as a whole, it is at times necessary to be guided almost exclusively by them . . . this will at least modify the symptoms and open up the way for other remedies.

In his *General Analysis* Boger cites a case of lichen planus in the selection of the remedy for which he was guided by two principles. To quote Boger, "We have Hahnemann's fundamental or central idea that the further a given symptom seems removed from the ordinary course of disease, the greater is its therapeutic value." "Pain in joints" "aggravated by covering" is a symptom of this kind — a symptom far removed from the ordinary course of the chief disease of the patient — lichen planus. We have again another statement : "Ranking close behind, or even at times taking precedence of the peculiar and general symptoms, must be placed the last appearing symptoms of a case." The modality of "pain in joints" was not only recent but also outstanding and definite. It was a symptom last to appear before homoeopathic treatment was instituted. Therefore, "pain in joints, aggravated by covering," was in this case, a symptom of the first importance in the choice of the remedy. The choice of the remedy for the case was therefore expected to be confined to the group emerging from these two rubrics.

32. Unmodified (Original) Symptoms. As opposed to the "last appearing symptoms," are another kind of symptoms which sometimes lead us easily to the curative remedy. They are the symptoms which first appeared in the history of derangement of health of the patient, ignoring the various modifications they have undergone on account of subsequent treatment with medicines of different systems. This applies in all cases irrespective of the type of complaint, whether it is an acute fever, a skin affection or a chronic condition. For example, in case of psoriasis of several years standing, the original symptoms of cracks and bleeding of palms and fingers aggravated by taking things out of the refrigerator, led us to think of petroleum, and the entire case when taken including the recent symptoms of "gnawing hunger that drives one to eat, yet causes pain or diarrhoea if one does eat" confirmed its choice which in turn, was justified by its curative action.

33. **Only Phraseology Different.** The new student of homoeopathy will form the impression that the principle of evaluation enunciated by Boenninghausen, Boger and Roberts are in many ways different from those laid down by Kent, Bidwell, Tyler and Miller. This is because of the different phraseology employed by each of the two schools, so to say (although it would be wrong to call them "schools" as they are not opposed to each other). It will be seen that behind the different phraseology we can clearly perceive many common, similar points. Both regard Mentals, if marked, as the highest ranking symptoms representing the patient. Even Kent says that if Mentals are not marked, we should go by modalities of temperature (if they are general), to which Boenninghausen attaches the highest value "because marked mentals are difficult to elicit." Kent's Physical Generals are only another name for the general Modalities of Boenninghausen. Even Kent allows the particular and common symptoms to be taken into account in the last stage of repertorial work if the first stage leaves us with four or five contending remedies. The concomitants of Boenninghausen are nothing but the strange, rare and peculiar symptoms of Kent.

34. For the practical guidance of the reader we shall now give a brief summary about the ranking of symptoms in order of their importance. This ranking holds true only if the respective symptoms are strong and well-marked. A strong particular will over-ride a weak General.

35. Ranking according to (when using) Boger-Boenninghausen's Repertory :

(1) Modalities
(2) Causation
(3) Concomitants

(4) Strange, rare and peculiar symptoms.
(5) Mental symptoms.
(6) Sensations
(7) Location
(8) Objective symptoms.

Symptoms No. 6, 7 and 8 bring the investigation in touch with diagnosis.

36. Ranking according to (when using) Kent's Repertory :

(1) **Generals** :
Mentals (emotions, intellect, memory), including cause of mental state, *e.g.* grief, disappointed love, mortification, etc.

(2) **Strange, Rare, Peculiar, Uncommon** Symptoms (including Key-notes)

(3) **Physical Generals** :

a. Modalities (time, temperature, open air, cicumstance, position, touch, pressure, etc.)
b. Cravings and aversions of food and drink.
c. Sleep and dreams.
d. Disorders of sexual function.
e. Causation (fundamental, *i.e.* miasmatic personal and family history).

(4) **Concomitants** : Complaints associated in time with the chief complaint.

(5) **Particulars** : Location, with sensation and Modalities (including Physical, proximate cause).

(6) **Objective Symptoms** :

Note : Our experience confirms Boger's affirmation :

"The prescriber has only to bear in mind the fact that the actual differentiating factor may belong to any rubric whatsoever." — depending upon how peculiar, characteristic and outstanding it is.

37. A Few Noteworthy Hints. Here are a few noteworthy hints from Margaret Tyler. We are giving them here even if some of them may be a repetition of what has been said already. The repetition will impress the points on your mind :

(i) The physician must realise that he is concerned not with diseases, but with sick persons. In a patient he must see a person who is suffering; an individual who deviates from the normal of the race, and from his own normal.

(ii) If you attempt to hunt for some named disease in the Repertory and Materia Medica, you are very unlikely to discover the curative remedy.

(iii) What you have to discover is the individual patient's remedy, the remedy that corresponds to his body and soul, the remedy for which his symptoms cry, symptoms inherent in himself — not those dependent on his pathological lesions, his "obvious morbid anatomy."

(iv) Be sure that the symptoms you take are peculiar to, and characteristic of the patient himself, and not merely secondary to disease. But remember, you cannot eliminate symptoms dependent on a disease which you have not diagnosed.

(v) Besides pathological symptoms, there are common symptoms; and these again will not help you at all, unless qualified.

(vi) A common symptom like extreme thirst during fever, becomes transformed into a "strange, rare and peculiar and therefore, a general," if qualified; *e.g.*, a raging thirst with no desire to drink.

(vii) Never start repertorial work with a common symptom. They will not help you one scrap. But if you can get something that qualifies, they may help you in your work.

(viii) Mental symptoms, if they are marked, dominate the case. They are of supreme importance, as they express the patient most absolutely, especially if they denote change from the patient's normal. In such cases the remedy should be in the same type as in the patient, *i.e.* only remedies in the higher types are likely to fit the case.

Evaluation of Symptoms

(ix) Do not risk missing your remedy from an ill-marked mental, or a very small rubric.

(x) When you have taken a case on paper, you must settle upon the symptoms that cannot be omitted in each individual. If you get such a marked mental, your remedy must be here, and you can use that rubric as an eliminating symptom.

(xi) After settling on the strongly marked mental as through the rubrics of the patient's symptoms in their order, *i.e.*, mentals first; then generals; then particulars with modalities, taking from each list only the remedies that appear in the first rubric.

(xii) To make sure that the symptoms are real and marked, and they do actually express the patient, you will have to ask many questions in order to elicit the few telling symptoms. Also make sure that you and your patient mean the same thing.

(xiii) Beware how you take rare and peculiar symptoms with only one or two drugs to their credit as eliminating symptoms. That is easy, but often fatal. They may or may not help you. But where there is nothing in the general to contradict, they are often invaluable to give the casting vote.

(xiv) Kent says, "Get the strong, strange, peculiar symptoms, and then see to it that there are no generals in the case that oppose or contradict."

(xv) If there are no marked mental symptoms, see if the patient is chilly, utterly intolerant of cold (or conversely he is intolerant of heat in any form). You may then limit your work by taking the rubric "worse by cold (or warmth)" as you work down your list.

(xvi) Kent says, "Don't expect a remedy that has the generals must have all the little symptoms. It is a waste of time to run out all the little symptoms, if the remedy has the generals."

(xvii) Finally, Kent says, "When looking over a list of symptoms, first of all discover three, four, five or six (as many as may exist) symptoms that are strange, rare and peculiar, work these out first. These are the highest generals . . . When you have settled upon three, four or six remedies that have these first generals, then find out which of this list is most like the rest of the symptoms, common and particular."

Self-Test

1. Since the diagnostic symptoms are common to many patients, one cannot use them for differentiation and for applying them to the sick individuals. Explain. (Para 3).

2. In what way does a knowledge of diagnosis and pathology help a homoeopath in selecting the remedy ? (Para 4 to 7).

3. Name the seven considerations (each one in not more than ten words) which Boenninghausen outlines for interpreting what constitutes a striking or characteristic symptom? (Para 12).

4. What are the reasons that lend importance to the concept of totality of symptoms in finding the curative remedy? (Paras 15 to 19).

5. In Kent's evaluation what are the types of symptoms that qualify as generals? What rank do they occupy in evaluation, and why? (Para 26, 27).

6. When does a particular or common symptom get raised in rank to a general? Give a few examples. (Para 27).

7. Give a few examples of peculiar symptoms. (Para 29).

8. What do you understand by 'Physical Generals'? Cite a few examples.

Study In Depth

On the Comparative Value of Symptoms in the Selection of the Remedy by Robert Gibson Miller.

Lesson 5

Taking the Case

> "Show me the examination of sick person and I will tell you if the man knows anything about our Materia Medica"
> — **Hahnemann**

1. If the case is not well taken, the remedy gets ill-selected; in the absence of the correct remedy, the patient's cure will not be in sight. If the patient does not get well, there is alround failure of both the patient and the physician. Therefore, a well taken case is much more than half the battle won.

2. How can we make sure of "taking the case well"? Firstly, by following a systematic procedure which automatically takes care of all the essential points, and secondly, by making it a habit to follow that procedure, so that the best results are achieved smoothly and quickly.

3. Unless we elicit all the essential information about the patient required in selecting the remedy, the time spent in case taking will be fruitless. The essential information is exactly that which we have learnt in the last lesson on evaluation of symptoms. It is said that the eyes do not see what the mind does not know. Now, as our mind knows what we want (after studying evaluation) our eyes and ears will be alert to catch everything relevant when taking the case.

4. **Difference Between Homoeopathic Case-taking and That in Modern Medicine.** It is well to take a special note here of the difference in the approach to case-taking adopted by physicians in modern medicine on the one hand, and homoeopathic physicians on the other. The allopathic doctor's primary aim in taking the case is to observe all the signs and symptoms which will help him to arrive at a diagnosis of the disease. For this purpose he uses his knowledge of symptoms peculiar to

different diseases but similar in some respects, *i.e.*, his knowledge of differential diagnosis, to fix the actual diagnosis. He then goes on to identify the cause of the disease, such as whether it is due to bacterial or viral infection, and of what type; or whether it is due to deficiency or excess of vitamins, nutrients like proteins or carbohydrates, insulin, hormones, acidity, or physiological imbalances or disturbed processes, or due to any structural changes which might call for surgery, and so on. He is not concerned with the past history of the patient (unless it is directly concerned with the present ailment; or with his subjective irritability, depression, fears, or sensations of heat or cold, burning, throbbing, etc.

5. We shall discuss "case-taking" under two heads, *viz.* (1) how to ask questions and (2) what to record and how to record it.

6. **How to Ask Questions.** Asking questions to get all the data (characteristic symptoms) we want, on which to base our prescription, is the most important task of the physician. Efforts should be made to continually observe one's own methods, as well as how the patients respond, for improving our technique of interrogation. A few guidelines are given.

i) It is advisable to first tell the patient and his attendants that much of the success for the treatment depends on the information given about his complaints freely and frankly especially how and when they are worse, and under what circumstances he gets relief. Ask him to tell you everything slowly (so that you can record). This done, listen, only listen, and refrain from interrupting him, (even if his answers are incomplete) unless he wanders off to irrelevant matters. Look at the patient in his eyes, listen and encourage him, this way, to talk freely, nodding occasionally to let him know that you are following him. Give him time to think and tell.

(ii) Observe the patient very closely to notice anything abnormal about his mannerisms, behaviour, fidgety restlessness of his hands or legs; his voice (hoarse or nasal), his cough hollow or hacking; whether he is slow, hasty or impatient; loquacious or taciturn; whether calm or anxious or hopeful; whether dull or

Taking the Case

sharp witted; whether he is free and frank or hesitates in giving answers; whether hard of hearing, etc.

(iii) When the patient has finished giving information spontaneously, you may find that there are a number of gaps; he may have stated a location without sensation or modality; a modality without sensation or location, and so on. Now it is your turn to ask questions to fill in the gaps.

(iv) When asking, confine yourself to one symptom at a time; he will be confused if two or three questions are mixed up. Get one point clear and then go on to the next.

(v) Do not rush the patient for a quick answer. A quick answer is apt to be wrong and defeat the object of case-taking.

(vi) Avoid asking leading questions that suggest answers. "Don't you feel hot in this sultry weather?" This is a wrong way. The right way to ask is : "Do you like hot or cold weather?" Some more typical questions would be : How does cold weather affect you (or hot, dry, damp weather)? Which positions are uncomfortable in — sitting or standing; lying on right or left side; or on back — Why? What about your craving for certain foods and drinks such as sweets, salted, sour, rich fatty foods, fruits, juices, eggs, milk — or aversion to any of these? What foods disagree with you, and in what way? How do you feel in tight-fitting clothes? What sort of fears do you have? (a) fear of water? (b) of animal? (c) of burglars? d) of falling? (e) of being alone? (f) of the dark? (g) of thunderstorm? (h) of financial difficulties? Tell me about any dreams you have, which repeat themselves. What foods or drinks do you dislike very much, cold or hot? What foods or drinks make you sick, disagree with you?

(vii) Avoid questions along the lines of a remedy; if any of his symptoms make you think strongly of a remedy, write it down in the margin for checking up later.

(viii) Don't jump to conclusions basing yourself only on partial answers of the patient. Don't be satisfied unless the patient himself gives a full description of how he feels.

(ix) Never substitute conjecture for actual observation, supported by examples and repeated occurrences, of say, anger at trifles, intolerance of contradiction, diarrhoea from milk, etc.

(x) Unless the patient is a child, imbecile, unconscious or in extreme pain or stupor. insist on getting the answers from the patient himself, and not from others. He knows more about his sufferings than anybody else can.

(xi) Make sure that what the patient says, what you take his statement to mean, and what the true fact is, are all identical. For example, the patient says, "I am worse when I get up in the morning." What does this really mean? Is he worse in the morning, or worse after sleep, or worse waking up while he is still in bed? You will have to cross-question him to get at the true condition by asking for instance, "Do you feel the same way when you get up from an afternoon nap on a Sunday?" Like this, the physician may have to question much and closely before recording the conclusion in a few words.

(xii) Lastly, seek the patient's co-operation in observing the details of his complaints (on the lines you have asked him) and telling you about them at the next visit. Explain to him that any sensations or complaints, even if most unimportant from his view point, must be reported to you, as the correctness of the remedy — and his speedy cure — depends on how fully and accurately he has given a picture of his disease or complaint.

7. **What to Record and How to Record the Symptoms.** It is essential to put on record all the information, we elicit from the patient. It is not advisable to trust one's memory for the minute and detailed symptoms we obtain to cover the totality of the individual patient. This record is indispensable not only in the process of selecting the remedy, but equally so when we have to follow up the case as it progresses towards cure, as we shall see in the lesson on management of the case.

Taking the Case

8. Only those symptoms rank high for purpose of repertorisation which the patient narrates (a) voluntarily (i.e. spontaneously) without being prompted, (2) which are intensely felt, as observed by the physician when the patient narrates his complaint, and (3) which are clear and unambiguous, not open to two interpretations. Therefore, when taking the case, all the symptoms which meet these conditions must be underlined or marked with two or three pulses (++ or +++).

9. Many physicians have prepared Case Record forms to meet their requirements. Some of them are very detailed, and some short, and only suggestive. The form recommended by us is given in Appendix 'A'. Yet, even this form may not suit all. We are therefore giving a few hints on how recording can be easy and smooth.

10. When a patient comes in our consulting room, the first thing we have to do is to build a rapport with him. For this we must first allow him to talk freely about his complaints (no writing down at this time). The patient must feel that he is talking to a doctor who is keen to understand and solve his problem.

11. Now comes the state of recording. Here is a practical outline, which will take the patient smoothly through the interrogation.

12. **Case-Taking Outline.** The simplest outline for case-taking we would suggest is (1) First, take the chief complaint, (2) next take the particulars, (3) third, Physical Generals, (4) fourth, Mental and Emotional state, (5) fifthly, Peculiar symptoms, (6) next, personal history, (7) family history and lastly (8) objective symptoms. The patient will find this order of eliciting symptoms easier to respond to than to take the Mentals or physical generals or even the objective symptoms first.

13. It is important to note that we record the patient's statements in his own words, as far as possible, reserving their interpretation to a later time when we are studying the case in all its aspects.

14. As we stated earlier, the patient is first encouraged to tell everything, without any interruption. While he speaks, notes of his statements should be recorded in one or the other of the

eight sections of the Simple Case Record mentioned in Para 12, leaving space in the right hand half of the paper to make additions.

15. When the patient has finished with his story, then the physician should go over his notes from the beginning and try to get more details for getting a complete picture. In other words omissions such as (i) the sensation of a given location, or (ii) a modality of a given sensation (burning better or worse from . . .?), or (iii) a causation of diarrhoea or headache, or (iv) whether he is averse to company or has fear of being alone, etc. should be made good by asking relevant questions. Record these answers in the right hand half of the Case Record.

16. Now, let us see how each of the eight sections should be got complete — without which study of the case will be very difficult.

I. **Chief Complaint.** For which the patient has come. Note the (i) location, sensations and modalities. Since when the complaint started? Can you attribute it to any (ii) cause (grief, suppressed anger, getting wet; or exposure to sun; or fall or injury etc.) (iii) any other complaint (concomitant) associated with this chief complaint?

II. **Particulars.** Though comparatively low in evaluation, the patient would be better disposed at this early stage to answer questions relating to various regions of body — and in the process, we will be able to elicit valuable concomitants. The best way to avoid any omissions in questioning is to question about each anatomical part from head to foot, including the related physiological functions. Any headache? Eyes and vision normal? What about ears, hearing? Throat : any difficulty in swallowing, or inflammation of tonsils? Nose : obstruction, constant colds? Mouth : aphthae, bad odour? Chest : breathing difficulty? Urine and stool — any difficulties? and so on, going up to extremities, sleep, skin, sweat etc.

III. **Physical Generals** : These are symptoms which affect the patient as a whole; when he uses "I" to describe the symptom. While the Physical Generals are most important in the selection of a remedy, they are also relatively easy to elicit and, given careful enquiry, are clear and definite. Some examples :

Taking the Case 81

a. (i)   Enquire about *aggravation* or *amelioration* as to time, periodicity; thermal state (agg. heat or cold); position; touch or pressure, etc. — If he is worse from heat or closed stuffy room and is better in open air, many of the remedies with the opposite modality (worse from cold or draft of air) are straightaway thrown out.

(ii)   Sleep : any complaints before sleep, during sleep or after sleep.

(iii) Do you feel full or heavy after food, a sort of distension of abdomen?

(iv) Any complaints before menses — how many days before? or after menses? — What are they? Are your complaints relieved with the onset of menses, or when the flow is established?

(v)   Enquire about similar modalities in relation to stool, urination, eructations, coition, expectoration, etc.

(vi) Perspiration — one-sided, on scalp during sleep; of palms, of soles; with flushes of heat, on uncovered parts; with aversion to uncovering, etc.

Cravings and Aversions. Any strong desire for (or aversion to) any food or drinks? — Sweet, sour, salty, fats, eggs or fried things, meat, milk, fruits, juicy or refreshing things, cold or warm drinks, cabbage, onions, coffee, tea, etc. (Repertory gives a long list — study it).

Sexual Function. Is your sexual desire strong, or diminished? Easy sexual excitement? Any complaints in this sphere?

Menses. Is it late or too early; profuse or scanty; dark or bright red, or clotted. Any painfulness during menses — location of those pains and their extension. Any leucorrhoea — is it thick, acrid, milky, profuse, offensive?

Sleep and Dreams. Any sleeplessness? What part of the night? Any cause for it? Is it due to thoughts and activity of mind? What are the thoughts? Are you sleepless, though sleepy? Are you sleepless for a long time after waking? Do you feel refreshed after sleep, or unrefreshed in the morning? Do you feel unusually sleepy during the day? Any dreams you see repeatedly? What are they?

IV. **Mental State.** By now you have developed a rapport with the patient. He would now be in a frame of mind when he does not mind answering even the most private questions like the sexual function or his relations with other members of his household (there should be nobody else in the consulting room at this time). What is your temperament — mild and yielding, or firm and unbending? How do you react to disappointments and frustrations — with anger, irritability, sulking, morosenses, or with taciturnity or weeping openly (or in the privacy of your room), or hatred of the person who gave you offence? Any anxiety over trifles? Can you forget insults soon, or do they trouble your mind for long? Happy in company or when alone? and so on. It is human psychology to justify one's actions. Our questions should therefore be so framed that if he is irritable or fault-finding for example, he is not to be blamed, but that is a "natural reaction" to the circumstances. "How do you react when you are hurt or humiliated? "might be a good way of getting an open minded answer from him, without being put on the defensive.

Mental symptoms, or states of mind, do not arise or exist in the abstract. They are invariably related to the various situations which the patient faces, or has faced, in his life. They are an expression of his reaction to those situations. Every patient does not react in the same way to the same situation. For example, grief may cause one to weep piteously, another to become taciturn, and yet another to be thrown in depths of depression, and still another to lose all appetite for food, or to lose sleep altogether, and so on. Irritability may be shown through several instances of violent anger, in which he strikes others, or even threatens to kill, or to commit suicide. Hence, it is useful to ask the patient about the environment at home, at his working place, in society, etc. and about specific occurrences which have upset him very much and the way he has reacted to them. Thorough familiarisation with the various rubrics in the chapter on mind in Kent's — better still in Vol. I of *Synthetic Repertory* by Dr. Horst Barthel — will suggest the kind of mental state of the patients to be inquired into. Strong well-marked mentals (repeatedly observed by patient and reported by attendants) obtained in this way will put the physician on the right track in his search for the similimum.

V. **Peculiar Symptoms.** These have been covered in detail in the previous lesson. Mention a few examples, and ask the patient if he has ever experienced such peculiar sensations or occurrences. (If the same modality or sensation occurs in different parts of the body at the same time, it could be regarded as a keynote. *Bryonia* has agg. from slightest motion anywhere; *Ars.* pains are burning, better from heat; *Theridion* has many complaints worse from noise).

VI. **Personal History.** Of serious illnesses suffered since childhood in chronological order, must be noted down — such as typhoid, pneumonia, jaundice, mumps, measles, tuberculosis, gonorrhoea or syphilis. History of vaccination (whether it took or not), prophylactic inoculations such as Triple Antigen (DPT), B.C.G. etc. should also be noted. In women, the history of miscarriages, ailments during or after pregnancy and labour; History of skin affections which were "cured" (driven in). They may leave a permanent mark on the constitution, and unless the obstacles are removed, the well selected remedy may not act.

Evolution of diseases. Diseases in individuals remain latent, exacerbate, change place from one organ to another or take a serious turn, depending upon their vital force, susceptibility, environment, exciting causes, nutritional state, mode of living (habits) and exposure to harmful influences and the wrong medical treatment undergone. In chronic diseases' all these aspects must be carefully examined. Susceptibility is shown by hereditary influences as well as the various illnesses the patient has suffered from childhood. The nature, course and progress of diseases vary from person to person. Personal and family history of serious illnesses is very relevant for this purpose.

VII. **Family History.** Serious illnesses suffered, such as tuberculosis, cancer, gout, heart attack, diabetes, venereal diseases, epilepsy, insanity, arthritis, etc. should be recorded not only in respect of the patient's father, mother, brothers and sisters, but even grandparents, uncles and aunts. Even with one common heredity, different members of a family may develop different tendencies. This valuable information is particularly useful in chronic cases.

VIII. **Objective Examination.** The physician has to be a very close observer for anything unusual, such as wrinkled forehead, movement of alae nasi, facial expression, dullness or drowsiness, stupor, moaning; arthritis deformans, intolerance of pain on touch or pressure; fear of being approached; nasal voice; incoherent speech; nails crippled or ridged; dull and has to be prompted by the attendant to answer, etc.

Wherever necessary, depending on the nature of the complaint, physical examination of the patient cannot be neglected — lumps, glandular swellings, painful spots, enlarged liver, lungs and heart; pulse; warts; ringworm, eczema and its discharges, etc. If necessary pathological investigations of urine, stool, blood, sputum,, or x-ray chest, barium meal, E.C.G., pyelography, blood sugar, P.V. exam. (by a gynaecologist), etc. should be obtained.

The value of objective symptoms lies in the fact that they cannot be distorted by non-observance (or design) of the patient. They are of particular importance in treating children who are not in a position to express their suffering. Close observation reveals the child's desires, aversions and mental disposition. In case of earache, the child will scream if we gently press on the ear; intertrigo may make the child to weep during stool or urination. Colic will make it flex its thighs on the abdomen, and cry. Photophobia will make it turn its face against light, and so on. Careful observation of objective signs and symptoms has helped many brilliant homoeopathic successes, especially with children.

17. **Understanding Sensations.** Kent's Repertory gives remedies against a large variety of sensations of pain, such as aching, boring, broken, burning, cutting, drawing, gnawing, pinching, pressing, scraping, shooting, sore and bruised, sprained, stitching, tearing, etc. While taking the case, therefore, it is helpful if we get the patient to describe the nature (and intensity) of the pain he experiences. What exactly those sensations mean is given below, so that we may understand their true meaning.

Throbbing or Pulsating. This usually indicates an inflammatory condition, and where the affection is serious, the pain may be severe. Inflammation usually produces an uninterrupted pain in a localised area and is worse by pressure. Severe inflammation may also be attended with fever, high pulse rate and severe thirst.

Taking the Case 85

Burning. This often indicates pressure, ulceration or inflammatory conditions. Where bone is affected, the pain may be excruciating in character.

Gnawing. It is generally a description of the pain of a stomach ulcer; this expression is also usually found in association with the growth of tumours, and great care should be taken where this symptom is given.

Aching, Sore, Bruised. When the pains are described with these words, they are apt to be the after-effects of the over-use of muscles, or of falls and injuries.

Stiffness. This may arise due to deposits of fatigue products in the tissues. In rheumatism also deposits or collection of synovial fluid may cause symptoms of stiffness with aching, usually localising in a particular joint or muscle.

Gripping, Colicky Pains. Irritation of such organs as the bowels, bile-ducts, bladder or ureters will cause this type of pain; the patient usually doubles up or flexes his thighs on abdomen for obtaining relief.

Burning Pains. If in the stomach or oesophagus, these pains are caused by an excess of acid in the gastric juice, which irritates the nerve endings in the stomach membrane. Burning pains are also felt after scratching of skin eruptions, or in the meatus during or after urination; or in the vertex, eyes or soles of feet. Generally, patients find no difficulty in describing "burning" pains.

Shooting, Lancinating. These pains are usually felt when they travel along the course of a nerve, leading to the inference of some irritation of a nerve.

Pains which come and go in the same part, either cramping or constrictive, relieved by warmth or pressure, indicate spasm of the affected part. Spasmodic pains, such as colic, cause the person to double by the severity of the contraction.

Note : The same sensation appearing in more than one place becomes a general, with a higher rank.

ACUTE DISEASES

18. The foregoing scheme for case-taking is especially suitable in the treatment of chronic diseases. In Para 72 of the *Organon* Hahnemann states that the "diseases of man resolve themselves into two classes" : acute and chronic. The acute diseases are self-limiting and always tend to recovery. They arise from such exciting causes as excesses of food, or insufficiency of food, chills, over-heating, dissipation, strains, etc. They may also be sporadic, arising from injurious microbes, affecting those susceptible; or contagious or infectious, as in epidemics. When left to themselves acute diseases terminate in a moderate period of time, in recovery or death. The nature of chronic diseases, which have "no tendency whatever to recovery, but have a continuous progressive tendency . . . even till death," will be dealt with in a later lesson.

19. The case-taking, the basis for the homoeopathic prescription, in the acute disease must confine itself to the acute state only and not go into the constitutional state of the patient. The objective signs and symptoms, mental restlessness or apathy, unusual irritability or torpidity, the nature of thirst or thirstlessness, the reaction to temperature (better or worse from the open air or draft), the side on which he is worse lying, partial heat or coldness of different parts of the body, the causation of the acute attack, the time of onset or aggravation and the concomitants such as constipation or diarrhoea, delirium, etc. will suffice as guides to the similimum.

20. Kent says in his *Lectures on Homoeopathic Philosophy* : A chronic patient may be suffering from an acute disease and the physician on being called may think that it is necessary to take the totality of the symptoms; but if he should do that in an acute disease, mixing both chronic and acute symptoms together, he will become confused and will not find the right remedy. The two things must be separated and the appearance of the acute miasm must now be prescribed for. The chronic symptoms will not, of course, be present when the acute miasm is running, because the latter suppresses or suspends the chronic symptoms, but the diligent physician, not knowing this is so, might wrongly gather together all the symptoms that the patient has had in a life . . . The symptoms of the acute attack are separate by themselves. What are called sequelae of measles, scarlet fever, are not due to the disease itself, but to a

Taking the Case

prior state of the patient. A psoric disorder may come up after scarlet fever or measles and must be treated as psora. These sequelae . . . are psoric and crop out at the weakest time, which is the convalescent period. The better the acute disease is treated, the less likely will there be any sequelae . . . but you cannot prescribe an antipsoric in order to prevent sequelae following the fever, while it prevails. Prescribe first for the attack, and the symptoms that belong to it.

21. Further, Kent says, "It is a fatal error for the physician to go to the bedside of a patient with the feeling in his mind that he has had cases similar to this one . . . and thinking thus : "In the last case I gave so and so, therefore, I will give it to this one." The physician must get such things entirely out of his mind . . . One of the most important things is to keep out of the mind, in an examination of the case, some other case that has appeared to be similar. If this is not done, the mind will be prejudiced in spite of your best endeavours. "I have to fight that with every fresh case I come to." Again, "Get all the symptoms first and then commence your analysis in relation to remedies. The analysis of a sickness is for the purpose of gathering together symptoms which are peculiar, for the peculiar things relate to remedies. Sicknesses have in them that which is peculiar, strange and rare, and the things in sickness that may be wondered at are the things to be compared with those in the remedy that are peculiar."

22. In conclusion, it may be said that thorough familiarity with the Repertory helps one to know the various types of symptoms found in remedies as well as in diseases. In turn, this knowledge helps you very much in case-taking. When a patient mentions some peculiar symptom you will not pass it by as unimportant, but will remember it is there in the Repertory and is important.

SELF-TEST

1. Why is it important to keep a record of the case taken? (Para 7).

2. What are the eight important heads under which symptoms should be elicited from the patient? (Para 12).

3. What is the difference between the case taking for chronic and acute diseases? (Para 20).

4. State at least three points to be remembered while eliciting mental symptoms (Para 16 — IV).

5. What are the factors that determine the susceptibility of an individual to diseases? (Para 16 — VI and VII).

STUDY IN DEPTH

1. *Genius of Homoeopathy* by Stuart Close — Chapter XII (pp. 167-182), "Examintion of the Patient."

2. *Organon of Medicine* — Aphorisms Nos. 83 to 104.

QUESTIONNAIRE

A form of questionnaire is appended as Appendix 'A'. If the physician keeps it before him every time he "takes the case," and elicits the patient's symptoms on the lines given therein, he will soon master the art of case-taking, so essential for selecting the similimum.

Lesson 6

Selection of the Remedy — Repertorisation

1. In the previous lessons we have learnt how to take the case as well as the relative rank or grading of the different symptoms. We now proceed to learn how to use the data which we have so carefully gathered about the patient and his disease, and find the similimum, the single remedy whose symptomatology matches that of the patient. Of the various methods followed by masters for this purpose repertorisation has been found to be the most dependable, systematic and easy one. We have already covered some ground on this subject in paragraphs 12 to 19 of Lesson 3.

2. **Repertorisation.** Dr. Margaret Tyler has rightly said in her booklet, *Different Ways of Finding the Remedy*, "Among the ways of finding the remedy is the elaborate repertory way, which yields excellent results in the majority of cases." Dr. Bidwell repeatedly emphasises in his book, *How to Use the Repertory* that "if our reasoning has been correct and if the technique of selection is without a flaw" (that is, if we have selected the symptoms for repertorisation after correct evaluation), "the remedy emerging from repertorial study must be the mathematically correct remedy," as is borne out by a reference to the Materia Medica as well as the cure which follows the administration of that remedy.

3. **Special Features of Different Repertories.** When we talk of repertorisation the first question which arises for consideration is which repertory should be used by a beginner. A number of repertories are currently popular and, while one could begin with one of them, we should not forget that the beginner grows in maturity as he gains experience and will feel the need to consult other sources, not one but several, in his

search for the similimum in a difficult case. After all, it is the pleasant duty of a conscientious physician to spare no effort to relieve his patient's suffering. We are, therefore, giving a brief outline of some of the most useful Repertories, so that the physician can turn to any or all of them when needed.

(i) **Kent's Repertory.** This is the most popular repertory used by the great majority of homoeopaths all over the world.

Chapters : It is divided into three broad sections, *viz.*

(1) Mind (pp. 1-95)

(2) Particulars, *i.e.* anatomical chapters from head to feet, including sleep, dreams, fever, and skin (pp. 96-1340).

(3) Generalities, *i.e.* symptoms of the patient as a whole (pp. 1341-1423).

Arrangement. Each chapter has rubrics of sensations and complaints, with many sub-rubrics under each rubric, all alphabetically arranged. After each main rubric, remedies are given in the order (S-T-M-E/L-s-t-m-e), *i.e.* side of the part, time of agg., Modalities of circumstances governing the sensation, and extension to other parts — followed by specific locations, *e.g.* forehead, occiput, etc. which in turn have the rubrics for S-T-M-E, where possible.

This arrangement has been found extremely useful as it gives the location (forehead), sensation (pulsating) and Modalities (agg. stepping and stooping) all on one page 157, revealing *Bell.* as the remedy, provided Generals agree, such as agg. bathing (1345) and Wet head (1421) or concomitant Photophobia (261). Such instances are legion.

Philosophy. As discussed earlier, in Kent's evaluation of symptoms, Mentals occupy the highest place, followed by Physical Generals, strange, rare and peculiar symptoms and lastly the particulars qualified by modalities. Such qualified particulars are scattered throughout the Repertory and are an invaluable aid to the prescriber. However, even a qualified particular, with the general not agreeing is useless. Example : Vertigo, morning, compels to lie down (96) has *Nit-ac.* and *Puls.* Of these *Puls.* will be useful only if the patient is agg. from warm air (1412).

Advantages. Very helpful in cases where we get strong Mentals, Physical, Generals and Peculiar Particulars (acute or chronic). Highly useful for treating mental or emotional disorders; and equally useful if Physical Generals and qualified Particulars are more marked than mentals.

Disadvantages. Nosological or pathological terms are not used, though conditions applicable to them are given. There is no section on circulatory, glandular or nervous system, as the book is not based on systems. However, parts of the systems are found scattered throughout under relative anatomical headings. Symptoms of the nervous system, such as analgesia, chorea, convulsions, paralysis, tremblings, etc. appear under generalities. Cravings and aversions to food and drink appear under "stomach," while aggravations from food are given under generalities. Nervous symptoms having to do with the spine appear under "back," such as opisthotonos, meningitis appears under two places, head (inflammation, meninges of) and back (inflammation, cord, membranes of). Dysmenorrhoea under genitalia (female), as well as under abdomen (pain, cramping). These are not great disadvantages; but they only point to the necessity for thorough familiarisation with the book.

(ii) **Boger-Boenninghausen's Repertory.** A much neglected repertory, but it offers a number of advantages which make it worthy of consultation according to the needs of the case.

Closely following the lines of Boenninghausen's *Therapeutic Pocket Book* (the first Repertory in homoeopathy), it has seven chapters, viz. (1) mind, (2) chapters on different anatomical parts, head to extremities, (3) sensations and complaints in general, (4) sleep and dreams, (5) chill, fever and sweat — each of these with detailed concomitants, (6) general conditions of agg. and amel. (7) concordances or relationship of remedies.

Arrangement or Presentation : Alphabetical order of symptoms in each chapter. Each chapter begins with remedies which cover different parts and sides of the concerned region, followed by sensations and complaints of that region, and ending with a section on agg. and amel., and, where applicable, concomitants applicable to that region.

Philosophy. Boenninghausen's Repertory is based on generalisation. He found that symptoms which existed in an incomplete state in some parts of a case (in provers and patients), could be reliably completed by analogy, by observing the conditions of other parts of the case. This is in accord with Hahnemann's dictum that the whole man is sick, and to get a picture of his "totality," we must combine the separate fragments (location, sensations, modalities and concomitants, including mentals and peculiar symptoms) into a whole. He did not regard any one of these as more important than the other repertories.

Advantages. This repertory is useful in cases where strongly marked mentals and qualified Particulars are not available in a case. The totality comprising the location, sensations, modalities and concomitants will yield a few remedies to choose from, after reference to the Materia Medica. Though Mentals in this Repertory are not as numerous as in Kent's, the Modalities of agg. and amel. are comprehensive, covering every conceivable modality. It also contains some compact rubrics : Pregnancy and related conditions (pp. 662); Childbed or Parturition (pp. 658); Infants, affections of (pp. 902-3); Sleep, character of pp. 986); Sleep, symptoms which prevent (pp. 982-4); Circulation (pp. 1006); Epigastrium (pp. 522-33); Remedies for various locations of upper extremities (pp. 805-8); also of lower extremities (pp. 842-5); Glands (pp. 937-40); Bones (pp. 940-44); heartbeat (pp. 1013); Concomitants of Heat (fever) (pp. 1063-76); of sweat (pp. 1088-99); Moon-phase agg. (pp. 1132). Directions of pain (pp. 892).

While Kent gives remedies in three grades **bold**, *italics* and roman types), Boger-Boenninghausen gives them in four grades : (CAPITALS, **bold**, *italics* and roman); these grades are based on their repeated occurrence in provings and confirmation clinically. The extra grade given in CAPITALS helps us with a further differentiation between the highest (boldface) remedies in Kent. Also contains a number of rubrics not found in Kent.

Disadvantages. Mentals are fewer as compared with Kent. Particular sensations (with remedies) are given in each chapter, and the modalities for that chapter are given separately. This contributes to the prescriber's difficulty, whereas in Kent particular sensations are given along with their modalities in innumerable number, which greatly facilitates our work.

(iii) **Concise Repertory by Dr. S.R. Phatak.** In this repertory all the headings — Mentals, Generals, Modalities, Organs and their sub-parts — as well as physiological and pathological conditions such as appetite, aversions, desires, nausea, vomiting, thirst, fever, pulse, etc. are all given in alphabetical order. In each rubric all important symptoms, their concomitants and modalities are given.

Advantages. Alphabetical arrangement helps in tracing the rubrics quickly. There are many rubrics which are not to be found even in Kent. Hence this book should be taken as a supplement to Kent. Very useful in bedside work. Time aggs. given in full.

Disadvantages. Being a concise Repertory, it cannot take the place of the exhaustive repertories like Kent's or Boger Boenninghausen's.

(vi) **Synthetic Repertory by Horst Barthel** : This is in three volumes, I-Mind; II-Generalities; III-Sleep, Dreams and Sex. They are presented in the same format as Kent's. The first volume on mind gives a number of additional rubrics not found in Kent. There are also a number of cross-references to allied rubrics; one has to see them to appreciate how extremely useful these cross-references are. This volume is a must for cases where Mentals of all sorts predominate. In volumes II and III also there are a good number of additional rubrics and remedies (e.g. cravings and aversions). The exact sources of rubrics and remedies (16 sources) are mentioned by using the numbering system. This set is indispensable for one who aims at being a proficient prescriber.

(v) **Boericke's Repertory by Dr. Oscar E. Boericke.** This is given at the end of the *Pocket Manual of Homoeopathic Materia Medica* by Dr. William Boericke. This is based on clinical conditions and clinical verifications of drugs in various nosological conditions. Consideration of totality of complete and characteristic symptoms — in the form of cause, type, location, sensation, concomitants and modalities — makes repertorisation easy, especially to those accustomed to nosological approach and are not yet adept with the symptomatic approach.

Remedies are given in two types : *Italics* indicate a frequently verified remedy; roman type, less frequently verified remedy.

Arrangement. Each section is divided into (i) Cause, (ii) Type, (iii) Location, sensation, concomitants, (iv) Modalities.

Analysis of Symptoms. For repertorisation take the Mentals, Physical Generals and Particulars.

Advantages. A case with few mental symptoms, characteristic particulars, and with known clinical diagnosis (or with more objective and pathological symptoms) can be easily worked out with this Repertory.

Disadvantages. For cases where the "totality of symptoms" approach is feasible. It is better to use Kent's Repertory, supplemented by reference to Phatak's.

(vi) **Kent's Repertorium General by Dr. Jost Kunzli.** Since Kent's death many important therapeutic observations have been made. Dr. Kunzli has brought Kent's Repertory up to date by the addition of innumerable rubrics and remedies from 72 reputable sources including the writings of Hahnemann, Kent, H.C. Allen, Boger, Hering, Clarke, Guernsey, Nash and Pulford. A special feature of this Repertory is his use of the "black dot" after a rubric or a remedy, to indicate that it is a reliable rubric, or a remedy, which Kunzli has found to be of particular use. The cost being rather high, prescribers may turn to this Repertory only after gathering sufficient experience with Kent's Repertory.

MORE ABOUT BOGER-BOENNINGHAUSEN AND KENT REPERTORIES

4. We shall, however, advise practitioners to first concentrate and master the use of the two Repertories, *viz.* Boger-Boenninghausen's and Kent's. Only then will they feel the need to refer to the other Repertories. We shall now briefly give the philosophical background of these two books.

5. Boger-Boenninghausen's Repertory is the product of Boger's augmentation of Boenninghausen's Therapeutic Pocket Book — the first Repertory in homoeopathy — without altering its form, plan or the philosophic base of its structure. In using this Repertory, precedence has to be given to Modalities and Concomitants. As the Modalities are not so difficult to elicit from the patients as the mentals, it is obvious that this feature makes

Selection of the Remedy — Repertorisation

for easier case-taking and easier repertorisation. However, probably seeing some point in Kent's criticism that Boenninghausen over-did the Generals by ignoring modalities of particulars (which he said should remain with Particulars only and should not be made Generals). Boger has given Modalities relating to each part of the body (head, eyes, stomach, etc.), in addition to the large General Modalities chapter. But even this presentation is not as complete as that given by Kent. For example, at page 604 we find stool "children in, agg." and at page 605 "fruit agg." It is difficult to make out whether these aggravations are of diarrhoea or of constipation. But in Kent at page 611 we find "diarrhoea, in children" and at page 613 "diarrhoea, fruit after". And Kent gives many more remedies. It is only this special feature which enhances the usefulness of Kent over Boger-Boenninghausen. Yet, Kent owed a lot to Boenninghausen's Generals which he has retained in his Repertory.

6. **Boenninghausen's Contribution.** A few words on Boenninghausen's contribution will not be out of place. He was the first to construct a Repertory, which was highly appreciated by Hahnemann. Breaking up the symptoms for construction of a Repertory was not an easy task. With his acumen and insight into the Materia Medica, supported by his clinical experience :

(i) He was the first to classify the symptoms into Location, Sensation, Modalities, Concomitants, and Mentals. This classification was a stroke of genius.

(ii) He solved the problem on the basis of analogy. He found that symptoms which existed in an incomplete state in some parts of a given case, could be reliably completed by analogy, by observing the condition of other parts of the case. (iii) He was the first to stress that aggravations and ameliorations have a far more significant relation to totality and the choice of the correct remedy often chiefly depends upon them. (iv) Boenninghausen had observed that the elements of disease (Location, Sensation, etc.) combine in ever varying forms according to the constitution and susceptibility of each individual patient. He found that the process of breaking up the symptoms in the Materia Medica, could be reversed to meet ever varying forms of disease, through analogy, by which the location in one part, a sensation in another part and a modality of a third part could be taken together to form a grand totality of the individual — even though this combination of symptoms had never been seen in provers. The successful prescriptions which emerge again and again from applying this approach, owe not a little to Boenninghausen's correct insight into the usefulness of breaking up the symptoms (for constructing the Repertory), on the one hand, and of synthesising them (for individual patients) to meet diverse types of totalities on the other. The Repertory constructed on Boenninghausen's lines, provides a surprising degree of elasticity and enables the prescriber to meet any syndrome, any group of symptoms, that may confront him in practice. (v) Not every remedy observed in the provings produced a given symptom equally intensively. The point had an important bearing on the applicability of one remedy against others. After a very careful study, he was the first to assign four grades to remedies denoted by different types.

7. Genius of Kent. The genius of Kent lies in the fact that he not only absorbed the full legacy of Boenninghausen, but made a few valuable contributions to it, because of which successful homoeopathic practice has become much more easy and certain of result than it could have otherwise been. These are his stress on the predominating role of Mental symptoms on the one hand, and the value of qualified particulars on the other, without neglecting the role of Physical Generals. Correct use of these elements transforms the prescriber from a therapeutic scientist to a therapeutic artist.

8. Scientific Method. Dr. J.T. Kent opens his short article, "Uses of the Repertory", with the pregnant words : "As homoeopathy includes both science and art, Repertory study must also consist of science and art . . . the scientific method is the mechanical method; taking all the symptoms and writing out all the associated remedies with gradings, making a summary with grades marked at the end." Of course, even the mechanical method must confirm to the tenets of the science, such as evaluation and graduation of symptoms according to their importance as characteristics, Mental, Physical Generals, strange and peculiar, etc. It is essential that we master the scientific method before we can ever learn the artistic method.

9. Artistic Method. Kent's observations on the artistic method of finding the similimum are given in his article "Uses of the Repertory."

Selection of the Remedy — Repertorisation

"There is an artistic method that omits the mechanical, and is better, but all are not prepared to use it. The artistic method demands that judgment be passed on all the symptoms after the case is most carefully taken. The symptoms must be judged as to their value as characteristics in relation to the patient; they must be passed in review by the rational mind to determine those which are strange, rare and peculiar."

These remarks sound very much like the scientific method, except that strange, rare and peculiar symptoms have been singled out for special mention. Kent further remarks :

"The artistic prescriber sees much in the proving that cannot be retained in the Repertory, where everything must be sacrificed for the alphabetical system. The artistic prescriber must study Materia Medica long and earnestly to enable him to fix in his mind sick images which, when needed, will infill the sick personalities of human beings. These are too numerous and too various to be named or classified. I have often known the intuitive prescriber to attempt to explain a so-called marvellous cure by saying : "I cannot quite say how I came to give that remedy but it resembled him" . . . Who can attempt to explain it? It is something that belongs not to the neophyte, but comes gradually to the experienced artistic prescriber. It is only the growth of art in the artistic mind, what is noticed in all artists.

"Such intuition belongs to all artists, but if carried too far it becomes a fatal mistake,and must therefore be corrected by repertory work done in even the most mechanical manner. The more one restrains the tendency to carelessness in prescribing and in method, the wiser he becomes in artistic effects and Materia Medica work."

10. Let us now summarise these views of Dr. Kent on the artistic method. He says, firstly, that it is something that does not belong to the neophyte, but comes gradually to the experienced artistic prescriber. Secondly, the artistic prescriber must study the Materia Medica long and earnestly to enable him to perceive the sick images of drugs and the corresponding sick personalities of human beings. Thirdly, the "intuition" which the prescriber develops from his long study of Materia Medica coupled with clinical experience, if carried too far, i.e., through misplaced overconfidence, may lead to fatal mistakes, and must therefore he corrected by Repertorial work done even in the most mechanical manner. In other words, failure to use the

Repertory even on the part of an artistic prescriber would amount to carelessness.

11. The new learner will find even the above hints on the artistic method to be far too general and vague. How should the neophyte start as a beginner, and which is the method that can give him high assurance of making successful prescriptions almost from the start, with the least possible expenditure of time and energy? Fortunately, Kent himself has provided us with an answer, though we shall have to read between his lines, exercise our intelligence and imagination for gleaning the true purport and meaning of his observations by drawing on the clinical experiences of artistic prescribers, and finding support for our conclusions in those experiences.

12. **Secret of Artistic Work.** Kent has wrapped the secret of his approach to artistic work in words which are expressed in flashes in his two articles, "Uses of the Repertory" and "How to Use the Repertory", probably because he was afraid of neophytes misusing it and getting into trouble.

13. In the second of these articles Dr. Kent examines the process of finding the remedy for "writer's cramp", firstly with the help of Particulars (i.e., specific rubrics such as "cramps in fingers", "numbness in fingers", etc.) and he remarks that "failure often follows" by relying on the Particulars "owing to the scanty clinical and pathogenetic record to which we have access; sometimes the scanty showing (of Particulars) presents just the remedy required, but oftener it does not." When the Particulars fail to give us a remedy, Kent advises us to use the General group of remedies at the head of the rubrics like cramps of hands and fingers; and numbness of hands, fingers and wrists (all without modalities such as "while writing"). He advises us also to use the general rubric "exertion" at page 1358 in Generalities. "This is using in proper manner a general rubric", he points out. It will be noted that this is Boenninghausen's method of using Generals. It may appear contradictory that in the very next paragraph Kent says "Our Generals were well worked out by Boenninghausen and much overdone, as he generalised many rubrics that were purely Particulars, the use of which as Generals is misleading and ends in failure . . . For example, 'aggravation from writing' is a rubric of Particulars . . . To make use of this modality for mental symptoms, when it is applied to complaints of the hand, is perverting

Selection of the Remedy — Repertorisation

the uses of circumstances. Aggravation from writing should be limited to the symptoms that are worse from writing and kept with them, as it is not a General. It is so done in my Repertory."

Kent also points out that Boenninghausen's arrangement whereby Generals can be quickly made use of to furnish modalities for individual symptoms, whether General or Particular, is preserved in his repertory "because of the success coming from the use of Generals in this way".

14. Now comes an important observation from Kent : "After cures have been made with remedies selected in this way (as in the case of writer's cramp with the help of general rubrics), such remedies may be added to the scanty list of particulars and in this manner our repertory will grow into usefulness. This is the legitimate use of clinical symptoms. It is the proper use of the general rubrics to the end that our scanty particulars may build up . . . The new repertory is the only one ever found that provides a vacant space for annotating just such information. If a large number of correct prescribers in the world would join in this extension, we could soon have a Repertory of comparatively extensive particulars . . . The author is devoting his life to the growth and infilling and perfecting of this work, and begs all true workers to co-operative by — noting such modalities of particulars as have come from Generals and have been observed in cures."

"The new Repertory is produced to show forth all the particulars, each symptom with the circumstance connected with it. It is in infancy and may remain so very long, unless all who use it unite to preserve their experiences in well kept records and furnish the author with such."

Kent further observers : "Many of the most brilliant cures are made from the general rubric when the special does not help, (because it is scanty — writer), and, in careful notes of ten years, would bring down (i.e., down to the list of Particulars in the Repertory — writer) many of the general rubric symptoms and furnish the best of clinical verifications. The longer this is done the more can the busy doctor abbreviate his case notes.

Again : "It is sometimes possible to abbreviate the anemnesis by selecting one symptom that is very peculiar containing the key to the case. A young man cannot often detect this peculiarity, and he should seldom attempt it. It is often convenient to abbreviate by taking a group of three or four essentials in a given case, making a summary of these, and eliminating all remedies not found in all the essential symptoms. A man with considerable experience may cut short the work in this way" . . . Further, "the strange and rare symptoms are so guiding . . . they include some keynotes which may guide safely   to a remedy or to the shaping of results, provided that the mental and the physical generals do not stand contrary, as to their modalities, and therefore oppose the keynote symptoms."

15. What is the main thrust of the above remarks which have been pieced together from Kent's two articles? We shall summarise : Firstly, Kent regarded it as his life's mission to collect clinically proved remedies for particular symptoms (with their modalities of course) and sought the co-operation of correct prescribers in the world, so that we could have a "Repertory of comparatively extensive particulars". He described the immense store of Particular symptoms (qualified) given in his Repertory as "scanty" because he knew that there is still greater scope (and need) for their augmentation. Secondly, he strongly felt that the Repertory will grow into usefulness by infilling of an extensive list of Particulars into Repertory. Thirdly, with this extensive list of clinically verified Particulars "with the modalities and circumstances connected with them", the busy doctor can "abbreviate his case notes". Fourthly, a young doctor may not be able to detect the one symptom which holds the key to the case, and in that event "it is often convenient to abbreviate his work by taking a group of three or four essentials, making a summary of these and eliminating all remedies not found in all the essential symptoms".

16. It is important to stress here that Kent regarded Mentals as belonging to the highest grade as they express the patient most absolutely. If one could not get any marked mental symptoms, he advised : "Get the strong, strange, peculiar symptoms, and then see to it that there are no generals in the case that oppose or contradict". The symptoms, in order of importance are : first Mentals, then Generals (pertaining to the man as a whole, including modalities, character of discharges, etc.) and lastly the Particulars (relating to a part or organ and not the whole man, but always qualified by modalities). In short, he

Selection of the Remedy — Repertorisation

advised : When looking over a list of symptoms first of all discover 3, 4, 5 or 6 symptoms that are strange, rare and peculiar. These are the highest generals and being strange, etc. must apply to the patient himself. Work these out first (i.e., using them as eliminative symptoms). When you have settled upon three, four or six remedies that have these first Generals, then find out which remedy of this list is most like the rest of the symptoms, common and particular."

17. Corroboration from Other Prescribers. Is this not what Sir John Weir meant when he said that we should learn to take the minimum number of symptoms with the maximum value? Perhaps he meant exactly this. Dr. J.H. Clarke says in his little booklet, *Grand Characteristic of Materia Medica* : "Fortunately there are many features of homoeopathy which tend to the simplification of practice and none knew this better than Thomas Skinner — to whom my friend Dr. John McLachlan rightly gives a place in the great Quarternary of Homoeopathic Empyrean — Hahnemann, Hering, Lippe, Skinner. I learned from Skinner many precious bits of practical knowledge most of which will be found their due place scattered through the pages of my *Dictonary of Practical Materia Medica*. When, for instance, we have a feverish patient who turns deadly pale and faints on any attempt to rise from the horizontal posture, we have no need to make an hour's search in Repertories to find the simillimum. The patient is crying out for *Aconite*. That symptom is a "grand characteristic" of the remedy in the phraseology of Dr. Skinner. Skinner gave me from time to time a goodly number of these . . . and I invite readers to insert particular Grand Characteristics from their own experience . . . Skinner's term *Grand Characteristics* has the same meaning as Lippe's *Key-notes* and Nash's *Leaders*. All indicate a method of simplifying a practice which is often very complicated — that of finding the similimum.

18. Dr. Pierre Schmidt, veteran homoeopath of world renown, calls these Particulars as "Cardinal" or "Pilot" symptoms. He says : "We always search for the cardinal symptoms. There is one symptom in every body which is so peculiar, so extraordinary that when you find this symptom, it leads you to the remedy. I call this the cardinal symptom, the pilot symptom. It is very rare that you do not find other symptoms fitting in with the remedy indicated by this cardinal symptom, *e.g.* running of nose during stool."

19. Dr. Sarabhai Kapadia, a firm practitioner of Hahnemannian homoeopathy in Bombay, is yet another physician who has found the "Particular" or "Cardinal" symptoms in Kent's Repertory of immense value. In a paper read at the All India Homoeopathic Convention, Calcutta, in October 1975, he says : "Apart from full repertorisation by referring to general rubrics . . . it is often beneficial to take the help of Particular rubrics. A particular symptom when authentic and complete with regard to sensation, location, extension and modality can become a key to that case in which it occurs. A 'particular' solves your case, like a small piece of paper, wrapper or the 'butt' of a cigarette which solves a murder case for a shrewd detective . . . Sometimes, you have already tried to select a medicine from Generals without results . . . In such circumstances Kent's Repertory is the richest and handy source of information for particular symptoms." He then gives 14 cases in which 'Particular' symptoms pointed to the curative remedy, which would normally have been missed. And he stresses : "You will not notice the remedies as important while reading the Materia Medica. You are not likely to come across *Iris* as an important remedy in cough, while it does suggest a condition like we meet in Eosinophilia" . . . In the same way I have learnt about *Tellurium* and some other medicines. Thus the Repertory can teach you Materia Medica in an entirely different context and make you see your remedies as new personalities.

20. By way of illustration, we are giving here the rubrics, with page numbers and remedies in the case reported by Dr. Sarabhai :

Fever, body pain — P. 161 — "Head, pain, forehead, above eyes, agg. sneezing" — *Echin.*

Hyperacidity — P. 590 — "Stomach, pain, drawing, extending to throat" — *Conium.* 1M. t.d.s. 4 days. — No other indications of Con. were present.

Intervertebral spaces reduced in cervical region, with Osteophytes : right-sided pain in forearm. "Pain, upper arm when lying on it" (p. 1054) and "Numbness of hand" (p. 1038). As the patient was relieved by warm bath, *Carbo-an.* was selected, and relieved the patient promptly.

Sciatic pain (Spondylosis) — "Pain with sensation as if thigh

Selection of the Remedy — Repertorisation 103

is broken, agg. while standing." (P. 1091). *Valeriana* 1M, 4 hourly, put him on his feet in a couple of days.

Sciatica (two cases) — "Pain in toes extending to hips" (p. 1081) : and "Shooting pain, toes to hip" (p. 1125) — The patient was proud and arrogant — *Palladium* B.D. for some weeks cured permanently.

Angina, high blood pressure, over-weight, tobacco addiction; also "Respiration difficult while walking on level ground, but not when ascending" (p. 772) — *Ranunculus bulb*, 1 M.B.D. improved the patient much, and blood pressure partly controlled in a couple of weeks.

Noises in head — old age, high blood pressure : "Head Commotion, painless, in" (p. 109) — *Causticum*, 1M weekly given, but the first dose itself relieved. O.K. in three months.

Calf muscles — Pain in, after eating : "Pain, sore, agg. after eating" (p. 1133) ; and "Pain, sore, cal.f, after eating" (p. 1172); The former rubric showed *Clematis* and latter *Bryonia*. As *Bry*. was not found indicated, *Clematis* B.D. for a week was given and it cured.

Eosinophilic Bronchitis — Elongated uvula with needle like point; ropy saliva : "Head, drawing pain on coughing" (p. 182)- *Iris-v*. This remedy relieved him from the first dose. Was kept under it for about 3 months; no recurrence even after 3 years.

Note : Some of the well-known indications of *Iris-v*. were absent and the remedy would have been missed.

Skin eruption (Hybrid between Eczema and Psoriasis) — "Salivation while talking" (p. 418), and reference to Boericke — *Iris-v*.

Eosinophilia — Rattling mucus in chest: "Expectoration, 10 a.m.." *Iris-v*. given for two weeks, cured.

Bronchitis Asthmatic; Eosinophilia, violent cough; pustular eruptions on knee : "Eruptions, knee, pustules, and psoriasis" (p. 1000); also uvula elongated; ropy saliva — *Iris-v*.

Nasal Catarrh and Obstruction — Deviated septum; agg. from cold; Uvula conical; ropy saliva while talking — *Iris-v*. 1

M.B.D. 90% better after a month. Reported after 5 months as fully cured.

Many more instances of these "Grand Characteristics" having abbreviated the labours of many artistic prescribers could be cited. A few more experiences of other prescribers are cited :

Menses, copious (frightening), agg. lying : Kreo. (725) — SMG.

Cough, violent, spasmodic perking of head forward and knees upward; (k. 810) : *Therid.* Dr. Ranjan Sankaran

Pain, cervical, riding in a carriage from : (900) — *Formica.* Dr. Jayesh Shah

Dreams of water, putrid (1245) : *Arg. nit.* — Dr. R.K. Chhaya

Extremities, own felt as if not his own legs : (1043) — *Agar.* Dr. R.K. Chhaya

Convulsions, epileptiform, with jerk in nape : (1353) — *Bufo.* Dr. R.K. Chhaya

Teeth, upper, right bi-cuspid (433) : *Cinnb.* — SMG.

21. **Two Repertories — One View.** It would be appropriate to state here that although there appear to be differences in the approach of Boenninghausen and Kent, the basic principles of evaluation followed by both are more or less the same. They are, in fact, complementary. Since evaluation of symptoms has to be repertory-oriented, to the philosophy and plan and special features of the Repertory we propose to use — it appears obvious that in a case where strong Mentals and qualified Particulars are wanting, and there are clear-cut Modalities and Concomitants, Boger-Boenninghausen would be more suitable; and Kent's Repertory where it is otherwise.

STEP BY STEP PROCEDURE FOR REPERTORISATION

22. We have so far studied a few of the essential steps before repertorisation, *viz.* taking the case, evaluation of the symptoms of the patient, or ranking them, for repertorisation as well as the philosophical approach to evaluation which suits

Selection of the Remedy — Repertorisation 105

each of the two Repertories : Boger-Boenninghausen's and Kent's. There are a few more steps to be taken, and we will describe them below :

(i) The first need is to develop thorough familiarity with the Repertory. This is best done by noting down in a notebook the pages of each chapter, as well as important subsections of the chapter. This must be done by the learner himself. These notes will be like the road map of a city, which will help you to visit any part of the city without costly, time-consuming detours.

(ii) After the case has been taken with all necessary details, make a list of the outstanding and characteristic symptoms (Mentals, Physical Generals, Peculiars and qualified Particulars), which qualify for repertorisation. Causation, such as concussion, fright, grief, mortification, delusions, suppressions, exposure to sun, rain, etc. should be taken as first class symptoms.

(iii) Keep a good number of slips handy, for use as bookmarks.

(iv) Next, find the Repertory rubrics corresponding to each one of the symptoms listed in (ii) above, note the page number against them in the list and insert a book-mark at the relevent page on your side of the Repertory.

(v) In selecting the rubrics, the following points should be borne in mind :

(a) While using Boger-Boenninghausen's Repertory, prefer a larger and general rubric to a smaller and specific one. For example take the whole rubric "Fearsome..." Instead of "Fear, eating after". Take "Thirst" in general instead of "diarrhoea, with", unless the specific small ru-bric is considered apt in a case, in which case remedies mentioned in both the large and small rubrics should be taken together. In short, do not sacrifice a general rubric to a local one, either in sensations or modalities. However, a regional modality or sensation, if strongly expressed by the patient, will have precedence over a general modality expressed indefinitely or half-heartedly.

(b) If it is felt appropriate to take two or more allied rubrics together to represent a condition, take them in as separate rubrics with their respective remedy-values. As one gains experience, one will be able to select the appropriate remedies with high marks from all of them together, as if from one rubric only.

(vi) Equip yourself with a graph-like chart for working out the repertorial synthesis of the rubrics.

(vii) Recording the Analysis. Our next objective is to minimise the time and effort involved in the detailed repertorial analysis. For this purpose, we resort to the device known as elimination. By this method we eliminate unsuitable remedies and confine our attention, at each succeeding step, to a smaller and smaller group of the most likely remedies. This method of "elimination" is described below :

(viii) **Combining Two Eliminative Rubrics.** There is a technique which greatly saves our time and labour in repertorial work. It is the use of eliminative symptoms. Suppose we have made a list of ten important symptoms, as described in (ii) above. Out of them we should choose the two most outstanding and peculiar symptoms which represent the patient's individuality, and which are indispensable for a study of the case. By comparing these two rubrics visually, we now make a list of the remedies which are common to these two rubrics, and make a note in the chart about the grade each remedy occupies. You will get a small number of such common remedies. This is the list of likely remedies, and one of them will be the remedy for the case, depending upon how the remaining rubrics "cast their vote". We now enter the grades (marks) for remaining rubrics, one by one confining ourselves only to the "likely group", and ignoring all other remedies even high ranking — which have been "eliminated" (thrown out) because they are not common to the first two rubrics.

The choice of the first two Eliminative Rubrics thus acquires crucial importance, for if we choose them wrongly, we shall be throwing out of consideration even the true similimum from the beginning. Remember, further, that as the two Eliminative Rubrics have been chosen as high ranking in the patient, they will also occupy high rank (grade) in the Repertory. So, we may not go wrong if we take only the top two grades in each rubric (in Kent), and top three in Boger-Boenninghausen. An example will make these points clear :

Selection of the Remedy — Repertorisation

Elimination Method — An Example

Case : A male aged 35 had stomach ulcer. He complained of stools consisting of slimy mucus. He had a strong desire for sweets. He was most uncomfortable in hot weather. He was very much frustrated and hurt by being bypassed in promotion. He used to repeatedly dream of snakes. (Repertorial working is shown below. All the remedies given in the Repertory for the first two Eliminative Rubrics only are given to show how to operate the Eliminative method.

TWO ELIMINATIVE RUBRICS FROM KENT

SYMPTOMS FOR REPERTORISATION

1. **Mortification** : (p. 68) : Arg-n., Aur., Aur-m., bell., bry., cham., **Coloc.**, **Ign.**, **Lyc.**, Lyss., merc., **Nat-m.**, nux-v., op., **Pall.**, **ph-ac.**, plat., puls., rhus-t., seneq., sep., staph., stram., sulph., verat.

2. **Desires sweets** : (486): Am-c., arg-m., **arg-n.**, ars., bry., bufo., calc., calc-s., carb-v., **Chin.**, chin-a., elaps., ip., kali-ar., kali-c., kali-p., kali-s., lyc., mag-m., med., merc., nat-a., nat-c., nat-m., nux-v., op., petr., plb., rheum., rhus-t., sabad., sec., sep., **Sulph.**, tub.

3. **Stool, mucus, slimy.** (639) : (105 remedies) Of these only the remedies found common to the first two rubrics are taken below in the Repertorisation Chart.

Repertorisation Chart

Rubrics No.	Arg-n	Bry.	Lyc.	Nat-m.	Sulph
1. Common Remedies	2	2	3	3	2
2. Common Remedies	3	2	3	1	3
3. _ _ _ _ _	3	-	-	-	3
4. Agg. Warm (1412)	2	2	2	2	2
5. Dreams of snakes (1243)	2	-	-	-	-
6. Stomach,Ulcers (531)	2	-	3	-	-

14/6

As you enter the marks of remedies against each rubric, make a mental note of the high grade remedies which appear more or less in one rubric after another. May be one such remedy has a strong relation to the case. This sort of guesswork trains the mind and makes repertorisation less mechanical.

(ix) Use of the pathological symptoms as eliminating (or confirmatory) rubric : Resort to this method is not encouraged, especially because very few remedies could be pushed in their provings, to the point of producing these symptoms without danger to the lives of the provers. Any remedy may cure a case, if indicated by its characteristics, even if not listed in pathological rubrics. Yet, the prescriber is sometimes left with no alternative but to fall back on their use when he is not able to get any characteristic symptoms of the patient. These rubrics can also prove useful in confirming the choice of a remedy already arrived at on the basis of totality. All this means that the absence of a remedy in the pathological rubrics should not, by itself, lead to discarding the remedy.

(x) It would be a good exercise if a few cases are repertorised by following each one of the above methods, and comparing the results. Such an exercise will help us to master the art of rapid and accurate repertorisation.

(xi) As we gain more and more experience, we would be able to find the curative remedy by taking only a very few, most characteristic, strange, rare or peculiar symptoms and comparing them visually — an ideal actually attained and repeatedly demonstrated by master prescribers. We should persist in our endeavours in that direction.

23. Synthesis, the Final Tally : The total number of marks obtained by each remedy in the analysis should now be written down in the column for "Totals". The number of rubrics covered by each remedy will then be written below the total marks for it, as a denominator. For example, 28/9 would mean 28 marks for 9 rubrics.

24. Judgement About the Similimum : The remedy carrying the highest number of marks and also covering all, or most of the rubrics, will normally be adjudged the similimum. If more than one remedy comes out equally strong, a close study of the complete Materia Medica will be more essential than ever for a decision between the competing remedies. In such cases, one

Selection of the Remedy — Repertorisation

should also look for factors which may not have entered into the repertorisation, such as the constitutional remedy of the mother or father, the nature of the patient's previous illness. It may sometimes be even necessary to enquire into additional symptoms which may lend support to one or the other of the competing remedies.

25. It is important to bear in mind that the similimum need not always be the remedy securing the numerically highest number of marks. The number of rubrics covered and the comparative rank of the remedies in respect of the outstanding symptoms must be taken into consideration. In short, the remedy selected must cover the marked and indispensable symptoms in the same rank (or intensity) as they occupy in the patient's case.

26. If an unusual or rare remedy comes through for even a couple of symptoms in a high rank, it is advisable to check up in the Materia Medica if it meets the other symptoms of the case. Not having been well-proved, it may not have as full representation in the Repertory as the Polychrests.

27. Quite often it will be found that repertorisation leads to the polychrests. It is unsafe to look on them with suspicion or distrust, *e.g.* on the ground that *Puls.* or *Lyco.* comes out again ! It should be remembered that polychrests have a wide range of action and their ranks are given in the Repertorial rubrics in the light of concrete clinical experience.

28. Materia Medica, the Final Court of Appeal : Because of human imperfections such as deficiences in case-taking, incorrect evaluation of symptoms, incorrect choice of rubrics or eliminating symptoms or even imperfections of the Repertory, we cannot take it for granted that Repertorial analysis will always lead us to the curative remedy. It is, therefore, imperative that the remedy should be studied in a complete Materia Medica both for its general correspondence, as well as for the chief complaint. The Materia Medica will always remain the supreme court of appeal.

SOME EXAMPLES OF REPERTORIAL STUDY OF CASES

29. We shall now show a few examples of repertorisation, some with Kent's and some with Boger-Boenninghausen's Rep-

ertories. Note the class of symptoms selected for repertorisation and the method of choosing the "eliminative group" of symptoms to save time and effort.

Case 1. "Stenosis of value of the heart-rheumatic" — Dr. H.A. Roberts — *Bryonia.*

Dr. H.A. Roberts, in a highly instructive article "The Finding of Homoeopathic Remedy in Heart Conditions", page 446 of *Homoeopathic Heritage*, Oct. 1977, stresses that the principles that should guide us in the selection of the curative remedy in heart conditions are not different from those applicable to other cases, viz., that we should take the whole condition of the patient into consideration, including concomitants, and not base our effort on the diagnosis. The following is one of the six cases detailed by him to illustrate his point, which we have repertorised with the help of Boger-Boenninghausen's Repertory.

Rubrics	BB Repertory
1. Agg. from deep breathing	1109
2. Aching Heart region (precordial distress)	773
3. Agg. from lying on left side	1130
4. Agg. from ascending steps	1107
5. Concomitants before menses	678
6. Agg. from cold air	1105
7. Agg. walking, while	1149
8. Knees	844
9. Cutting pains	891
10. Agg. from cabbage	1119

	Symptom Numbers										
	1	2	3	4	5	6	7	8	9	10	Total
Aco.	4	1	3	2	-	3	1	-	-	-	
Bell.	3	1	1	1	-	3	-	x	x	x	
BRY.	4	2	3	4	2	2	4	2	2	4	29/10
Merc.	3	1	1	3	3	3	2	2	4	-	
Phos.	3	2	4	2	3	3	3	2	3	2	27/10
Rhus.	4	1	-	2	1	4	2	4	1	-	

Comments. The diagnosis of this case was "Stenosis of valve of the heart of Rheumatic origin," but this point had no role in the selection of the remedy. The totality of the symptoms alone led to the selection of the curative remedy, *Bryonia*. This selection by Dr. Roberts has been confirmed here by the repertorial analysis with Boger-Boenninghausen's Repertory. As to the method, remedies common to the first two rubrics were taken as the eliminative group.

Case 2. Prolapsus of Uterus — Sepia. Dr. J.T. Kent

Mrs. K., a married woman, 28 years old came to me from the country, with what a gynaecologist had called a prolapsus. She was a tall, slim woman, otherwise in a good health. She was wearing a Hodge pessary. She could not walk or stand long without her "ring". She came to my office in a carriage. I removed the ring and gave her *Sac. Lac.* At the end of a week I had noted the following symptoms. The symptoms noted and the repertorisation done with the Kent's Repertory are given below:

Rubrics	Kent
1. Urine retarded, must wait long for the urine to start	660
2. Lump in rectum	628
3. Empty feeling in stomach	487
4. Bearing down in pelvis (uterus)	735
5. Pressure on vulva ameliorates	736
6. Crosses limbs (to prevent uterus from escaping)	735

Symptom Numbers

	1	2	3	4	5	6	Total
Caust.	3	2	2	-	-	-	
Nat-mur.	2	2	2	3	-	-	
SEPIA	3	3	3	3	3	3	18/6
Sil.	2	2	1	2	-	-	

Comment : Common remedies in the first two grades have been taken as eliminative.

Note : Nos. 1, 2 and 3 are Concomitants; 4 a Local sensation and No. 5 and 6 are Modalities.

The above case has been worked out with Boger-Boenninghausen's Repertory, as follows :

Rubrics

	Page Nos.					
	1(629)	2(613)	3(517)	4(663)	6(665)	Total
SEPIA	3	4	3	4	2	16/5
Caust.	3	1	1	-	-	

Comment : Common remedies in the first two rubrics have been taken as eliminative.

Case 3. Epilepsy — Causticum — Dr. Glen Bidwell.

Boy, age 14; epileptic attacks for three years. First attack followed fright caused by other boys, make-believe to hang him. Attacks increasing in frequency until at this time they occur every two weeks. The following symptoms were given. Attacks begin by running around in circle, then falls down unconscious Attacks are more frequent in cold dry weather and during new moon. Involuntary urination during the attack. Boy complains of always being cold; wants to keep warm in both summer and winter. He is very touchy; everything makes him cry; seems depressed all the time. Appetite either ravenous or wanting. Aversion to all kinds of sweets, of which he was previously very fond. The repertorial analysis done by Bidwell with Kent's Repertory is given below :

Rubrics Kent

1. Agg. from fright (complaints from)   49
2. Sadness, mental depression   75
3. Agg. from cold, dry weather   1349
4. Aversion to sweets   482

Symptom Numbers

	1	2	3	4	Total
Acon.	3	3	3	-	
Arg-nit.	2	2	-	-	
Aurum	2	3	-	-	
Bell.	2	2	-	-	
CAUST.	2	3	3	3	11/4
Coff.	2	2	-	-	
Cuprum	2	2	-	-	
Gels.	2	3	-	-	
Graph.	2	3	-	-	
Hyosc.	2	2	-	-	

Selection of the Remedy — Repertorisation

	1	2	3	4	Total
Ign.	3	3	-	-	
Lyco.	3	3	-	-	
Nat-m.	3	3	-	-	
Nux-v.	2	2	3	-	
Phos.	3	2	-	-	
Phos-ac.	3	2	-	-	
Puls.	3	3	-	-	
Rhus-t.	2	3	-	-	
Sep.	2	3	1	-	
Sil.	3	3	2	-	

Bidwell's comments. "We have arrived at the solution of the case by four steps and have used all general symptoms. Now, you may ask, why did we start with the rubric "complaints caused by fright?" First, this is a general symptom and we are working from the generals to particulars. Second, this condition was caused in this boy by fright. This mental shock was so profound that it caused the whole condition of this patient to be changed. It not only produced the epileptic seizure, but affected his desires as well. The second symptom is another general — sadness and depression, a mental condition produced by a derangement of the patient's most internal condition, the mind. Another general condition is the modality that the attacks are worse in cold dry weather ... We find only five remedies covering the first three symptoms ... In order to decide which of these will cover our case we will take the general aversion to sweets. Here we find that *Causticum* is the only remedy which covers our rubrics . . . Turning to our Materia Medica we find that the pathogenesis of *Causticum* not only contains the rubrics taken, but the remaining symptoms of our case as well... Our records show that after two doses of this remedy the attacks lessened during the first month to one; the second attack, a very slight one, did not follow for seven weeks, and now, after an interval of a year and a half, there has been no sign of a return, so we may safely say the boy is cured."

The above case will now be worked out with Boger-Boenninghausen's Repertory, just to show that if case-taking, evaluation and repertorisation are correctly done, the curative remedy emerges. A beginner may feel unsure of himself if he takes only four symptoms as Bidwell has done; and so, in the present analysis we show that if we take all the characteristic symptoms of the case to cover the totality, not only the same similimum emerges, but we also have the satisfaction and assurance of not going wrong by the omission of symptoms. By the way, "agg. during new moon" is not found in Kent's Repertory.

Rubrics	Kent
1. Agg. from fright	1116
2. Agg. from cold, dry weather	1105
3. Agg. from new moon	1132
4. Aversion to sweets	475
5. Involuntary urination	627
6. Epilepsy	896
7. Sad, melancholy	215
8. Weeping	221

Symptom Numbers

	1	2	3	4	5	6	7	8	Total
Acon.	4	4	-	-	-	-	-	4	
Ars.	2	2	1	2	2	2	4	3	18/8
CAUS.	3	4	3	4	4	4	2	3	27/8
Puls.	4	3	-	-	4	x	4	4	
Sep.	2	2	3	-	4	3	4	3	
Sil.	3	2	4	-	2	3	2	1	

Comment. It will be observed that Causticum emerges as the leading remedy even after the first three rubrics; subsequent rubrics confirm its choice. The common remedies in the first two rubrics were taken as eliminative.

Case 4. Varicose Veins — Lachesis — Dr. P. Sankaran

Mrs. L.C., aged 62 years, complained that six years back she started having pain and stiffness in the lumbo-sacral region which later descended into the left leg. Now, there is pain and swelling in the left ankle which sometimes disappears from the left and appears in the right ankle; sometimes it exists in both legs together; often painful, sometimes painless. Pain and heaviness in leg, agg. motion, and amel. by rest and agg. when legs hang down. Occasional pain in epigastrium piercing to back. Sweats on palms and soles even in winter; sweat offensive. Feels hot in legs and body; wants to place the legs on cold floor and also sleep on cold floor; likes cold in general. Dislikes noise

Selection of the Remedy — Repertorisation

made by children. Recently has developed fear of thunder. Nowadays nervous; fears every little thing; fears something may happen, and trembles. Nervousness has started after death of husband of heart-failure. Constipation; no sensation for stool.

Previous history. Menses were generally very profuse; during menopause had much bleeding and other troubles. Also had blood pressure with headache and vertigo; vertigo was agg. looking up.

Family history. N.A.D. physical Exam : Has varicosities in both legs : also oedema, more in left leg. Wt. 115 lbs. B.P. 150/100. The symptoms were evaluated and repertorised as follows with Kent's Repertory :

Fear of thunder being a mental symptom and the latest to appear was taken first. This was combined with another mental, the fear that something may happen.

	Rubrics	Kent
1.	Fear of thunderstorm	47
2.	Fear of misfortune	46
3.	Sensitive to noise	79
4.	Agg. from warmth	1412
5.	Side left, then right	1401
6.	Perspiration, offensive	1298
7.	Varices, lower limbs	1223

Symptom Numbers

	1	2	3	4	5	6	7	Total
Lach.	1	1	2	2	3	2	2	13/7
Nat-mur.	1	1	2	2	-	-	-	8/5
Phos.	3	1	2	2	-	2	-	10/5
Sulph.	1	1	-	2	-	3	2	9/5

Comment. Common remedies in the first two rubrics were taken as "eliminative". "Lach. also covered the haemorrhagic tendency discovered in previous history.

After *Lach.* 30 was given there was a quick amelioration without any initial aggravation. There were one or two relapses and every time *Lach.* 200th put her all right. She is now well for the last 2 years.

This case, worked out with the same rubrics, with the help of Boger-Boenninghausen's Repertory is given below :

Symptom Numbers

	1	2	3	4	5	6	7	Total
Bry.	2	3	2	1	-	-	-	
LACH.	2	2	1	4	4	1	4	18/7
Nat-c.	3	3	2	1	-	-	-	
Nat-m.	2	3	-	2	-	-	3	
Nit-ac.	2	3	1	1	-	-	-	
Petr.	3	2	2	-	-	-	-	
Phos.	4	4	4	1	-	4	1	18/6

Comment. *Phos.* does not cover the important rubric No. 5. Even in Dr. Sankaran's analysis with Kent's Repertory this symptom has "vetoed" other remedies except *Lach.*

This case stresses the advisability of taking the fullest totality possible in order to avoid erroneous selection. In this case the "descending direction" of symptoms (Lumbo-sacrum to left leg) carries one mark for *Lachesis* in Boger-Boenninghausen. For Haemorrhagic tendency, *Lach.* and *Phos.* both have 4 marks in Boger-Boenninghausen and for agg. from grief, sorrow (husband's death)" *Lach.* has 3 marks and *Phos.* has only one. Then again, "Agg. from warm air" is prominent in this case, and for this Kent gives 3 marks for *Lach.* and 2 for *Phos.*, whereas Boger-Boenninghausen gives 4 for *Lach.* and 1 for *Phos.*

Case 5. Mr. R., age 42 — Unsteady gait — Agaricus — Dr. B.D. Desai.

This case of unsteady gait with vertigo of two months' standing came for treatment, after the patient failed to get any relief from other systems of medicine.

	Rubrics	BB Repertory
1.	Stumbling, uncertain gait	868
2.	Uncertain, unsteady gait	855
3.	Mind, intoxicated, as if	208
4.	Reeling, staggering gait	916
5.	Agg. after motion	1132
6.	Vertigo	239
7.	Hips — lower extremities	842
8.	Weakness	873

Selection of the Remedy — Repertorisation 117

Symptom Numbers

	1	2	3	4	5	6	7	8	Total
AGAR.	3	2	2	4	4	2	4	2	2/38
Arg-n.	3	1	-	-	-	x	x	x	
Bar-c.	3	2	-	-	x	x	x	x	
Cocculus	1	2	1	4	2	2	3	x	14/7
Secale	1	2	-	3	-	2	x	x	
Stann.	1	1	-	-	4	1	3	3	13/6.

Comments. As there are four different rubrics on the chief complaint; it was thought advisable to take common remedies from them first. A modality and three concomitants gave a massive vote for *Agaricus* which effected a smooth and speedy cure.

The following is the working out of the same case with Kent's Repertory :

Rubrics	Kent
1. Ataxia	953
2. Awkwardness	953
3. Incoordination	1017
4. Agg. after motion	1374
5. Vertigo, Agg. motion	101
6. Extremities, Hip weakness	1229

Symptom Numbers

	1	2	3	4	5	6	Total
AGAR.	2	3	2	2	2	1	12/6
Calc-c.	2	3	1	-	-	-	
Cocculus	2	1	1	3	2	-	
Heli.	2	3	-	2	-	-	
Lach.	2	3	-	2	-	-	
Nux-v.	2	2	1	3	1	-	
Plumb.	2	1	2	2	-	-	
Sil.	2	1	-	3	2	1	
Stram.	2	1	2	1	-	-	
Sulph.	2	1	2	3	-	-	

Comment. Common remedies in the first two rubrics were taken as the eliminative group.

Case 6. Mr. B.S.T., age 46 — Ankylosis of spine (dorsal) Lyco. — Dr. Bhanu D. Desai.

Rubrics	BB Repertory
1. Agg. from sitting erect	1141
2. Agg. from rest	1137
3. Agg. from lying down	1128
4. Agg. from 4 A.M. (Boger's Synoptic Key)	
5. Spine, dorsal	788
6. Stiffness	792
7. Memory weak	211

Symptom Numbers

	1	2	3	4	5	6	7	Total
Carb-v.	2	2	2	-	3	4	3	16/6
Cham.	2	3	4	-	2	-	x	
Coloc.	3	3	2	1	1	-	-	
Conium	3	4	4	3	2	-	4	20/6
LYCO.	3	4	4	3	4	1	4	23/7
Saba.	2	4	3	-	2	-	x	

Comment. The most striking modalities were first taken up and remedies common to the first two noted as the eliminative group.

Lyco. 30th for a week, and then 200th at infrequent intervals cured the patient in 2 months.

The above case worked out with Kent's Repertory is given below :

Rubrics	Kent
1. Agg. sitting	1401
2. Agg. rest (Amel. by motion)	1374
3. Agg. lying down	1371
4. Agg. 4 A.M.	1342
5. Back, stiffness	946
6. Memory weak	64

Selection of the Remedy — Repertorisation

Symptom Numbers

	1	2	3	4	5	6	7	Total
Caps.	3	3	3	-	-	-	-	
Duls.	3	3	2	-	-	-	-	
Euphr.	3	3	3	-	-	-	-	
LYCO.	3	3	3	3	2	3	-	17/6
Puls.	3	3	3	1	2	2	-	14/6
Rhus-t.	3	3	3	-	3	2	-	14/5
Sulph.	3	3	2	-	3	2	-	15/3
Valer.	3	3	2	-	-	1	-	

Comment. In these analyses *Lycopodium* has come on top with a narrow margin. This shows the need, especially in the case of beginners, for eliciting fuller symptomatology, and in this case the choice of *Lyco.* would have been reinforced with additional symptoms such as "Desire for sweets", "Agg. from fats", "Easy satiety", or "Proud and obstinate nature", if we cared to enquire about them.

Case 7. Melancholia, neurotic — Sepia — Dr. Tomas P. Paschero.

This is a case reported by the famous Dr. Tomas Paschero in the "British Hom. Journal", Vol. LIII, No. 2, April 1964, and which Dr. Jugal Kishore has used to demonstrate a case analysis with "Kishore Cards" (a very useful, comprehensive Card Repertory). It relates to a woman aged 31, suffering from exhaustion, extreme irritability and intolerance, weeping, frigidity, etc. This condition developed on account of her mentally retarded son aged 5 who had encephalitis when a year old. The first dose of *Sepia* 200 caused an aggravation; *Sepia* 1M after 2 months caused a rash on the face. *Sepia* 10M given forty days later modified her apathy and her attitude towards her son was totally changed. She became tender, affectionate with him, with her husband and her other two children, and also herself became tranquil. The case is worked out with Boger-Boenninghausen's Repertory.

Rubrics	BB Repertory
1. Wet, drenched, etc. aggaravates	1152
2. Spring aggravates	1142

3.	Desires sweets	477
4.	Anxiety (after stool) in abdomen	545
5.	Weakness, exhaustion	935
6.	Agg. in morning	1103
7.	Agg. on rising	1137
8.	Averse to loved ones (family)	193
9.	Agg. from consolation	1112

Symptom Numbers

	1	2	3	4	5	6	7	8	9	Total
Calc.	4	3	-	1	4	4	3	1	-	
Lach.	3	4	-	-	1	3	4	-	-	
Lyco.	3	3	4	1	4	2	3	1	-	21/8
Nat-m.	2	2	1	-	4	4	3	-	2	
Rhus-t.	4	2	2	1	4	4	3	-	-	
SEPIA	4	2	1	2	4	3	2	3	2	23/8
Sil.	3	2	-	-	3	2	3	-	4	

The working out of this case from Kent's Repertory, with the same rubrics as above, is given here :

Symptom Numbers

	1	2	3	4	5	6	7	8	9	Total
Apis.	2	2	-	-	3	-	-	-	-	
Bell.	2	2	-	-	1	-	-	-	-	
Bry.	2	1	2	-	-	-	-	-	-	
Calc.	3	1	2	1	3	3	-	2	-	
Colch.	2	2	-	-	2	3	-	-	-	
Hepar.	2	1	-	-	3	-	-	-	-	
Lach.	1	3	-	-	3	3	1	-	-	
Lyc.	2	2	3	-	2	-	-	-	-	
Puls.	3	2	-	-	2	-	-	-	-	
Rhus-t.	3	2	2	-	3	3	3	-	-	
SEPIA	2	1	2	1	3	1	1	3	3	17/9

For acquiring a mastery of repertorisation the reader is advised to read "How to Find the Similimum with Boger-Boenninghausen's Repertory" By Dr. Bhanu Desai, and work out the seventy five exercises given in it.

Selection of the Remedy — Repertorisation

30. **Learning from repertorisation.** In an earlier lesson we have stated that we can learn the Materia Medica from every case of repertorisation. What are the lessons we learn from the above seven cases? First, that for the same set of symptoms both the Repertories (Kent's and Boger-Boenninghausen) lead to the same remedy. This shows that the Repertories are both well constructed and dependable. Second, the symptoms selected for repertorisation belong to the classes of Modalities, Mentals, Sensations, Concomitants and Locations. Causation in Case 3. In Case 4 the pathological condition (Varicosis) has been taken more as a confirmatory symptom than as a guiding one. Thirdly, the "diagnostic" label has no place in selection of the remedy. Fourthly, each case treated successfully with a single remedy at a time impresses the remedy on our mind its characteristic or guiding symptoms. *Bryonia* has the highest rank for "Agg. deep breathing", "Agg. ascending" and "Agg. from cabbage." *Sepia* (Case No. 2 and 7): Look at its vast range from Prolapsus to Melancholia, its peculiar sensations of Lump in rectum and empty feeling in stomach; and above all its most outstanding "aversion to loved ones" for which there are few remedies and that too in lower rank. *Causticum* : Each of the eight symptoms repertorised from Boger-Boenninghausen (Case 3) is an unforgettable characteristic of *Causticum. Lachesis.* It is worth nothing its marked agg. from warmth, and its equally characteristic, and rare, direction of symptom going from left to right side tilts the balance in favour of *Lachesis* in Case 4. *Agaricus* : Case 5 brings before us a group of remedies with marked action on the cerebro-spinal system in which *Agaricus* holds an important position. *Lycopodium* : This is a polychrest ("broadspectrum"), as wide-ranging and deep acting as "*Calcarea-carb., Sepia, Nux vomica, Causticum* etc. Only a few facts of its range, however, are revealed in Case 6, and of them the importance of time modality is noticeable. Apart from such concrete lessons from practice, there is also the deeper knowledge of remedies we gain from every repeated reading of them, as is necessary after repertorisation, but before administering, to satisfy ourselves that the selected remedy truly fits the case.

31. **Precautions in Using Particulars** : In his preface to the Repertory itself Kent says, "All the useful symptoms from the fundamental works from our Materia Medica, as well as from the notes of our ablest practitioners" have been included in it; and "many unverified (inconsistent) symptoms have been omitted, while clinical matters have been given a place if they were

consistent with the nature of the remedy". Since Kent himself regarded his list of Particulars as "scanty", it is obvious that the limitations, in the first instance, arise from their incompleteness. This is a matter for the research-minded leaders in the profession to rectify. The second precaution is against the indiscriminate use of the Particulars by the prescribers. Note Kent's remark quoted above that he included clinical matters which were consistent with the nature of the remedy. This means that in selecting a Particular remedy the physician should make sure that it is "consistent with the case," that is, with the other characteristic symptoms of the patient especially General. Sarabhai noticed *Iris-v.* against several rubrics in the "Cough and Expectoration" section of the Repertory before he concluded that that group of symptoms suggest a condition such as we meet in Eosinophilia. Similarly, he found *Tellurium* very useful in Spondylosis "when referred neuralgic pain are aggr. by coughing, laughing and sneezing, etc." In short, a Particular should be found at least in a small group of rubrics, which together "suggest a condition", to justify its selection. The prescriber should guard against the temptation of ignoring this essential requirement. The third precaution in using the Particulars is that the physician must develop a strong power of observation in taking the case without ignoring the smallest details, and translating the detail in the language of the Repertory, which means locating it in the repertory. This capacity can be acquired by constant thumbing through the pages and absorbing mental impressions of every little rubric in the Repertory.

32. Limitations of Repertories : A close examination of Kent's as well as Boger-Boenninghausen's Repertories will reveal to the advanced practitioner that each one of them has some incomparable features as well as deficiencies. Space forbids a detailed listing of these differences. The wise prescriber would, therefore, do well to consult both these Repertories (as well as Dr. S.R. Phatak's "Concise Repertory" and the Repertory in Boericke's Materia Medica) at least in difficult cases. The result will be greater accuracy of prescriptions as well as greater mastery of the Materia Medica.

33. More Exercises for Practice. As in any sphere of activity, constant practice alone helps towards mastery. The more one uses the Repertory for each case, by closely following the steps outlined above, the more he will master the art of selecting the "minimum symptom groups of the maximum value" and finding the similimum with the help of the Repertory. At the same time, he will also master the peculiar genius of the remedies and become a master prescriber. When confronted with the need to know the remedy for a case at the bed-side (urgently), or even a chronic difficult case, the Repertory will then, only then, like a faithful servant at your beck and call, reveal it to you in no time — just by thumbing through the pages. Using the Repertory as your habitual guide in prescribing is the only way to find the correct remedy in emergencies when, as Tyler says, you would give your very soul for a drug that could save.

34. To help the reader to develop practice in repertorisation a few cases are given in Appendix I. The learner should make an earnest effort to find the remedy through repertorisation either with Kent's or Boger-Boenninghausen's Repertory, and resist the temptation of referring to the solutions given in Appendix K.

SELF-TEST

1. State the class of symptoms which should be selected for repertorisation, according to their order of importance, while using (i) Kent's and (ii) Boger-Boenninghausen's Repertory?

2. What are the distinguishing features of Kent's Repertory and Boger-Boenninghausen's Repertory? What is the difference between their philosophical approach, as reflected in the construction of their chapters on "Mentals", "Modalities", "Sensations and Complaints" and "Concomitants"?

3. What is the advantage of combining two "eliminative rubrics" while repertorising? Is there any exception to be made in respect of remedies not coming in the group?

4. Why is it necessary to refer to a complete Materia Medica after repertorisation has led us to one, two or three remedies?

5. How can we learn the Materia Medica from repertorisation? Give examples.

Lesson 7

Selection of Potency and Repetition of Dose

1. The most important task facing the physician after selecting the most suitable remedy, called the similimum, is the choice of potency (or strength) in which to administer the remedy. How often the dose should be repeated, i.e., whether the remedy should be given as a single dose or at frequent intervals or infrequently are questions which follow next. We shall deal with the question of potency first.

2. **The Need for Potentisation.** As we have seen before, Hahnemann first started with the administration of crude drugs, as was his wont as an allopath. But when he observed that they invariably produced aggravations he was forced to "dilute" the remedies, and he found that these dilutions cured the cases gently and speedily. Thereupon he went on experimenting with various potencies, and these experiences were reflected in the revision of relevant paragraphs in successive revised editions of the *Organon*. He is reported to have used the 30th potency mostly and rarely the 200th. Hahnemann's observations on this subject (vide paragraphs 112, 128, 156, 157, 159 and 160 of the *Organon*) are worthy of careful study.

3. In his *Chronic Diseases* he emphasises : "No harm will be done if the dose given is even smaller than I have indicated. It can hardly be too small if only the antipsoric was selected correctly in all respects for the carefully examined symptoms of the disease and the patient, did not by his actions disturb the medicine in its action." Addressing those who still disbelieved in his "small doses" as too small to be trusted, and even ridiculed them, he cried out : "What would they have risked if they had at once heeded my words

Selection of Potency and Repetition of Dose

and had first made use of these small doses? Could anything worse have happened than that they might have proved ineffectual? They could not have injured anybody? But in their unintelligent self-willed use of large doses in homoeopathic practice they only passed again through the same round-about route, so dangerous to their patients, which I, in order to save them the troubles, had already passed through with trembling, but successfully, and after doing much mischief and having wasted much time they had eventually, if they wanted to cure, to arrive at the only correct goal, which I had made known to them long before faithfully and openly, giving to them the reasons therefore."

4. **Advantages of potentisation (dynamisation)** : Boenninghausen states in his *Lesser Writings* (pp. 102-3) : "Since I, among living homoeopaths, have had the greatest and most extended experience with high potencies, . . . I consider myself sufficiently equipped to give here the advantages of these higher dynamisations as compared with the lower potencies, and even with the thirtieth potency. They have induced me to use the higher dynamisations almost exclusively, not only in chronic, but also in acute cases, not only with men, but with animals of all kinds, and everywhere with the most favourable results. These advantages as observed also by others, are especially stated in brief hereunder :

(i) The sphere of action of medicine continually enlarges, the higher the dynamisation is carried : consider especially those remedies which in their raw state excite few symptoms, *e.g.*, Calcarea, Silicea, Natrum-mur., Aurum met., Argentum-met., Alumin-met. etc. The immediate consequence of this is that they correspond to an ever-increasing number of ailments as their homoeopathic similia, and therefore in chronic ailments they hasten the cure.

(ii) In acute disease the after-effects or curative effects appear more quickly . . . There is nothing worse to be found than the exclusion of high potencies from the treat-ment of acute, and even of the most acute cases. One has only to witness their rapid effects to be convinced.

(iii) By continual dynamisation, remedies get more and more withdrawn from the laws of chemistry. A dose of *Phosphorus* highly potentised can lie in a paper envelope in a desk and if taken after a year, will show the full medicinal power, not of *Phosphoric acid*, but of the undecomposed

Phosphorus itself. If protected from wetting and strong-smelling substances, they prove their undiminished virtue even after twelve or more years.

(iv) The higher the dynamisation used, the less the damage or interference from a defective diet which, especially in cities and in the higher social ranks, frequently spoils the best cures.

(v) The avoidance of toxic or physiological effects and of all the dangerous concomitant symptoms which lie outside the symptomatic sphere of the disease in question (*i.e.*, side effects in present-day parlance). How great this advantage is, must be manifested to every one who knows the injurious, even poisonous, effects of even the smaller but unpotentised doses.

5. **Methods of Potentisation.** Hahnemann might not be technically the original discoverer of the Law of Similars. Hippo-crates and Paracelsus might have had glimpses of this law, though they all had failed to take the next step of determining what symptoms the remedies produced. But had it not been for the discovery of the powers of dynamisation, the homoeopathic art of healing would not have become as practical and magically effective even in chronic or desperate cases as it is today. The sole credit for discovering the hidden powers of dynamisation belongs to Hahnemann and none else. When he witnessed the fearful aggravations from crude doses of the "similar" remedies, he started the procedure of "reducing" the dose, and the small dose was first called "dilution". To this process of dilution, Hahnemann had added another far-reaching condition, *viz.*, at first two, but later ten forceful strokes, called succussion, given to the dilution at each stage. In hitting upon this idea of friction or succussion he drew inspiration from the somewhat analogous phenomena in the physical domain, *viz.*, the generation of heat of at least 5000°F. from the violent friction of the flint down the steel (when striking fire) so that the fused steel flies out into infinitesimally small balls in the form of "sparks".

6. In the fifth edition of the *Organon* Hahnemann laid down clear instructions for making potencies on the centesimal scale. According to this method, one drop of the strong tincture of a soluble drug is put in a small bottle with ninety-nine drops of alcohol, and this vigorously succussed. This becomes the first centesimal potency. Subsequent potencies are prepared in the

Selection of Potency and Repetition of Dose   127

same way — always one drop of the preceding potency in ninety-nine drops of the attenuating medium, to form the next higher potency. Boyd of Glasgow has proved that every single succussion, upto forty, alters the potency (releases the latent power; then it remains constant, till furthur potentised by taking one drop into fresh ninety-nine drops of alcohol.

7. But how can we make use of many insoluble substances and divide them into finer and finer sub-divisions involved in succussion? With insoluble substances, such as gold, silica, carbon, lycopodium, etc., Hahnemann made the first potencies by trituration (one part of the substance in ninety-nine parts of sugar of milk, triturated in an agate mortar for a couple of hours). One part of its first centesimal trituration is again ground up with ninety-nine parts of sugar of milk for the same period, to make a second centesimal potency, and a third potency is made in the same way. That gives the substance, as one in a million. And he shows that after these three triturations all substances become soluble in alcohol or water and potencies can now be run up in the usual way.

8. **Range of Centesimal Potencies.** In the early years homoeopathic physicians used to make the potencies by their own hands in all ranges, such as 30, 200, 500, 2,000, 48M and so on. There was no regular scale of potencies. It goes to the credit of Dr. J.T. Kent that he brought order out of chaos. "After long observation in the range of potencies", he says, "I settled upon the octaves (as there are "octaves" of musical notes) in the series of degrees as the 30th, 200th, 1,000th (1M), 10M, 50M, 100M (CM) and often needed the DM and MM. The degrees must be far enough apart, or there would be failure." As everyone is aware, the potencies now available are all made in these series. In our discussion, "low" potencies would mean Mother Tincture (Q) to 12c. ; "medium" would mean 30c. and 200c. ; and "high" from 1M upward, the "highest" being CM, DM, MM, etc.

9. **Fifty-Milliesimal Scale of Potencies.** About the year 1840, roughly four years before his death Hahnemann modified the preparation of potencies to the 50 milliesimal scale obviously after satisfying himself through experiments with their greater advantages. He incorporated instructions about the method of making them in paragraph 270 of the revised Sixth edition of the *Organon*. However, as the edition remained with his widow and thereafter went into the hands of her daughter, it became available to the homoeopathic world only in 1921, about 80 years late, through the

efforts of William Boericke. Meanwhile, during the long interregnum, Drs. Hering, Kent, E.E. Case, C.M. Boger, Adolph Lippe, Nash, and other pioneers achieved marvellous results from the centesimal scale of potencies. As the working of these 50-milliesimal potencies is quite different and because of paucity of wide experience with them even now a majority of homoeopaths all over the world are using the centesimal scale of potencies. In India Dr. Ramanlal P. Patel has written *My Experiments with 50-millesimal Scale of Potency*. It is claimed on their behalf that (i) they are less liable to produce medicinal aggravations even in highly sensitive patients and (ii) they can be repeated every day in acute as well as in chronic diseases. These potencies are prepared in the scale of 1 : 50,000 as distinct from the centesimal (1 : 99) and the decimal (1 : 9). The 50-millesimal potencies are denoted by a `O' prefixed as follows : O/1, O/3 - O/30. The centesimal potencies are denoted thus : 30c. or plain 30, 200c. or just 200, and so on. The decimal potencies are shown with `X' (ten) suffixed, thus : 3x, 12x, 30x, etc.

10. **Scientific Basic for the Power Developed in Dynamisation.** Two effects of drugs are commonly known — firstly, the pathogenetic, which is synonymous with the term toxic ; and physiological when the doses are massive but not so high as to be toxic. Both these "doses" and their "effects" have nothing to do with curative action from the homoeopathic point of view, because homoeopathic remedies are never used in physiological doses. Even low potencies are not used with an eye to physiological effect.

11. The third effect of remedies, *viz.* the *dynamic* action, is known only to the homoeopaths. This dynamic power is developed through the process of dilution and succussion. What is the secret of this power? Various explanations have been offered by different thinkers to prove the effects of dynamisation at which we have to marvel. Boenninghausen reveals his penetrating intellect when he stated that this mysterious principle (of dilution with succussion releasing latent power) eludes our grasp, and must not be measured by the rule applied to ponderable substances. He pointed out that "in its evolution and propagation it is rather akin to the imponderable principles like light, heat, electricity, magnetism". It must be realised however, that if this dynamic principle in medicine is "hard to understand" so are many things that are generally accepted by the scientific world. The wonderful discoveries of radioactivity in matter, the wireless radio, electronics, etc., are discoveries which have almost paralleled this discovery by Hahne-

mann which preceeded them all. Our acceptance of the concept of the electron, and our present-day concept of the minuteness of matter are a further recognition of the infinite divisibility of matter.

12. **Dr. T.K. Bellokossy, M.D.** offers a very convincing elucidation of the micro-magnetic mode of transmission of power from one potency to the next higher, ad infinitum, and we quote relevant portions from his article in extenso (Journal of American Institute of Homoeopathy, May-June, 1966) for the benefit of readers. Condensation will not do justice to the subject or the readers. Says he :

13. "In all matter, two neighbouring atoms form a magnetic dipole. If all the dipoles in a material are aligned in the same direction, we have a perfect magnet. Every magnet sends out a magnetic field and if we bring a non-magnetic iron bar in this field, it will be magnetised ... Similar phenomena ensues if we place an iron bar in an electric field and this is called electro-magnetism. There is no difference in principle between these two modes of magnetisation (natural and electro). These same energies are used in homoeopathic therapeutics with the only difference that, instead of rubbing two objects, we rub and triturate powdered drug materials. We thus produce electric fields around every particle of the powdered drug and the more we triturate, the stronger the electric fields we produce, and the more potentised becomes the triturated material ... When the particles of Sac. Lac. are brought into the spheres of the numberless electric fields of the drug particles, they become magnetised, thus becoming carriers of the medicinal energy. When the last molecule of the drug fails to appear in a still higher potency, no more electric fields are formed, but the magnetic fields in the Sac. Lac. remain. From now on, all the still higher potencies come not from electric but from magnetic fields of the previously produced magnets of saccharum, or of the alcohol. There can be no end to this process as every magnet (micro-m.) can always give another micro-magnet without any loss of intensity. My highest potency is the DMM and it is just as powerful as any other.

14. "Life is an infinitely intelligent interaction of electro-magnetic energies carried by chemical materials. Without these energies the materials are nothing. To pay all attention to chemical materials and neglect the energies is like wanting to fly in a plane without a pilot and without fuel. Potency or dynamisation are the only proper terms for these micro-magnets we use ... those who speak of division, surface enlargement of the drug and increased

surface tension, think only in terms of chemistry, not of physics. There would be no homoeopathy if homoeopathic remedies acted chemically.

15. "Some think that a high potency is too small (chemically); but a high potency can be much more effective than a low. Our dose is only one, regardless of potency; only one or two pellets of a low as well as a high potency. The most horrendous mistakes are made by repetition of low potency remedy by those who cannot emancipate themselves from similar allopathic practices. In chronic diseases we administer only one dose. In acute, we repeat, and as soon as by close clinical observation we find that results have started to appear, we stop the remedy. Prescribing 3x or 30x is poor homoeopathy. The 3x may be too low not to be toxic to a sensitive, and a 30x is too low to be any good in inveterate deep-seated troubles.

16. "Because of their electro-magnetic power, administration of the remedies by mouth, dissolved on a clean tongue, is simple and practical. In emergencies Hahnemann showed even olfaction (two strong whiffs of the remedy) to be effective. The electromagnetic waves affect all the tissues of the body in an instant. The waves do not propagate in the manner of chemical contacts through the circulatory, lymphatic or nervous system but with the speed of light through every cell.

17. "**Guy Buckley Stearns** was the first to demonstate that the iris of the eye responds if the similar remedy is brought near the eye. This proves that the remedy radiates energy in the form of Hertzian waves. Trituration and succussion create emission of alpha, beta and gamma rays. Alpha rays correspond to very low, and the gamma rays to very high potencies. It is a fact that the gamma rays are much more penetrating, and this explains why high potencies are effective in the treatment of chronic, inveterate and deep-seated diseases. This is being confirmed by 100 year's practice of thousands of physicians. These are the tools which Hahnemann bequeathed to us for the treatment of sick people at a time when nuclear science was far from being born.

18. "The patient is oversensitive to the similar drug, a condition which we call allergy today, and every homoeopathic remedy is and should be an allergen. An asthmatic, sensitive to the fur of a cat, will instantly come down with an attack. No chemicals, only the waves of some energy from the cat were sufficient for the morbid effect. Since the body cures diseases with its own vital energies by

Selection of Potency and Repetition of Dose 131

overcoming the therapeutic artificial diseases, it is only natural that for this purpose we employ allergic diseases as they are stronger by far than any natural or chemical non-allergic diseases. By adjusting the potency, the size of the dose and its repetition to the reactive powers of the patient, we can always keep allergic effects under control.

19. "In order to prove and explain that the statement (in Kent's Materia Medica that "the worst failures are homoeopathic failures") is not true, I tell the layman that the homoeopathic remedy is not different from a spark in its action. To light a fire we don't need more than a spark with which to touch the inflammable material, but if we throw the spark on a rock, the rock will not burn; the spark will die out; the rock will suffer no harm. So is the homoeopathic remedy; it dies if it does not fit the treated case, and there is no harm to the body. Homoeopathic failure is only lack of benefit, a loss of time and not a positive harm as seen in allopathic drugging . . . But I am much opposed to hundreds of pills of low potency being dispensed, and the buyer taking them for months and years. This creates toxic effects and produces provings . . . loss of time, waste of money . . . harmful to the cause of homoeopathy. In sensitive patients crude drugs and low potencies, whether similar or not, have no allergenic powers but a toxic one. Their action is chemical, not dynamic, therefore not penetrating deep into diseased cells. On the other hand, too high potencies may do harm and even be dangerous. How? Because their power is more penetrating and finer, resembling gamma rays. Their administration does not do much harm to healthy cells, yet it does stir up the sick cells too much, arouses the body to a too violent battle of the faulty function in the pathological tissues, that is, causes excessive reaction (not drug aggravation). When the pathology of the patient is too extensive and the potency too high, this reaction may usurp all the life forces so that none are left for the functioning of the circulatory and respiratory centres in the medulla and the patient may go into collapse of anaphylatic shock. Hence the warning against too high potencies in cases with too much pathology. Poor prescribers do not see such accidents because they never find the similimum."

20. **Selection of Potency for Administration.** Having seen what potentisation is, how it is done, and having known the "secret" of its power, we shall now turn our attention to the problem of deciding on the choice of potency in each given case. In other words, when should we use the low, medium, high or the highest

potency? Let us remember that the physiological action of a drug is the exact opposite of its curative effect; and when the remedy is "similar" to the diseased patient, even the "smallest dose" acts on the same tracts or tissues on which it is known to act when given to the healthy. Therefore, if given in large doses it is apt to increase suffering and distress, by its medicinal effect, whereas the homoeopathic cure is to be achieved without drug effects. For this reason we should be wary of using very low potency, and especially the crude drugs. On the other hand, we should be careful to see that we do not, in the words of Dr. Bellokossy, "Stir up the sick cells too much or cause excessive reaction of the body which may usurp all the life-forces in the battle."

21. Two factors occupy a prominent place in deciding the choice of the potency :

(i) The degree of "similarity" of the remedy.

(ii) The vitality of the patient to absorb a high potency with an excessive reaction.

22. As regards the first factor, the power of the drug over disease lies solely in its similarity. Dr. Roberts says that just as there is a law of cure (similimum), there is a law of dosage (minimum). How can we know the degree of similarity (or special susceptibility to the action) of the drug before its administration? He answers : The near similitude or exact similitude is revealed by how nearly similar the characteristic symptoms of the drug are to those of the diseases. "The greater the number of characteristic symptoms of the disease that are found to correspond to the drug the less the quantity and the higher the potency that can be used."

23. The second factor of susceptibility of the patient (i.e. whether his vital reaction will be strong or feeble), follows as a corollary. This susceptibility has several aspects :

(i) Some patients are oversensitive to the smallest quantity of some drugs.

(ii) There is an equal insensibility (sluggishness) to even large quantities of drugs in others.

(iii) Advanced pathology.

(iv) Enfeebled constitution; as in old age or after prolonged illness.

(v) Infants and weak children.

(vi) Nature of the disease, i.e., whether it is acute, serious acute, sub-acute or chronic or even incurable.

(vii) The nature of the drug, i.e., whether it is superficial, or deep acting, short or long acting, whether it is an organ remedy (to be given in mother tincture).

(viii) Whether there are any obstacles to cure, miasmatic, iatrogenic, environmental, etc.

24. We shall now give, in brief, the advice given by master prescribers based on their own experiences. In the final analysis, the question of potency to be used is an open question and each prescriber is advised to experiment, draw his own lessons, and develop his confidence in using varying potencies in various conditions, keeping in mind the general guidelines given below. Let the prescriber "dare to be wise" and develop his ability to assess the beneficial power of various potencies from the low to the highest.

25. Comments of the masters are given below in six parts :

(i) High and higher potencies.

(ii) Medium and high potencies.

(iii) Low potencies and crude drugs.

(iv) General comments.

(v) Kent's general guidelines.

(vi) Kent's specific directions.

(i) **High and Higher Potencies (1M and above) :**

26. **Roberts and Stuart Close** : The greater the susceptibility to the remedy (i.e., greater the number of characteristic symptoms of the drug in the case), the higher the potency required.

27. **Douglas Borland** : The more acute the disease, the higher the potency.

28. **Elizabeth Hubbard** : High potencies needed in diseases manifestly of psychic origin. Functional diseases too, with subjective symptoms, respond well to high potencies. Acute disease even with pathological changes will also need high potencies. Cases with marked mental symptoms need high potencies.

29. **Jugal Kishore** : Higher potencies are best indicated in sensitive, nervous, intellectual, impulsive and zealous people.

30. **Templeton** : For ready results in acute cases one must go high. In case of collapse, when it is a question of life and death, high is needed.

31. **Wilbur K. Bond** : In early functional states with not much pathology as yet present, high and higher potencies can be nicely tolerated.

32. **Pulford** : The higher potencies range from the 10M for the chronic curable cases.

33. **Yingling** : There is no question but that the crude or very low potency will cure when homoeopathic . . . but experience completely establishes the fact that the high and higher potencies act more promptly and efficiently and will cure cases, especially of chronic diseases, that the crude cannot touch. It is erroneous to suppose that the high potencies excel in the treatment of chronic cases and are not efficient in the acute states of disease. My experience goes to prove that the high potencies are more reliable and efficient in the acute cases and will abort sickness or restrict it to a few days, whereas the crude would require many days or weeks to accomplish the same . . . I have seen the most profuse haemorrhage cease and the most distressing pains change like magic into regular labour pains after a single dose of high potency of the similimum.

34. **R. Gibson Miller** : Frequently potencies, especially the higher ones, will act inspite of these substances (*i.e.*, cosmetics, perfumes, tobacco, alcohol), even when they (cosmetics, etc.) are distinctly antidotal to the drugs in the crude form. Who has not

Selection of Potency and Repetition of Dose

seen one or two doses of high *Phosphorus* or *Sepia* act promptly; or after the usual interval, when given to excessive smokers?

35. **Jugal Kishore** : Those exposed to continual influence of drugs, or those drugged with crude medicines or low homoeopathic potencies may require high potencies to initiate curative action.

36. **R. Gibson Miller** : While in acute cases it is true that almost any potency at all removed from the crude substance will, in the majority of cases, prove curative if properly indicated, yet I have no hesitation in stating that the medium and high potencies act much better in such cases, and induce a positive action much more quickly than do the lower potencies. Accordingly, while in acute cases the exact potency is not, as a rule, a matter of vital importance, it is very different when we come to deal with chronic disorders.

37. In chronic cases, the almost unanimous experience of those who use the medium and higher potencies is that such potencies induce, as a rule, not only a much quicker positive reaction, but also an infinitely deeper and more lasting one, with the result it is not necessary to wait so long for the reaction as when using the lower one . . . yet, at times, little or no positive action can be obtained, at least at first, from the higher potencies, and only the lower or lowest bring response.

MEDIUM AND HIGH POTENCIES
(30TH, 200TH AND 1M)

38. **Borland** : When there is general similarity in addition to local indications, medium and high potencies.

39. **Stuart Close** : Medium and higher potencies for children; for sensitive and intelligent persons; for persons of intellectual or sedentary occupations and those exposed to excitement.

40. **Elizabeth Hubbard** : In acute crises of chronic disease (such as cardiac asthma) medium or low potencies would be preferable. In chronic prescribing, it is safe to begin with 200th.

41. **Jugal Kishore** : Idiots, imbeciles, and the deaf and dumb have low power or reaction to high potency energies.

42. In certain malignant and rapidly fatal diseases like cholera, we may require material doses of medicines like *Spirit of Camphor*. Of course, exceptions are there, when high potencies have aborted such diseases . . . In the advanced case of cerebral syphilis *Lyco*. 200 did not make any impression, but the 30th was always able to relieve. He also got better results from *Senega* in low than in high potencies.

Low Potencies and Crude-Drugs
(Mother Tincture to 12c)

43. **Borland** : In treating purely local conditions, remedies with affinity for the organ or tissue may be used in low potency. Low potencies in pathological conditions and sensitive patients.

44. **F. Hubbard** : For sensitive people we have to use low and gradually increase.

45. **Jugal Kishore** : Lower potencies evoke better response from persons of coarse fibre, sluggish, dull comprehension, torpid and phlegmatic individuals.

46. **Jugal Kishore** : The greater the pathology, the lower the susceptibility. Thus, in cases, for example, of advanced tuberculosis or pathological condition of the heart with congestive failure, or advanced nephritis and in malignant growths, the treatment should be started with low potencies. The injudicious use of high potencies sometimes spell disaster. It is often observed that in such low grade conditions there are very few characteristic symptoms and one has to fall back on the so-called organopathic remedies and that in low potencies.

47. **Wilbur K. Bond** : In diseases of great pathology or with more end results present, or in the aged where vitality is sadly weakend, one should favour the low potencies, perhaps given a little more often.

General comments on Potencies

48. **High potencies work surprisingly better** : Though I used to be a strict low potency man (and had some excellent results with the Mother Tinctures), unprejudiced experiments have convinced me that the high potencies work, and they often work suprisingly better than the low potencies. (W. Gutman).

Selection of Potency and Repetition of Dose

49. Stuart Close : There is as great an advantage in having a large scale of potencies as there is in having a large number of remedies. Different potencies act differently in different cases and individuals at different times and under different conditions. All are, or may be, needed. No one potency, high or low, will meet the requirements of all cases at all times.

Stuart Close's guidance on "Homoeopathic Posology" in his penetrating work, *The Genius of Homoeopathy* is worth studying closely. His comments are very briefly summarised :

A living organism offers resistance to everything which tends of injure or destroy its normal functioning. Resistance is manifested by suffering, pain, fever, inflammation, changed secretions and excretions, etc. When the similar or homoeopathic drug is administered in disease, little or no resistance is encountered, because the sphere of its action has already been invaded and its resistance overcome by the disease. Susceptibility to the similar drug is, therefore, greatly increased. The reason for the small homoeopathic dose lies in the fact that disease has rendered the affected part abnormally sensitive. A larger dose will produce pathogenetic symptoms, and a severe aggravation; this must be avoided.

The question of dosage is entirely one of susceptibility. The higher the susceptibility, the higher the potency. We must learn how to judge the degree of susceptibility if we would be successful homoeopathic prescribers. Susceptibility varies in different individuals according to age, temperament, constitution, habits, character of diseases and environment. It also varies in an individual to a remedy at different times. It is, therefore, as necessary to individualise the dose as it is the remedy, and the whole scale of potencies must be open to the prescriber.

The law of similars, in terms, is equivalent to the third law of motion, "action and reaction are equal and opposite". The task then, is to discover the quantity of the "disease force", so that we could determine the quantity of the "drug force." How can we determine these relative forces? Grauvogl provides the answer : Will a chemist who wishes to ascertain how much potash a certain spring contains, forthwith add a given quantity of acid empirically to the given quantity of mineral water ? No, if he knows the art of experiment, he must begin with the smallest quantity of acid, highly diluted and add it, drop by drop, and count every drop till the experiment is concluded. Precisely the same rules might guide us in finding the dose in any particular case of disease.

The provings of medium and higher potencies have thrown up finer and most characteristic symptoms, revealing the more and more developed individual peculiarities of the drugs. In other words, the higher potencies have revealed the enlarged sphere of action of the drugs. This fact has a great practical bearing on potency selection, *viz.*

Low Potencies. Diseases characterised by diminished vital action require the lower potencies.

Certain malignant and rapidly fatal diseases, like cholera, may require material doses or low potencies. Hahnemann's famous prescription of *Camphor* in drop doses of the strong tincture, given every five or ten minutes, which saved thousands of lives is an illustration.

In terminal conditions when the susceptibility is so low and the patient does not react to well selected remedies, nor to intercurrent reaction remedies given in potentiated form and small doses, you may have to resort to the crude drug and increase the dose to the point of reaction. It takes more to drive an automobile up a hill than it does on the level. The similia principle as to remedy and dose is as true in terminal conditions, in chronic diseases marked by gross pathological lesions and symptoms, as it is in any other kind of cases. The homoeopathic physician should not, at such a crisis, abandon the principle of similia and resort to the routine measures of allopathic practice based on theoretical assumptions. On such critical occasions give the drug that is really homoeopathic to the case, but give it in the stronger doses required at that stage of the case to excite the curative reaction. The high potency man should not overlook the need for material doses in such cases.

Low Potencies. When the symptoms are not clearly developed and there is a scarcity of characteristic features; or where two or three remedies seem about equally indicated and as such susceptibility and reaction are low.

Medium and High Potencies. Diseases characterised by increased vital action respond better to high potencies. Give high potencies when the symptoms clearly indicate one remedy, whose

Selection of Potency and Repetition of Dose 139

characteristic symptoms correspond closely to the characteristic symptoms of the case.

Higher Potencies. These will be called for when the symptoms are the finer, the more peculiar and more characteristic of the remedy, showing a higher degree of susceptibility.

Intercurrent Remedies. Sometimes cases do not at all respond to the indicated remedy. If due to previous drugging, it may be best to cease all medication for a few days and resume with a low or medium potency. It has been found that in such cases susceptibility can be increased and new symptoms of the disease brought to light by giving remedies like Opium, Carbo veg., Laurocerasus, Sulphur and Thuja and other remedies. The Nosodes, Psorinum, Syphilinum, Medorrhinum, Tuberculinum are also to be remembered where these latent diseases are revealed by existing symptoms or previous history. A single dose of the Nosode in moderately high potency will clear up the case for selecting a new remedy.

50. **Wilbur K. Bond.** There is no such thing as the ideal potency for all. I have seen the CM work wonders. I have seen the tincture run up to 3rd work wonders. If you think you have the right remedy and nothing happens, do not despair; you may not have the right potency, the right vibration frequency . .

51. **C.E. Wheeler.** It frequently happens that the high will relieve more effectively (otherwise they would have never come into use), but it also happens now and then that low potencies succeed when the high have failed.

52. **Kunkel of Kiel.** When I wish to act chiefly, and primarily in a local manner, I give low potencies; when I wish to act in a more general and lasting manner, I give the higher one.

HIGH TO LOW OR LOW TO HIGH

53. **Hutchinson.** If high potencies fail, we should try low.

54. **Lutze F.H.** Considers that the initial dose should be a high potency and the later ones lower potencies. He says : "I myself followed the usual method adopted by most homoeopaths (going from lower to higher potency) until I saw in Hahnemann's Materia Medica Pura that he advises us to begin with the higher potencies and then follow with the lower. (From my experience) I have come to the following conclusion: that "Hahnemann is right as usual." He

starts with a high potency and "as he improves, he can stand lower potencies better, should repetition still be needed."

55. **W.E. Jackson.** Don't be afraid to use the lower potencies in the beginning, especially in a malignant condition. As you go along you will use the higher potencies. Don't push too hard, because you will push your patient into the grave. (Grimmer : I have confirmed Dr. Jackson's observations several times, and I am very careful . . . I have been guilty of trying to hurry a cancerous proposition).

56. **J.T. Kent.** If the remedy fits the symptoms any potency will do all the curing it can in two or three doses at long intervals. It is better to begin low and go higher and higher. Each change of the potency brings new and deeper curative action. Cure is not accomplished by going high at once. In many chronic diseases the patient must be kept under the remedy a long time and the remedy must be managed, so that the curative power is not thwarted. In this way the cure is always mild, gentle and permanent.

57. **J.T. Kent.** In chronic diseases for the first prescription the single dose dry on the tongue will be found ever the best. After several doses, given at long intervals, have acted well, the action grows feebler and feebler, and the symptoms still call for the same remedy. At such time, a series of doses will show a stronger and deeper action, and this is even true if the potency given is much higher. It becomes safe to follow this procedure, whereas it would not have been good practice (to give a series of doses) with the first doses. **30th Potency is Good to Start With.**

58. **H.A. Roberts** : It is a hopeful sign when the younger physicians begin with the use of the fairly low potencies, say the 30th or 200th, and they progress upward. In this way one learns for himself the use of potencies and their dynamic action, and he will soon learn to use the higher potencies with skill and with much satisfaction.

59. Is there a specific (perfect) potency for a particular case?

60. Ellis Barker : States that one must select not only the right remedy but also the right potency. He gives a case in which *Plumbum*, the indicated remedy, given in the 3, 6, 9, 12, 15 and 29th potencies failed. Only the 30th helped. He again tried higher and low potencies but all failed to help except the 30th.

Selection of Potency and Repetition of Dose

61. **Caroll Dunham** : Is of the opinion that cases frequently occur in which a remedy will act only in a certain potency, high or low. He quotes Chapman of London, a very keen observer, making a similar remark, furnishing striking illustrations from his own practice. In an epidemic of dysentery Dr. Wells found that *Nux vomica*, the genus epidemicus, had no effect in Q, low or medium potencies, but had immediate effect in the highest potencies, and a single dose of the 400th sufficed in every case.

62. **A. Pulford** : The following exhortation by Pulford, veteran homoeopath of America, deserves careful attention and testing out in practice :

(i) The true similimum when combined with the correct potency becomes the perfect similimum.

(ii) In each and every case, no matter how serious or complicated, the perfect similimum can carry it completely through without the aid of any other agent, irrespective of miasmatic theories, and in the great majority of cases without a single repetition.

(iii) The perfect similimum acts promptly, continuously and without aggravation.

63. "These bold statements", he asserts, "are hard to believe, yet not made without good and sound reasons". He then cites a number of cases to prove his thesis (*Homoeopathic Heritage*, July 1979), and then formulates the following general rules :

Potency	Nature of Case Suitable for	Nature of Effect
Lower potencies below 30x	Good for pathogenetic and physiological purposes.	Palliation and temporary relief, not curative.
30x to 200th	Acute cases which do not not rest on, nor are part of a deep chronic malady.	Low curative
200th to 10M	Sub-acute cases, all of which rest on some deeper dyscrasia.	Medium curative

Contd...

Contd...		
Lower potencies of medium range (30th, 200th, 1M)	Sub-acute cases, in which the chronic malady on which it supervenes is not active.	Curative
Higher potencies from 10M up	For chronic curable cases	Curative
Lower potencies	For all incurable cases	To avoid dangerous reactions.

64. E.E. Case. Case, the master prescriber, almost echoing Pulford says : "I prescribe a potency of a remedy that I know is indicated and get unsatisfactory or no result; then I prescribe the same remedy in a lower or higher potency and get immediate results ; this experience repeated a number of times leads me to believe that there is a homoeopathicity in the potency as well as in the remedy. Years ago I had given *Calcarea-carb.* in the 200th and the 1M to a patient with no results. On the advice of Dr. Wells, I then gave him 40M. It cured the patient rapidly. My rule is when a remedy holds only for a short time, to give a higher potency and generally with good results.

CURING BY LYSIS OR CRISIS

65. Douglas Borland was a great prescriber in the London Homoeopathic Hospital and his views expressed in his well-known book *Pneumonias* are worth studying as a guide to action. He says:

66. "When you are dealing with acute disease there are two courses you can adopt. One is "play for safety", restrict your prescription to low potencies repeated four hourly — thus you can avoid the complications of disease, make the patient comfortable and reduce the mortality rate. But by this you do not reduce the duration of disease. In a case of pneumonia the crisis may come from the seventh to the tenth day. This is curing by lysis."

67. "The second method is to administer high potencies, something above a thirty, and start off giving the drug every two hours. You thus give a number of stimuli in a comparatively short time in order to obtain the crisis. In six hours, you ought to find the temperature coming down, in twelve hours it will probably come

down to normal, and in twenty-four hours it certainly ought to. Thus you abort the disease. It does not run its normal course and you have an anticipated crisis. By doing this you cut-short the duration of an acute illness and still further diminish your complications, as well as the stress the patient has to endure; you are less liable to get any sign of weakness developing. This precipitated crisis is attended with a certain amount of stress or risk, although this is not likely when the crisis occurs early in the disease rather than after seven or ten days of continuous fever. You do not get a collapse because you have a perfectly healthy patient to start with.

68. "In using lower potencies, your matching of the symptoms of the drug and the disease need not be so accurate, as it does when you are using higher potencies. The lower potencies produce a modifying effect without necessarily covering the whole case. But I am sure, once you have experienced the power of the system of crisis through higher potencies, you will never go back to the other. I think it is worthwhile acquiring a more detailed drug knowledge (which this system requires) in order to obtain the better results."

How Many Doses in the First Prescription?

69. **R. Gibson Miller** : The concensus of opinion of masters is that in chronic cases of people of ordinary constitution, the best procedure is to give a single dose, and then wait at least ten or fifteen days, before concluding that one dose is insufficient to produce a positive effect.

70. **Quinton** : The 30's which are "medium", are of great use when appropriately prescribed, and may in certain cases be repeated frequently, violent reactions with them being rare. He has reasons for believing that "repetition" lessens the tendency to aggravations.

71. **Kent** : The single dose in all sensitive people (anticipates the change of symptoms) and must be the safest for general practice. The axiom should be kept in mind. When the symptoms change, the remedy must be discontinued, as it ceases to be homoeopathic.

72. **Rudolph Rabe** : The finest cures are made with single doses of the high and highest potencies.

73. **A. R. A. Acharya** : "Repeat the dose until there is a marked change" is a general rule. In acute conditions nature is fighting vigorously and quick and sustained help is necessary, and so we repeat the dose at frequent intervals and, when improvement sets in, doses are repeated at longer intervals.

74. **Wilbur Bond** : As a rule, the average chronic case, I start on the 200 or 1M, 5 doses 12 hours apart. If a remedy is going to "hit", it will do so in 48 hours.

75. **Double Dosage.** C. Gordon holds that a certain potency may be the most similar to a diseased individual at a certain time. A patient who needs a 50M will be unaffected by a 30 and one who needs 12th may be killed by a 1M, (compare Pulford's "Perfect similimum"). He believes that Dishington's discovery of "plus dosage" or "double dosage" has proved its value beyond all questions. This consists in giving, instead of the familiar single dose, two doses of different potencies 24 or 48 hours apart, *e.g.*, *Phos.* 200 (I) followed in 24 hours by *Phos.* 1M (one dose). This is particularly useful in chronic cases, and gives deeper and quicker results. This double dosage may be repeated in some potencies at the second prescription, and go higher for the third and fourth, and higher again for the fifth and sixth.

76. **Ascending Series of Three Potencies.** T. S. Iyer advises (following the practice Kent and Tyler are reported to have favoured) that it will be much simpler if the medicine is given in three distinctive potencies, in the ascending order in the general series of 6, 30, 200, 1M, 10M, 50M, CM, DM, and MM. The doses are taken on three consecutive days, as in that case, the combined action of the three doses is very effective and continuous for a long time. For example, in chronic cases, a dose each of the 30th, 200th and 1M may be given on three successive days in the mornings, and these allowed to act for a long time till some change is noted. He says that this procedure has been tried and found to be much more effective than the single dose in a high potency, or the daily repeated doses in low potency. For acute diseases, the potencies to be used are 6 (or 12), 30, 200 and in some cases 1M according to the age, susceptibility of the patient and nature of the disease.

KENT'S GENERAL GUIDELINES

77. A few master-prescribers have been quoted above in order to give the student an idea of how experiences regarding potencies

Selection of Potency and Repetition of Dose

have varied widely, and also have converged in many respects. We shall now close this discussion by setting out the specific, clear and unambiguous advice of J. T. Kent who carried forward Hahnemann's tradition as a great experimenter, close observer and an inspiring teacher, no less than the master of the art of homoeopathic prescribing that he was. We are quoting from his *"Lesser Writings"* below :

78. The similimum, the curative power or force, is not essentially the curative drug. The similimum may be found in *Aconite* 200th when *Aconite* 3x failed . . . I have seen *Arsenicum* 200th fail in a case so clearly indicating Arsenic . . . but the 10M cured it promptly. The remedy was *Arsenicum* but the simillimum was *Ars.* 10M. I have seen this same *Ars.* 10M cure when the 2x, 6x, 30, 60, and 200 had failed. (p. 427). The similimum may be found in the lowest attenuations, but is positively found for all curable diseases in the high and highest genuine potencies."

79. "The nearer we come to the perfect similimum, the less medicine we need give . . . This proposition may be stated again in other words. It is the opinion of our best prescribers that the similimum will cure most cases best if given high and in one dose, or at most a few doses. Indeed, experience tells us that the higher potencies are always best; this is experience, however, and not law. But the converse of this proposition is not true." (p. 214)

80. Very sensitive persons should not be given too high a potency. For oversenitiveness it is best to begin not higher than 1M. This can be repeated two, or sometimes three times, and then a higher potency used. Each potency can be used two or three times with benefit. Sometimes we will need to begin again at the lowest potency and go through the series. Then you will perhaps cure the patient without change of remedy." (. 455)

KENT'S SPECIFIC DIRECTIONS

81. The physician who knows how to use the various potencies has ten times the advantage of the one that always uses one potency, no matter what that potency is. After thirty years of careful observation and comparison with the use of the various potencies it is possible to lay down the following rules :

(i) Every physician should have at his command the 30th, 200th, 1M, 10M, 50M, CM, DM and MM potencies, made carefully on the centesimal scale.

(ii) From the 30th to the 10M will be found those curative powers most useful in very sensitive women and children.

(iii) From the 10M to the MM all are useful for ordinary chronic disease in persons not so sensitive.

(iv) In acute diseases the 1M and 10M are useful.

(v) In the sensitive women and children, it is well to give the 30th or 200th at first, permitting the patient to improve in a general way, after which the 1M may be used in similar manner. After improvement with that ceases, the 10M may be required.

(vi) In persons suffering from chronic sickness and not so sensitive, the 10M may first be used, and continued without change so long as improvement lasts; then the 50M will act precisely in the same manner, and should be used so long as the patient makes progress towards health; then the CM may be used in the same manner, and the DM and MM in succession.

82. By this use of the series of potencies in a given case, the patient can be held under influence of the similimum, or a given remedy, until cured. When the similimum is found, the remedy will act curatively in a series of potencies. If the remedy is only partially similar, it will act in only one or two potencies; then the symptoms will change and a new remedy will be demanded.

83. Many chronic cases will require a series of carefully selected remedies to effect a cure, if the remedy is only partially similar; but the ideal in prescribing is to find that remedy similar enough to hold the case through a full series to the highest. Each time the patient will say that the new potency acted as did the first one received. The patient can feel the medicine when it is acting properly. (pp. 207-8)

84. A few more observations from Kent :

(i) There is a wonderful latitude between the tincture and the CMs and in my judgement the selection of the best potency is a matter of experience and observation and not as yet a matter of law.

(ii) For many years I have found the 30th strong enough to

Selection of Potency and Repetition of Dose

begin with... but no single potency is equal to the demands made upon it by the disease of different individuals.

(iii) The nature of disease makes a difference; patients who have heart disease, or who are suffering from phthisis are apt to have their suffering increased and the end hastened by the highest potencies; they do better under the 30th or 200th.

(iv) Sometimes, very sensitive patients will do well on a high potency if they have been prepared for it by the use of a lower one.

(v) I have not used *Sulphur* as an intercurrent "to awaken the susceptibility when the remedy ceases to act", as we are told to do. This is because the indicated remedy will not so often cease to have curative effect if the potency is properly varied. I have seen patients making no improvement on repeated doses of the right remedy, just because their susceptibility to that potency had been exhausted, but the curative result was obtained simply by changing the potency without changing the remedy.

(vi) Any potency, no matter what it is, high or low, will cease to act after a time. That shows at once the usefulness of knowing about more than one single potency of a medicine. (p. 348)

85. **Remedies which seem to act better in mother tinctures or low potencies.** They are, Apocynum-cannabinum, Sabal-serrulata, Ornithogallum, Adonis, Avena-sativa, Blatta-orientalis, Hydrocotyle-asiatica, Cactus, Crataegus, Senega, Syzygium-jambolanum, Sumbul, Turnera, Uva-ursi, etc.

86. The Nosodes should always be given in 200th or higher potency.

87. **Caution** : Beware of giving the following remedies in high potencies in the conditions mentioned against them :

Kali carb. in advanced arthritis or gout. *Silicea* for abcesses in dangerous locations like the lungs. psorinum in a deep psoric case like asthma. *Arsenicum-alb.* in the last stage of acute diseases, say pneumonia. It may hasten demise (euthanasia). *Hepar-sulph., Sulphur* and *Silicea*, to patients with encysted tubercle in lungs. *Phosphorus* to tuberculous patients. *Calcarea-carb.* should not be repeated often in old people, though children may need it, and tolerate it, frequently.

Administering the Dose — How and When

88. How to administer. In paragraphs 288 to 292 of the *Organon* Hahnemann says : "The tongue and mouth are most susceptible to the influence of the medicine; the interior of the nose is especially so; the rectum too: also parts destitute of skin, wounded or ulcerated spots. Even those organs which have lost their peculiar sense, *e.g.*, a tongue or palate which has lost the faculty of tasting, or a nose that has lost the faculty of smelling: even the external surface of the body covered with skin and epidermis is not unsusceptible to the powers of medicines, especially in a liquid form.

89. Boenninghausen. His case is a telling example. He had not had a stool for thirteen days; the pains in the sides of his bowels were dreadful. He says: "All those signs gave clear indication that I was suffering from a crossing of the bowels (ileus). *Nux-vomica* by olfaction, then a whole drop of 12th, *Cocculus* 6th, all failed to relieve . . . Determined not to quit until I had either found the suitable remedy, or was delivered by death from my torments, I studied till it was midnight when I found in *Thuja* the characteristics of my ailment . . . I immediately smelled once with each nostril at the pellets which had been moistened a year before with the 30th dilution . . . In five minutes the pains began to diminish and in ten minutes I had a most copious discharge of the bowels and fell into a refreshing sleep."

90. Bellokossy : The mode of administration *per os* is simple and practical. The electro-magnetic field of the remedy sends out electro-magnetic waves which affect all the tissues of the whole system in an instant — not in the manner of chemical contacts, but with the speed of light, through every cell.

91. Kent : It has been supposed by some that by giving one or two small pellets a milder effect would be secured, but this is a deception. The action or power of one pellet, if it acts at all, is as great as ten. If a few pellets be dissolved in water and the water is given by the teaspoonful, each teaspoonful will act as powerfully as the whole of the powder if given at once.

92. When to Administer the Dose. Kent says : "It is an old settled rule that nearly all follow. To give a deep acting remedy in

Selection of Potency and Repetition of Dose

the midst of great suffering would be to court an aggravation, increase the suffering and to use up the curative power of the remedy uselessly. The dose when repeated would often fail to act. Better nurse the case to an opportune moment to give the medicine — that is, after the excitement has passed, e.g. after the menstrual suffering is over; or after the chronic sick headache; or after the paroxysm of intermittent fever — that will be the best time to give the medicine.

93. **Fortier Bernoville** : If the application of medicines is untimely, there are aggravations and the diseased condition of the patient is prolonged . . . For constitutional remedies it is better to apply them one or two hours before the time of aggravation . . . *Ricinus communis* in a case of cholecystitis acts towards 4 p.m. if the patient has taken his meal at 1 O'clock. This is the moment of the elimination of urea in the urine . . . The aggravation of *Natrum mur.* and *Gelsemium* is due to the solar influence, between 10 a.m. and 3 a.m . . . *Rhodo.* and *Phosphorus* are to be applied before the storm...or earlier before the great heat preceding the storm; if given during the storm, during the fall of the barometer, they will not act very well. For seasonal aggravations we have two medicines : *Lachesis* and *Nat-sulph.* Do not be too late or too early; apply 15 days before their seasonal aggravation (of asthma or rheumatism).

94. It is also believed that certain remedies should be preferably given at certain times for the best results, such as *Sulphur* in the morning, *Nux-vomica* in the evening, *Ignatia* and *Sepia* at night, etc.

REPETITION OF DOSE

95. There are two types of repetition of dose. The first type aims at evoking the primary positive reaction or response; and the second type aims at continuing the action of the first prescription the effect of which, after a lapse of time, is seen to be wearing off. In our discussion on potencies under the heading "General Comments on Potencies" we have already discussed some aspects of repetition involved in the first prescription. A few more aspects of this question will now be presented before bringing this lesson to a close. (The second type which may be called "secondary repetition" or "second prescription" will form a part of the next lesson on management of the case).

96. We shall recapitulate, briefly, the advice of the masters given earlier. Kent advises a single dose especially in chronic cases and so does Gibson Miller and Stuart Close. Quinton and Acharya

find starting with a medium potency like the 30th and giving it repeatedly, say, three times a day, till a response is produced to be a better way to provide sustained help to nature in fighting acute conditions vigorously and avoiding aggravation. Wilbur Bond's practice in the average chronic case is to start on the 200 or 1M and give five doses, 12 hourly. Gordon has found the "double dose" in two successively higher potencies given 24 or 48 hours apart of "value beyond question". T. S. Iyer recommends Tyler's practice of giving three doses in ascending series, on three successive mornings obviously in chronic cases. Borland advises aborting an acute illness by precipitating a crisis with repeated doses of high potency. Kent's advice is specific and clear for all conditions.

97. What is the reason for this division of opinion and practice as to whether the single remedy should be given in one, two, three or more doses in the first prescription? Let us remember that after all, our object is to produce a favourable response in the patient in the form of positive signs of amelioration of his complaints, whether acute or chronic. The opinion on the number of doses becomes divided because we cannot say before hand how much of the "drug force" has to be applied to overcome the "disease force", without disturbing the "vital force" too much.

98. We have some idea of the "drug force" in the form of the potencies; but it is difficult to measure the "disease force", and the "vital force" as they vary from one case to another. If only we could know in advance the strength of the "disease force" we would have been able to decide on the most important question: How long a period must be allowed to elapse for the manifestation of a positive action". The most practical answer to this question, which has in fact become an absolute rule is that when favourable reaction sets in, the administration of the remedy must cease : and no repetition or change of remedy is permissible until the favourable reaction has spent itself — therefore, we may give one or more doses, till a response is produced.

99. There are various factors which come in the way of the remedy in a single dose, and which delay or nullify its action. In many ordinary acute diseases, the period that is required for a positive action to show itself will, as a rule, be of short duration; sometimes the action is almost instantaneous, and the improvement, as experienced by the patient and observable by the physician, is so sharply defined that the physician has little difficulty in deciding when to stop the remedy. But diseases differ largely in

Selection of Potency and Repetition of Dose

regard to intensity of suffering, plane of action and their normal duration. Patients also vary in their responsiveness to remedies; some are oversensitive and prove every remedy, while others are sluggish. It must be confessed that in dealing with a case for the first time it is not easy to determine how to classify the patient.

100. The rapidity of response to the remedy is not infrequently diminished in cases that have been long drugged allopathically, or by unsuitable very low-potency remedies of homoeopathy, and in such cases it becomes necessary to repeat the remedy frequently before a positive action can be obtained.

101. The pace of the disease also profoundly influences the rapidity of response. In very violent disease with severe suffering, the positive action generally manifests itself very quickly. In such cases of sudden onset, fast pace with expected briefness of duration, Gibson Miller advises that a single dose (in high potency) may be all that is necessary though, at times, it may be necessary to repeat the remedy frequently, say, every four, eight or twelve hours. Similarly, frequent doses may be needed in very acute cases of fever when the increased metabolism, so to say, "eats up the remedy" fast; that is, when the "drug force" has to be applied repeatedly to overcome the "disease force". (cf. Borland).

102. Kent advises that in severe acute sickness, in robust constitutions, several doses in quick succession are most useful. In typhoid with high fever, the best work is done by repeating the remedy until the fever begins to yield, which is at times several days. In a remittent fever the remedy may be repeated until the fever shows signs of falling. While the fever is rising in robust constitutions, the remedy may be repeated with advantage, and in some cases it is positively necessary.

103. In chronic cases, Kent advises that the very high doses seldom require repetition, if clearly indicated, to produce a long curative action.

104. It is unsafe for the beginner to indulge in the desire to repeat too much. The higher the potency, the greater the aggravation caused by the kind of unrestricted repetition.

105. In the case of patients who are less sensitive in nature it is necessary to give repeated doses before a primary reaction can be induced.

106. **Positive, favourable reaction.** How do we know that the remedy given has started acting and producing a favourable reaction? The most important indication of such reaction is the general feeling of the patient, a sense of well-being and comfort that is the very antithesis of disease. The improvement spreads from the centre to the circumference. The indication is so unmistakable that even if the patient paradoxically declares that his headache or backache is unchanged yet he feels better in himself. Other indications may be the passing of suppressed urine, or stool, or he goes into a gentle soothing sleep as compared with earlier restlessness, or he smiles and asks for a sip of water or milk, etc. When this happens in acute cases, we know with absolute assurance that positive reaction is taking place, and no more medicine is required so long as the ameliroation continues. Let us be warned against continued or hasty repetition of doses in our excessive zeal or anxiety to hasten the cure, as such action has many times turned back the flowing tide and "converted what seemed certain victory into disaster." In homoeopathy there is no need for "some more of a good thing" as it defeats itself and actually hinders cure.

SELF-TEST

1. What are the advantages of potentisation? What is the difference between the working of a potency and a crude drug on a sick person? (Para 4, 10)

2. What are the three scales of potencies and which of them is most popularly used, and why? (Para 9)

3. What is the secret of the power, or the secret of dynamic action of drugs? In homoeopathy, why do we reject the chemical action and take advantage of the dynamic action of remedies? (Para 13, 14, 15)

4. What is the basis for the statement that "every homoeopathic remedy is and should be an allergen"? (Para 18)

5. What is the explanation for the very high potencies being harmful or even dangerous, if not used with discrimination? What are the types of cases in which we should not use them? (Para 19)

6. Which potency (low, medium or high) should be used in the following conditions :

　　(i)　Sensitive, intelligent people. (Para 29, 39)

Selection of Potency and Repetition of Dose

(ii) Chronic cases with advanced pathology. (Para 46, 47)
(iii) Serious acute conditions. (Para 30, 33)
(iv) People who are sluggish and of dull comprehension. (Para 41, 45)
(v) People who are very sensitive to almost every remedy, i.e., they "prove" the remedy. (Para 43, 44)
(vi) Chronic curable cases. (Para 36, 37, 40)
(vii) People who are exposed to various drugs, perfumes, tobacco, etc. (Para 34, 35)

7. What is the best potency to start with, in the case of beginners, and how often can it be repeated? (Para 56, 70)

8. What is the difference between a remedy which is the similimum and a remedy which is only partially similar, so far as their action in different potencies is concerned? (Para 82, 83)

9. What is the general rule of repetition in acute conditions? (Para 73, 101)

10. What is the rule respecting "when to stop administration of the remedy" and "when repetition of remedy is permissible"? (Para 98)

STUDY IN DEPTH

"Homoeopathic Posology" (Chap. XIII - pp. 183-211) in the *Genius of Homoeopathy* by Stuart Close, M.D.

Lesson 8

Management of the Case

1. After what we believe to be the curative remedy has been selected and administered, there arise the problems of following up or managing the case till it is really cured. It may be said without exaggeration that in tackling these problems the physician is called upon to display the following variety of skills :

(i) Thorough knowledge of the principles and philosophy of homoeopathy.

(ii) Close observation.

(iii) Capacity for fine discrimination to ascertain the true state of health of the patient (as against apparent signs).

(iv) An infinite capacity to wait and watch, when necessary and resist the temptation to repeat the dose or change the remedy and, above all,

(v) Great courage of conviction in the power of the similimum (and the remedy and potency he had selected) when faced with a difficult situation. Of course a sixth dimension of,

(vi) Knowledge of disease processes, prognosis and pathology lends firm support to the foregoing qualities required of a physician. And all of them are acquired by study, practice and observation, and drawing appropriate lessons from each case. A proper knowledge of,

(vii) The diet and regimen which will aid progress towards cure and also,

Management of the Case

(viii) Of the different obstacles to cure which need to be removed, are two more aspects of managing a case, which cannot be neglected. In what follows we shall see how, at different stages, a demand is made on one or the other of these skills on the part of the physician.

2. Criteria of Cure. To begin with, let us be clear in our minds as to what really constitutes a cure or recovery ? Is it just a matter of subjective feeling on the part of the patient or physician, or the removal of the most annoying symptoms? According to the philosophy of Homoeopathy, it is neither of these. The symptoms are nothing but the external manifestations of the struggle between the vital force and the inimical disease force. While the disease force marches forward in the direction of attacking the vital organs more and more, the vital force tries to counter the attack by throwing the invader from the vital organs (to save them first) to the less vital parts like the skin, extremities, or in the form of discharges which rid the body of harmful toxins. Drawing on his long experience and meticulous observation, Hering formulated three rules which are fulfilled when the symptoms take the direction of cure. When the remedy is acting curatively, the patient's symptoms are relieved:

(i) From within outwards, i.e., the mind and other more important organs like the lungs, heart, etc. are relieved first, and relief in the periphery follows later.

(ii) From above downwards, which again means that the more vital organs which occupy a higher level, like the brain, heart, lungs. etc., feel the relief first.

(iii) The symptoms come, only to go by themselves, in the reverse chronological order in which they appeared in the patient; i.e., the carpet is rolled back, the latest symptom is the first to go, than the one which preceded it, and so on. Hering perhaps got his hint from Para. 253 of the *Organon.* The correctness of *Hering's laws of the direction of cure* has been time and again confirmed by the experience of various therapeutics, and these laws provide us with a sure and clear guide in deciding whether a remedy given is acting curatively or otherwise. The only thing required of the physician is to observe the patient's condition closely, compare his present symptoms with those he has recorded while taking the case and making the prescription, and decide whether the difference between these two states follows any one or more of these laws of cure, or not.

3. **Remedy Responses — When, what types, why they arise and what to do with them.** After the carefully selected remedy has been administered in what we consider to be the correct potency, the physician is confronted by four questions :

(i) What is the period required for the positive action to show itself, so that once the reaction starts he may refrain from any repetition of doses till the response comes to a halt; and secondly, how long does such curative action last?

(ii) What are the types of responses he meets with?

(iii) Why do these responses arise, that is, what is the real meaning of the responses in relation to the patient's illness.

(iv) What action should he take in answer to the responses? We shall discuss these points one by one.

4. **Period Required for Positive Action.** This period varies within very wide limits depending upon several factors, such as :

(i) Correctness of the prescription.

(ii) The degree of potency used.

(iii) The nature of the case in hand, i.e., whether it is acute sub-acute or chronic.

(iv) The vitality of the patient.

(v) The nature of the remedy, i.e., whether it is short and superficially acting, or deep and long acting.

5. The more closely the characteristics of the drug and the diseased patient match, the more prompt is the positive action.

Management of the Case

6. What holds true of the correct remedy applies with equal force to the correctness of the potency. The lower potency than required by the case may bring a slower reaction; the crude drug may cause a medicinal aggravation; and a higher potency may cause aggravation of the symptoms.

7. In many ordinary acute diseases, the period that is required for a positive action to show itself will, as a rule, be of short duration; sometimes the action is almost instantaneous, and the improvement, as experienced by the patient and observable by the physician, is so sharply defined that in this class of cases there will be little difficulty in deciding when to stop the remedy. (Gibson Miller)

8. However, the pace of the disease profoundly influences the rapidity with which the primary response manifests itself. In very violent diseases with severe suffering, the positive action will manifest itself very quickly, and such cases may not call for more than one or two doses in high potency to produce a favourable action.

9. Where the pace of the disease is slower and the suffering much less acute, it may be necessary to repeat the dose several times before reaction occurs.

10. In continued fevers the entire course of the disease is slower, and it is not reasonable to expect that one dose or a few doses will be sufficient to produce a reaction. It is necessary in the vast majority of such cases, to repeat the remedy every few hours for at least two or three days, before positive action is manifest. We may recall Borland's similar advice mentioned in the last lesson.

11. As far as chronic cases are concerned, the consensus of opinion of the masters, based on their accumulated experience, is that in people of ordinary constitution, the best procedure is to give a single dose and then wait at least ten or fifteen days before concluding that one dose is insufficient to produce a positive effect. In many long-standing, chronic cases, where the suffering is not very acute, it may be necessary to wait three weeks or more. Gibson Miller warns that it is in such cases that we are apt to go wrong in our over-eagerness to cure. We must realise that, once reaction has begun, any interference will most likely bring it to a stop, for action and reaction are contrary and opposite.

12. Where the disease has progressed considerably and the vitality of the patient is low, it is often dangerous to repeat the dose frequently in our anxiety to produce a positive response, because the reaction induced by the doses rapidly following one another, may be too violent for the strength of the patient to bear.

13. On the other hand, the vital reactivity of the patient may have been blunted by a number of factors and until that "load of resistance" is overcome by repeated doses, the desired response may not come forth. The response may become sluggish in those who have been drugged allopathically, or from the case becoming confused by administration of inappropriate, though somewhat similar, potentised remedies. The response may be tardy also when the sphere of action of the remedy administered coincides only partially with that of the disease.

14. Remedies are classified in different categories, such as acute and chronic; short acting, medium acting and long acting; and lastly superficial and deep acting. Remedies listed according to "duration of action" are given in Boger-Boenninghausen's Repertory. Such "durations are also given in Gibson Miller's "Relationship of Remedies", as well as Clarke's "Clinical Repertory". A chart giving the various depths of action of remedies will be found at Appendix "I". Dr. Kanjilal while giving this chart points out : "None of the charts give the time taken by the respective drugs to start their action, and we may take it for granted that the longer the duration of action the later is the onset of action."

15. It should be remembered that the physician's eagerness to have clear guidance on this point is prompted solely by his anxiety to know whether the remedy, though carefully selected and given, is really the similimum and the potency is really appropriate. Kent furnishes a cogent and clear guidance on this point, much more than all the preceding theoretical disquisition, though it is not irrelevant. Kent's reasoning is simple and direct. He says, "The remedy is known to act by the changing of symptoms. If the prescription is accurate, it commences to act immediately, to effect changes in the patient, and these changes are shown by signs and symptoms. The inner nature of the disease appears to the physician through the symptoms; and he has to watch, observe, weigh and judge from the changes what to do, and what not to do. If a prescription effects no changes, it

is not related to the case and to patiently wait for a response to a foolish prescription is but loss of time."

16. Dr. Koppikar makes yet another and, in a way, original contribution to an understanding of this aspect in his book *Clinical Verifications and Reflections*. He suggests the name "latent period" for the long or short time taken by drugs to start showing effects on the body, to differentiate it from "incubation period" used in natural diseases. He says that the time required for the medicine to start showing visible effects be compared to the incubation period of infectious diseases. After all, the drugs we give are only artificial diseases which are exactly similar to the natural diseases they cure. So they too must have an incubation period. This period varies from drug to drug and also depends upon the dose . . . and the type of case to be treated. For example, in the treatment of typhoid, Kent says : "I very commonly give in vigorous typhoid patients medicine in water, because it is continued fever . . . and the slightest sign of action of the remedy causes me to stop it always." It is obvious from this that Kent does not expect to see any action of the remedy for several days. Again, in his essay on typhoid fever, Wells writes, "When as sometimes happens in typhoid fever, this period of what may be called latent medication is protracted for days or even weeks, and the course recommended requires more than common firmness and the exhibition of much of that quality called nerve, there can be no doubt but that he who has not these qualities or is unwilling to use them is not fit for the responsible duty of treating such cases."

17. Dr. Koppikar cites a case of Osteoarthritis of both shoulders which showed absolutely no change for six long weeks after one dose of *Aurum-met*. CM, but in the seventh week every vestige of the complaint disappeared. In a case of caries of the clavicle, remaining uncured after two operations, *Silicea* CM single dose produced no change for three long months after which, one day a bit of the sequestrum came out and that ended the trouble. Such experiences, he concludes, "Taught me that a long, long time must be allowed for the dose to show its effect." He holds that this need to allow enough time for the remedy to act and cure does not refer to cases where there are two or three different aspects which might require two or three remedies to cure : nor to cases where a definite visible action of the remedy shows that it is working. It refers specially in those cases where one single picture of the case is presented to start with and continues

apparently unchanged as if no medicine has been taken. In such cases, there is every likelihood of our repeating the remedy or changing it, or even being hurried by the patient to do so, in our anxiety to show some results. Thus we do a wrong thing by trying to hasten the cure.

18. As for the "duration of action", all the masters of the art are unanimous. Reiterating Hahnemann's precaution to avoid "Hastiness is not allowing each dose sufficient time to develop and exhaust its action", Dewan Harish Chand points out that "There can be no arbitrary time-table for this whether on the basis of the remedy or the potency or the type of disease. The duration of action mentioned in the books may at best be suggestive, and to my mind only poorly suggestive, especially for the beginner who cannot comprehend such long action of our remedies . . . the duration of reaction is mostly, if not entirely determined by the patient . . . in my practice I am always guided by the duration of reaction in a particular individual, rather than any arbitrary rule of the thumb." He then summarises by quoting the forceful words of Drs. Margaret Tyler and Sir John Weir in "Repertorising" : "Get the right drug, the stimulus needed, and you will find the reaction of the organism deep enough in all conscience, and long-sustained. Then "keep your hands off." Wait long for a second very definite cry, before you dare to interfere. You may have to wait months — then wait. Remember, it is the patient who has to cure himself, the drug cannot cure him, the drug is only the stimulus that starts the vital reaction . . . So long as curative reaction is in progress, it is senseless, `criminal', to interfere. This is the way to crush your work, to vitiate your experience, to break your heart. When the patient begins to slip back, that is the first possible moment to repeat, or to reconsider the case. It is safer to be a little late than a little soon.

19. Dewan Harish Chand continues : "I still very vividly remember the lectures of Sir John Weir that I heard in 1946-47 during my initial training in homoeopathy. He related a number of cases where patients had been quite well after a single dose for as long as a year or more and then returned for fresh medication because of a return of the same symptoms. From my own practice of more than a quarter century, I could give numerous such instances to dispel any doubt about the long, and often very long, reaction from a remedy in chronic diseases. ("Follow up of the Case" — *Hahnemannian Gleanings*, April 1975).

Dr. J. N. Kanjilal narrates similar experiences in *Hahnemannian Gleanings*, February 1971.

20. **What Are the Types of Responses.** The commonest types of responses are of two kinds : (i) Aggravation, (ii) Amelioration. When the patients report either of these, the physician has to exercise his judgement to find out the real condition. It may appear strange but it is true that many times even educated patients are not able to report correctly. He may have steadily improved from the day of the first dose till yesterday, but today the effect of the medicine having worn off, he may find a return of the symptoms, though milder, and he will refer to this only without referring to the earlier relief. It is a good practice, therefore, to ask how he felt over the entire period and even going over individual complaints, and day by day too. Such an enquiry is always helpful. Then again, the relief may be in peripheral complaints at which the patient is happy, while in reality he is weaker, and the symptoms are taking an inward (unfavourable) course. If on the other hand, an aggravation is reported, we have to see whether it is an aggravation of the disease or aggravation of the symptoms, which latter may be called medicinal aggravation. Aggravation of the disease means that the patient is growing weaker, the symptoms of the disease are growing stronger, and the disease is not being healed by the innermost. But in a true homoeopathic (medicinal) aggravation, though the symptoms appear to have aggravated, the patient is growing better. He says, "I am feeling better." We must judge whether the patient's report, either way, is corroborated by his detailed symptoms as compared with those we have recorded while taking the case and administering the remedy. This comparison alone is the physician's most satisfactory evidence in arriving at his judgement whether the remedy is acting curatively or otherwise. When in doubt, wait till you get sufficient evidence to form a judgement.

21. There is a clue to differentiate whether the aggravation pertains to the disease or it is a homoeopathic (medicinal) aggravation. In medicinal aggravation the symptoms become suddenly worse after the remedy is given : whereas the aggravation of the disease is gradual and progressive, manifesting such symptoms as belong to the advanced stage of the malady. Change of remedy would be urgently called for in an aggravation of the disease; and if the medicinal aggravation be severe an antidote may be necessary.

22. There is one peculiar kind of aggravation, especially in chronic cases, which need to be watched over long periods with just placebos. Dr. Kanjilal cautions us thus : "In treatment of chronic cases, especially very chronic ones, it is my oft repeated experience that one dose of similimum is followed by not only one set of homoeopathic aggravation followed by amelioration, but by a series of such sets of aggravations and ameliorations with gradually lesser and lesser intensity and at longer and longer intervals, through a course of many months, sometimes more than a year, when I have to keep in touch with the patient only through placebos. I have bitter experience from my own cases as well as from those of my colleagues of the deplorable results of knowingly or unknowingly ignoring this phenomenon and fact. Gibson Miller comments on much the same phenomenon by writing in his essay, "The Repetition of the Remedy". "It is by no means uncommon to have the improvement in chronic cases interrupted by short secondary aggravations, and before repeating, it is necessary to make sure that the recrudescence is truly permanent and not simply temporary.

23. In chronic cases, owing to the complex nature of miasms and the possible distortion caused through previous inappropriate treatment, the progress of cure is often apparently erratic. Hence it is not always easy to determine whether real improvement continues to take place. In such a state of affairs, however disturbing it may be to the patient, so long as the symptoms progress from within outwards, in the reverse order of their original appearance and from above downwards, we may rest absolutely assured that there is as yet no call for any repetition.

24. **Misconceptions About Aggravation.** Judging from the way the patients enquire anxiously about the possibility of aggravation, it seems that people know more about the aggravation than about homoeopathy itself. Is homoeopathic aggravation an essential part of the treatment? No, if we take the words in Para 2 of the Organon to mean what they say, *viz.* "The highest ideal of cure is rapid, gentle and permanent restoration of health and annihilation of the disease. In the . . . most harmless way . . . " Why then do we find references galore to "aggravation" in any literature on homoeopathy? The fourth observation on "prognosis" in Kent's *Philosophy* visualises a class of cases which progress towards cure without any aggravation when the curative remedy is combined with the correct potency, and there is

Management of the Case

no organic disease. It is the highest order of cure in acute affections, "yet the physician sometimes will be more satisfied if in the beginning of his prescribing he notices a slight aggravation of the symptoms." Why is there so much attachment to "slight aggravation"? For the answer we must go to Para 45 of the *Organon* in which Hahnemann says that "the stronger disease annihilates the weaker" and to Para 48 in which he says that "the malady can be removed solely by an agent that is similar in symptoms and is somewhat stronger." Naturally the stronger force will cause "immediately after ingestion — for the first hour, or for a few hours — a kind of slight aggravation (for a considerable number of hours where the dose has been somewhat too large)" vide Para 157. We have seen earlier how Hahnemann was forced by the aggravations to "dilute" the drugs, so that in Para 159 he says : "The smaller the dose is, so much the slighter and shorter is this apparent increase of the disease during the first hours." Finally, in Para 160 he says: "The dose can scarcely ever be made so small that it cannot overpower the natural disease, and we can therefore understand why such a dose always, during the first hour after its ingestion, produces a perceptible homoeopathic aggravation of this kind."

25. Dewan Harish Chand says that "I have not had the aggravation so frequently in my practice . . . In fact, on the basis of the general impression I have, not only in my own work but also in discussion with colleagues with long experiences, I would put it nearer 25% . . . If the patient does not notice it, we have to consider it as not having occurred; and when it occurs for "an hour or more" with general improvement felt in the intervening period, it can easily be missed." He further asserts that "looking through the clinical cases reported by masters, in books and in numerous journals, one fails to find a reference to aggravation in a large percentage of patients, acute or chronic." Even Kent says : "In acute diseases, we seldom see anything like striking aggravations unless the acute disease has drawn near death's door . . . When the chronic disease has not ultimated itself in tissue changes, you may get no aggravation at all."

26. To our mind the reasons for which homoeopathic aggravations are rarer now, as compared with Hahnemann's times, appear to be three-fold. Firstly, whereas Hahnemann mostly used the 30th potency, the potencies nowadays commonly used are much higher, going up to CM or higher. Secondly, on account of allopathic drugging that is so common, the sensitivity of

people appears to have been blunted. But most important of all, the reasons seem to lie in the fact that homoeopathic practitioners rarely follow the "single dose" and it has given place to the "double dose" or the "ascending scale of dose", etc., and even more frequent repetition "till response is produced."

27. Why the departure from the unit dose has lead to a reduction in the phenomenon of aggravation generally is perhaps explained by Dr. Koppikar's likening it to "anaphylactic shock". Koppikar cites three cases, of which two were fatal and the third was barely saved, because he repeated *China* 200 in the first case, *Apis* 200 in the second case and *Kali carb.* 1M in the third case about 10 to 13 days after the first dose of the same remedy. To find an answer to this problem he searched among clinical cases in our literature but in vain, because doctors rarely report their "failure". At last he found that, in the sixth edition of the *Organon*, Hahnemann has stated that "it is impractical to repeat the same unchanged dose of the remedy once, not to mention its frequent repetition . . . The vital principle does not accept such unchanged doses without resistance." He advised that the potency should be altered slightly every time the remedy is repeated; but he did not mention anything about the time lag required to produce the oversensitive state.

28. Koppikar then found Kent's observation in his *Philosophy* that "if we examine into the effects of poisons, we find those who have once been poisoned by *Rhus* are a dozen times more sensitive than before. Those who have been poisoned by *arsenic* are extremely sensitive to *arsenic* after they allow the first effects to pass off. If they continue to keep with the first effects, however, they become less sensitive . . . In other words, sensitiveness to a medical agent (poison) is dulled and hypersensitiveness does not supervene if they continue the medicine. In homoeopathic treatment an aggravation is expected because the remedy selected is extremely similar to the disease and the patient is therefore highly sensitive to it. Therefore, a second dose about the tenth day from the first dose may partake of the effect of an anaphylactic shock. Just as a guinea pig collapses when a small quantity of horse serum is injected subcutaneously on the first and the tenth day, in man, anaphylaxis may appear in a sensitive person on a second injection, if he had a serum injection ten days to six months earlier. It takes a minimum of ten days after the first injection to develop this hypersensitiveness to the same serum.

Management of the Case

29. While studying in college, Koppikar says, "He had learnt that a second injection of a small quantity within twenty-four hours of the first one, would prevent the development of this supersensitiveness. He thereafter stopped giving a single dose for any case. Instead, he has been giving on the first day, two or three doses at intervals of three or four hours . . . Kent and others also used this method which is called "Single Collective Dose." Koppikar says, "I have never seen any upset by subsequent repetition in such cases, and I find this an absolutely safe method. Hahnemann's advice to change the potency, ever so slightly, at each repetition, which permits even daily repetition in chronic cases, is also aimed at preventing severe aggravation or "anaphylactic shock". (This is done by the "Plus Dosage" method in which 2 or 3 globules are dissolved in 3 ounces of water. Out of this two or three teaspoonfuls are taken for a dose, after which the same quantity of fresh water is added to the bottle, and the contents vigorously shaken, thus raising the potency slightly).

30. **Why the Responses, and What to Do.** We shall now examine the two remaining questions, *viz.* (i) why do responses, whatever they be, arise, and (ii) what is their real meaning; and how should the physician deal with them? Kent has thrown a flood of light on these questions in "Prognosis after observing the action of the remedy". (Kent's *Philosophy*). Of this chapter Dr. Kanjilal states, "Of all the teachings of Kent, this chapter giving twelve observations after homoeopathic prescription is decidedly the most important. Kent's name would be ever remembered if he did not do anything but left only this lecture to his progency . . ." Dewan Harish Chand has further elucidated the points in his paper "Follow up of the Case." We now present those ideas in the form of a Chart so as to make them easy of grasp and to facilitate quick reference.

31. **Chart :**

	Nature of Response	Cause of Response	What to do?
I.	Amel. with very slight agg. or even without an initial agg., with recovery of patient.	Remedy is curative and potency exactly fitted the case. No organic disease present.	This is the highest order of cure; do not interfere till symptoms return.

Nature of Response	Cause of Response	What to do?
II. In chronic cases old symptoms return in reverse order of appearance.	The remedy is deep acting, and has attacked the disease in its inmost nature.	The old symptoms will disappear by themselves in a short time. If some old symptoms persist, they rank high for the next prescription.
III. There is no change in the symptoms.	Remedy may be wrong.	If so, retake the case and find the correct remedy.
	Potency is wrong.	See, if looking to the disease force and the patient's vitality, you must try higher or lower potency before giving up the remedy.
	Patient may be sluggish in reacting.	Give a high potency to jog him, and then follow with a medium one.
	Remedy given is slow-acting in a chronic case.	If it is a high potency, wait for a month; if medium (200 or 1 M), wait at least 15 days.
	Any interference with remedy action?	Check up and remove interference.
IV. Agg. is quick, short and strong followed by quick improve-	Remedy and potency both correct. Reaction is vigorous.	Best results will follow such initial homoeopathic agg.

Management of the Case

Nature of Response	Cause of Response	What to do?
ment, it being long-lasting. (In Acute : agg. in the first few hours. In Chronic : agg. in the first few days).	No tendency to organic changes in vital organs, though may be in parts not essential to life.	Hands off, till symptoms return.
V. Agg. is long (may be weeks) and severe but finally there is slow improvement.	Prognosis good. Case was almost incurable, vitality being low. You have got him before the trouble has gone too far, as organic changes were just threatening to come. The potency was too high.	All will be well if remedy is not repeated too soon. Wait till patient has sufficient strength to react to another dose. In doubtful cases of low vitality, better start with lower potencies only — being prepared to antidote if it takes a wrong turn. If incurable, try to palliate.
VI. Immediate amel. followed by long agg.	Case is incurable and remedy acted unfavourably. Or Remedy was superficially acting and palliative only. Or Remedy though similar to the most pronounced symptoms, did not cover the whole case. Or Amel. is too short	Find the true similimum without ignoring concomitants. Select a deep-acting remedy to cover the whole case, and go up carefully from 200th.

Nature of Response	Cause of Response	What to do?
	becuse of conscious or unconscious interference with the action of remedy.	
VII. Too short an amel.	If an Acute case, patient is in a desperate condition.	Try low potencies in repeated doses or palliate with 50 Millesimal potencies.
	If Chronic : Organic changes present, and patient is in bad shape; Or There is interference by wrong diet or regimen.	
VIII. Full time amel. of symptoms without any increase in patient's strength.	Patient is too weak for restoration of health.	Patient can only be palliated with low or medium potencies given repeatedly in water till vitality is restored.
	Organic changes present.	
	Full cure is not possible.	
IX. Long agg. with slow decline of patient's strength.	Marked organic changes present.	Try to palliate with short acting remedies in lower potencies.
	Potency is too high for the feeble reaction of the patient, and the remedy was too late.	Do not give a deep-acting remedy when organic disease is present.
X. New symptoms, not in the provings of drug given	Prescription is wrong.	Retake the case including the new symptoms and select a new remedy

Management of the Case

Nature of Response	Cause of Response	What to do?
(and not a return of old symptoms) have come up.		corresponding to new totality. However, if the new symptoms are very troublesome, antidote the remedy given and after waiting for a while, proceed to retake the case, etc.
XI. Marked improvement, but in the wrong direction i.e., symptoms have gone from periphery to the centre, and vital organs are being affected.	Prescription is wrong, and not based on totality of symptoms.	Antidote the remedy at once and retake the case. Otherwise, organic changes will take place.
XII. Patient develops symptoms of the remedy given without improvement in his disease symptoms.	Patient is oversensitive. Cure mostly not possible.	Case is hard to treat even for an experienced homoeopath.
XIII. Patient gets a proving of every remedy given.	Patient is very sensitive, and very difficult to cure.	You are dealing with tubercular miasm; give the Nosode.
XIV. Favourable response followed by new drug picture.	Tubercular miasm.	Give Tuberculinum.

F-14

Nature of Response	Cause of Response	What to do?
XV. A severe agg. in curable cases and sound vitality — caused unnecessarily by high potency.	Too high a potency say, a CM, was given.	Even during agg. patient feels better as it is only medicinal agg. and not of the disease. Agg. will pass off if left alone.
	Or Too low a potency given repeatedly.	If agg. is severe antodote it and follow with a medium potency, limited doses.
XVI. To avoid agg.	In very feeble vitality.	Give a single dose of a really high potency and watch the minutest sign for direction of symptoms (E.W.H.)
	Strong vitality but with marked tissue changes.	Try medium potencies in repeated doses, or the 50—Millesimal, potencies.

32. The Second Prescription. The physician's duty does not end after the first prescription, not even after the second or subsequent prescriptions. It only ends after a cure is accomplished. Thus, more than one prescription may be necessary in most of the cases. In homoeopathic literature the "first" prescription is the one which has brought about a change or reaction. Even if several prescriptions have been made, none of them qualify to be called the "first" prescription if they proved their unsuitability by their failure to evoke any response. Then again, even the third, fourth, fifth and subsequent prescriptions are called "second", since they are second to the immediately preceding prescription. This is because no prescription is, or ought to be, made unless it is based on symptoms which, in turn, have come forth from the preceding prescription.

Management of the Case

33. Great care is, therefore, necessary in making each "second" prescription. Hahnemann is said to have taken the case in full each time before making a prescription. Kent has said: "If the medicine is not very similar, only partially similar, it yet may be similar enough to cure, but you will not see the same results as you do when you make accurate prescriptions. When you do so, you are doing best work . . . If you will observe the work of ordinary physicians, you will notice they give two or three remedies to get their patients through, where the master gives but one."

34. Roberts writes : "In chronic conditions, no prescription, either first or second, can be made without careful, thorough study of the case and the sequence of symptoms. It is only by working out the case with the Repertories that we are able to see clearly the indicated constitutional remedy in the light of the symptoms that have been cured or relieved. It is only then that we can administer another remedy intelligently and with confidence." Margaret Tyler cautions against hasty prescribing by saying. "If you take a lot of trouble with a case (when you know how), it will give you very little trouble afterwards. Conversely, if you take very little trouble to begin with, it will give you endless trouble, many times repeated. You have fouled the clear waters with a wrong prescription, and how are you going to peer into the depths? . . . One bad prescription leads to several, perhaps to a hopeless mixing up of the case." And what is true of the "first" prescription is also true of the "second".

35. In the chart given on p. 191 we have mentioned the different types of responses we have to deal with after each prescription and what to do with them. What we have given under the heading "What to do" is nothing but the second prescription itself. Yet, this question needs to be discussed in a little more detail in a somewhat different way, so that the ideas get fixed in our mind. After carefully observing the symptoms which arise following the first prescription and coming to a judgement about their nature, the physician has the following eleven courses open to him :

(i)   Repeat the same remedy in the same potency.

(ii)   Repeat the same remedy in a higher potency.

(iii)   Repeat the same remedy in a lower potency.

(iv)   Administer a complementary of the last remedy.

(v)   Administer a cognate of the remedy.

(vi) Administer an entirely new remedy — Change of remedy.

(vii) Succession of remedies or zigzagging.

(viii) Change of plan, according to uppermost miasm.

(ix) Wait and watch.

(x) Antidote.

(xi) Intercurrent.

36. Repeat same remedy in the same potency :

(i) The symptoms ameliorate and after sometime the patient returns with the same image, though less intense — or even without the characteristic symptoms or concomitants. Then the remedy and potency, which were correct, may be repeated to give him the full benefit of the same.

(ii) The patient feels the improvement, and the symptoms are changing according to Hering's "law of direction of cure", relieving the vital organs and going to the periphery; then also the same prescription may be repeated but only when we notice that the progress has slackened.

37. Repeat the same remedy in higher potency. When after considerable amelioration there is no complete relief inspite of repetition of the same remedy and potency, and such repetitions do not give long-term benefit, we may go to the higher potency; and thus go from medium to high and from high to higher and highest, in order to give the patient the benefit of the full range of potencies.

38. Repeat the remedy in the lower potency.

(i) When immediate amelioration is followed by wrong aggravation, and we have reason to think that it is an incurable case, and if the symptoms still point to the same remedy, a lower potency of the same remedy will palliate (and even antidote the unfavourable action of the high potency given earlier). For example : A patient had a dose of *Sulphur* 50 M (though it was intended to give 10M). The patient who had left the town shortly thereafter returned to her home-town a year later "to die of tuberculosis". The doctor then gave her a dose of *Sulphur* 30x and in two weeks' time she was out of bed and doing her house-work.

Management of the Case

(ii) When in a serious acute case the amelioration is too short, and the patient is in a desperate condition, we may give the same remedy, if still indicated, in lower or medium potency in repeated doses, either dry on tongue or in water, or by the "Plussing" method.

(iii) If it is a case like the one just mentioned in (ii), but it is chronic, and organic changes are present, we may palliate with lower potencies, or try the 50-Millesimal potencies.

(iv) When there is full-time amelioration, and yet the patient is not gaining strength, we can only palliate with low or medium potencies given repeatedly, till vitality is restored, whereafter the higher potencies may be resorted to.

(v) When long aggravation is followed by a decline of the patient, it is obvious that marked organic changes are present. The symptoms have settled in one vital organ, and we can only palliate with low potency or even a crude organopathic drug. If there is gradual improvement we may then consider ascending the scale of potencies.

(vi) There is no change in the symptoms even after administration of the best selected (indicated) remedy. This may be due to sluggish reaction of the patient, in which event, an initial dose of high potency to jog him up may be followed by medium or low one to continue healthy reaction.

39. **Administer a complementary remedy.**

(i) When a remedy has given considerable relief, but no further progress is witnessed inspite of its being tried in all ranges of potencies, yet symptoms remain the same. How to change the remedy when symptoms are same? Here a remedy which bears a complementary relation to the preceding one is called for. A complementary is like a close, loving friend who is always welcome, and will help in completing the work of the remedy given earlier.

(ii) In a serious case like Asthma or Pneumonia, after *Arsenicum* is given for the acute condition, we should follow up with a deep-acting complementary remedy like *Thuja* or *Kali-carb.*, or *Sulphur* or *Psorinum* or some other deep-acting anti-psoric or anti-sycotic remedy according to symptoms. (Asthma grows on a sycotic soil).

(iii) The second prescription must sustain a friendly complementary relation to the last one. No intelligent prescription can be made without knowing the last remedy.

40. Administer a cognate of the last remedy. Sometimes in chronic cases, the cure is not accomplished by a single remedy owing to the deep-seated nature of the chronicity. There are some remedies which work well in a cyclic order. One remedy always leads to one of its cognates, i.e. when the symptoms change they lead to the cognate. The cure is accomplished with the pattern of remedies one following the other. The difference between a complementary and cognate remedy is very delicate. In the complementary remedy the symptoms usually remain the same, but when the cognate is to be used it is called for by the change of symptoms which themselves point to it, if only we are careful to observe. A knowledge of the cognates helps us in this. A cognate should not be employed unless indicated by the symptoms. While complementary is like a friend who is welcome at all times, the cognate is like a relative who is not welcome unless particularly called for. For example, a bilious fever in a *Sepia* constitution is likely to call for *Nux-vom.*, and as soon as that bilious fever or remittent fever has subsided the symptoms of *Sepia* come out immediately, showing the cognate relation of *Nux-vom.* and *Sepia*. Some of the remedies which work in a trio in cyclic order as cognate, are given below :

(i)   Puls — Sil. — Flour-ac.

(ii)   Sulphur — Sarsap — Sepia.

(iii)   Colo. — Caust. — Staph.

(iv)   Arsen-alb. — Thuja — Tarent.

(v)   Allium-cepa — Phos — Sulph.

(vi)   Carb-veg. — Ars. — Mur-ac. (have saved many from jaws of death. "Corpse revivers").

(vii)   Sulphur — Calc-c. — Lyco. (Hahnemann's Anti-psoric trio).

(viii) Lyco. — Carb-veg. — China (Flatulent trio).

Management of the Case

(ix) Acon. — Ars-alb. — Rhus-tox. (Restless trio).

(x) Bell. — Hyos. — Stram.

(xi) Thuja — Staph. — Nitric acid (Trio for condylomata).

(xii) Nit-ac. — Benz-ac. — Sepia. (very foul odour of urine).

(xiii) Camphor — Cuprum — Verat-alb. (Asiatic cholera).

(xiv) Sepia — Caust — Gels. (Ptosis of eyelids).

(xv) Caust. — Rhus-tox. — Sulph. (Rheumatism and paralysis)

(xvi) Carbo-an. — Conium — Bromine (glandular affections).

(xvii) Ignatia — Natrum-mur. — Sepia (ladies, mental upsets).

(xviii) Acon. — Spongia — Hep-sulph. (Boenninghausen's Croup Trio).

41. Administer an entirely new remedy

(i) If a remedy, though believed to be well-selected, has no effect (better or worse), it is obvious that the case has not been well taken, or the symptoms on which the prescription is based do not represent the characteristic totality. The only course left is to retake the case after sweeping off the cob-webs and fixed ideas in our mind, and select a new remedy which will be the similimum. When the last remedy has not acted at all, it makes no difference whether the newly selected remedy is incompatible with or inimical to the first one.

(ii) Dr. S.R. Pathak is reported to have said that changing the remedy for the second prescription (i.e. after the first prescription has acted beneficially) is akin to deciding on a surgical operation. We must not forget that "the medicine that has partly cured the case often finishes it . . . may be in different potencies."

(iii) In re-taking the case and considering a new prescription we would do well to bear in mind that "the last appearing symptoms must ever remain as the best guide to the next remedy, and a remedy having it as a characteristic will most likely have all the rest of the symptoms. But if the last appearing symptom is an old symptom of the patient, on its way to final departure, the first prescription was the right one, and there is no need to change it."

42. **Zig-zagging (using a succession of remedies).** We sometimes find constitutional conditions which require, for a complete cure, a succession of remedies, with one remedy following another as the symptoms change. This may amount to a process of zig-zagging the case or like peeling the onion, as Elizabeth Hubbard said, beginning at the top layer, i.e., the most recent symptoms being the guide to the remedy. We peel off layer after layer with each prescription. This process may be necessitated by two reasons, either because of lack of knowledge of our remedies, or because the case does not unfold before us fully at a time, or unfolds part by part. As regards the remedies, Kent affirms, that it is very rarely the case that among the provings of our remedies there is none which corresponds to the characteristic features of a case. It was rarely so in Hahnemann's days, and it is certainly very rare today with our voluminous Materia Medica. Yet, Kent concedes that there is one thing we can depend upon, *viz.* the image of the patient's illness becomes more simple when we have done our best to prescribe one remedy after another, of course based on symptoms. In these difficult cases, he continues, when we have zigzagged the patient for a number of years, we will find his symptoms become more definite and striking and more clearly understood and after a lapse of sometime we find we have little trouble to grasp the case and make rapid progress.

43. **Alternating conditions.** We are apt to play the zig-zagging game, unwittingly though, when we meet with alternating complaints without knowing them to be such. It is not uncommon for a patient's malady to have two sides, one side being manifested at one time and the other side at some other time. You may find that *Euphrasia* is more sharply related to the eye symptoms than the antipsoric that fits the whole case, and that *Pulsatilla* fits the stomach symptoms much better than the antipsoric that fits the whole case. "But remember", warns Kent, "that there is one antipsoric that is more similar to the whole patient than these special remedies because it is better fitted to the generals. The oftener you prescribe for different groups of symptoms, the worse it is for the patient . . . it may make him incurable. Do not prescribe until you have found the remedy that is similar to the whole case, even though it is clear in your mind that one remedy may be more similar to one particular group of symptoms and another remedy

Management of the Case

to another group . . . These alternating one-sided complaints are sometimes dreadful to manage, when everything is thrown to the surface or the extremities".

44. Change of remedy according to uppermost Miasm. We have already had a glimpse, in a previous lesson, of Hahnemann's discovery of the three Chronic Miasms, one or more of which are at the bottom of chronic deep-seated diseases. We shall learn more about them later in this lesson. Meanwhile, we have to note that for the purpose of the "second prescription" we must take into consideration the miasmatic condition facing us at each prescription. It should be borne in mind that, even in a case suffering from mixed miasms, one miasm is generally submerged under another at any one time. For this reason, after one miasm (represented to us by symptoms) has been removed by the similimum, the second raises its head; when this happens, our plan of attack should be changed accordingly to meet the symptoms of the miasm which is showing up just now. We cannot expect to remove any miasm with a single dose of any remedy; but by attacking each miasm when it raises its head, we continue the process of "peeling the onion" till all the layers of disease are removed.

45. After the administration of a miasmatic remedy, if there be any need, the previously given constitutional remedy may be tried again from the lower potency to the higher ones. After every change of potency the patient responds well and he is lifted to a higher level of cure.

46. Wait and watch. The following are some of the more important conditions or circumstances under which the physician would do wisely not to be hasty with a prescription but to "Wait and watch". Any premature interference may spoil the case.

(i) When long aggravation is followed by slow improvement, it is clear that the remedy has taken hold of the case and is bringing order in the economy. It should be allowed to act at its own pace without any interference whatsoever, until we are doubly sure that the improvement has really come to a halt. By that time the patient's strength will also improve.

(ii) When the patient is having medicinal aggravation, as is shown by his feeling better in himself, there is no need to be too anxious to relieve the aggravation, which in any case will pass off of its own accord. If after waiting for a sufficient length of time, we find that the aggravation is too severe and does not subside, then only would we be justified in antidoting it.

(iii) When the patient continues to improve after the administration of the remedy, there is absolutely no ground for even repetition of the dose on the ground of "a little more of the good remedy will speed up cure". Nothing could be more ill advised.

(iv) When in a chronic case a slow but deep-acting remedy has been given in high potency, (provided we have taken every care to see that it is the similimum), the remedy should be given full time to act, and we should hold our patience. Pertinent in this connection are the cases cited earlier in this lesson by Kanjilal, Dewan Harish Chand and Koppikar, under "Duration of Action".

(v) When strong aggravation is followed by quick improvement, such improvement is generally found to be long lasting. Better follow the policy of "Hands off — till symptoms return, and return definitely".

(vi) When the patient is getting better, as shown by the directions of cure (from within, outward, etc.), there are apt to be temporary "secondary" aggravations as pointed out earlier by Kanjilal and Gibson Miller. We should leave them severely alone, prescribing a Placebo if need be. The greatest sufferings might be involved sometimes, during the progress towards permanent recovery. If they are disturbed or palliated (out of misdirected sympathy) by inappropriate medicines, the patient will never be cured.

(vii) And lastly, whenever in doubt, wait. Nothing is lost by waiting, and taking the time to observe, study and think. Only correct action though a little late can save; wrong action will always do harm.

ADVANCING THE FRONTIERS OF HOMOEOPATHY

47. The approaches of Drs. Maganbhai Desai and Sarabhai Kapadia to the question of repetition of doses in high potencies beat a new, nay, an unconventional track. Very few will take the courage to follow their method. In justification of their stand, Dr. Sarabhai

Management of the Case

says : "The approach of Hahnemann is perfect but the work is not over. It is our responsibility to carry on further with this work by elaborating the approach like so many of our old masters have done after him." Another reason is the more or less uniform success which the experiment of using high potencies in repeated doses over a prolonged period, has met with. This successful method, therefore, deserves careful study and adoption in practice in suitable cases.

48. Most of the classical homoeopaths even today follow Hahnemann's advice in the 5th edition of the *Organon* about the repetition of the dose, *viz.* to keep "hands off" so long as improvement continues. In the 6th edition, however, he introduced the 50 millesimal scale and allowed its continued repetition to speed up the process of cure even when improvement is observed. The question before Dr. Maganbhai was why we should not repeat the doses in high potencies of the centesimal scale even when improvement was going on? The correct answer to this question could not be found otherwise than through actual experimentation. Dr. Sarabhai himself was successfully treated for his migraine headaches with high potencies of various remedies in repeated doses. Dr. Sarabhai was thus closely watching his work and was intimately involved in these experiments. After passing out of college and starting practice, Dr. Sarabhai has been using this method of dosage in his own practice since 1953, and he has also found it useful.

49. Dr. Sarabhai recalls that Dr. Maganlal Desai tried this method in various acute conditions, particularly typhoid in the thirties during his practice in Calcutta. He thus became clear about the advantages of repetition of high potencies in acute cases. He observed that a typhoid case of Zincum will recover and survive on infrequent repetition, but may still retain paralytic effects. However, if repeated doses of high and the highest potencies of Zincum are given during the acute phase, and if reactions of convulsions and increased fever are undergone during the action of such repeated doses, full cure is the ultimate result, with no trace of paralytic effects. Dr. Borland has also reported the advantages of repetition of high potencies in pneumonia (curing by crisis). Therefore, there is not much of an argument about such repetition in acute cases.

50. When Dr. Maganlal started with the use of repetitions of high potencies in chronic patients, he migrated from Calcutta to Surat (Gujarat State) in 1942. It was during this period that Dr. Sarabhai came under his treatment for his chronic migraine, and

later followed him closely, and himself adopted the practice of using high potencies in repeated doses in chronic cases. Sarabhai explains the working of this Posology :

"It is now clearly known that when adapting to a morbific influence of a miasm or a drug, the living organism either tries to absorb and live with the same by some adjustment ("Syntoxis"), or tries to destroy the same ("Catatoxis"). Syntoxic adjustment tolerates latency of 'disease' and very often involves some inner compromise; whereas catatoxis may involve some suffering and symptoms caused by the process of destruction and elimination of the morbific factor. The living organism is resourceful with syntoxic processes as well as catatoxic processes. However, as patients are eager to obtain relief from inconvenience and pain quickly, modern medicine tends to trade with such drugs which give prompt relief, and thus induce and maintain syntoxis. However, real and total elimination of morbific influence is possible only when catatoxic processes get their due sway. Then only there is true recovery from the susceptibility to the disease.

51. The chronic patient has two courses open to him. He may choose a superficial sense of well being and absence of symptoms through syntoxis. The living organism then has only declared a 'truce' with the morbid influence or the influence of crude drugs, and this background is capable of developing complexes and subsequent diseased states whenever an exciting cause favours such development. However, for true and lasting health it is necessary to root out these influences and eliminate the susceptibility through catatoxis, which is achieved by the repetition of high potencies. Hering's laws of direction of cure guide us all the way in this process. It is obvious that the catatoxic process requires complete co-operation from the patient, who should be willing to face aggravations.

52. As for the remedy, it goes without saying that it should match the patient's susceptibility through symptom similarity. Both the remedy and potency must match susceptibility. The remedy should be selected on the presenting symptoms linked with the "background" of past history. Often past history is given importance in the style of Burnett. A patient reacts to a potency so long as he is susceptible to it; when he stops reacting, his susceptibility in that range is exhausted, and we thus go to higher and higher potencies till susceptibility is eliminated and the deviated vital force is restored to normalcy. (For detailed study, read Dr. Sarabhai's paper mentioned in the "References" at the end of this book).

Management of the Case

53. Antidote. Antidotal action would become necessary in the following circumstances :

(i) If the new symptoms which come up after the administration of a remedy in an incurable case (a knowledge of the disease will settle this) are very troublesome and distressing, we have to antidote that remedy and after allowing some time to pass for allowing the symptoms to settle down, retake the case for consideration of another more suitable remedy.

(ii) If a remedy brings about marked improvement in some symptoms, but in the wrong direction — for example, rheumatism of joints yields place to, or is followed by complaints in the region of the heart, i.e., if the complaints go from the less vital to the more vital organs —an antidote is urgently called for; otherwise, organic changes might ensue. The antidote may be the same remedy but a very low potency, in some two or three doses. The case may be retaken for a new remedy after the symptoms are stabilised.

(iii) When severe aggravation follows the administration of remedy in too low a potency, given repeatedly and that in a curable case with sound vitality, the same remedy in a high potency will antidote the unfavourable action.

54. Intercurrrent remedies. It so happens occasionally that a patient does not react to the best indicated remedy. The administration of certain remedies has been found to help the patient to shake off this "lack of reaction." Such remedies are: Carbo-veg., Conium, Cuprum, Opium, Laurocer., Med., Phos-ac., Psor., Sulphur, Syph., Tuberc., etc.

55. Relationship of remedies. Ideally, in simple cases especially, only one remedy properly selected should prove curative. However, most cases, especially the chronic ones, are not so simple and we have to steer them towards a cure by removing one layer after another with different remedies. The pioneers of homoeopathy found in the course of their practice, that remedies are related to one another in different ways and these relationships either help forward or hinder or undo the action of the remedies which preceded them. When one remedy has to be followed by another, and then by some other, their mutual relationship acquires significance. Excellent data about these relationships is given in R.

Gibson Miller's *Relationship of Remedies*. The chapter on "Concordances" in Boger-Boenninghausen's Repertory also is very useful and the method of using it is explained in Bhanu Desai's "How to find the Similimum with the Boger-Boenninghausen's Repertory," as well as H. A. Robert's introduction to the *Therapeutic Pocket Book* of Boenninghausen.

56. **Complementary relationship.** Sometimes an indicated remedy does not remove all the symptoms, because it may not cover some one or two items of the totality, though it might cover all the rest of the case. The complementary remedy makes good this deficiency as it not only covers this want, but it also does not disturb the action of the previous remedy in the patient. It thus carries forward the action of the earlier remedy which has not the same depth. For example, *Belladonna* may meet successfully an acute case of sore throat or tonsilitis, but *Calcarea-carb.* its complement has no capacity to so act by virtue of its slow, sluggish nature. But when we meet with this recurring condition calling for *Bell.*, and the child makes no further improvement, *Calc-c.* by virtue of its deep action will carry forward the action of *Bell* and complete the curative process.

57. Most complements are also antidotal to the same remedy if given too early before the action of the earlier remedy is over. In the example given above, it is only when symptoms of *Bell.* have subsided will *Calc.-c.* act as a complement. Another example, *Sulph.*, will act as complementary to *Merc-sol.* in dysentery only when the acute symptoms of *Merc.-sol.* have subsided. This timing of remedies is important.

58. **Some examples of complementary action.** Boenninghausen's personal case of *Thuja* requiring to be followed by *Conium* and and *Lycopodium*; Boenninghausen's croup powders of *Aconite, Spongia* and *Hepar-sulph.* all in the 200th potency, given in rotation at specific intervals; when *Arsenic* has overcome the crisis of extensive hepatisation in double pneumonia, the patient will die unless *Sulphur* is given in twenty-four hours. (Kent). After *Causticum* helped a case of Hemiplegia in every respect, the remaining aphasia was not set right till Baryta-carb. was exhibited.

59. **Acute-chronic relationship.** When an acute illness improves with a remedy, the chronic of that remedy will set the economy in order and prevent recurrence; conversely, when a chronic patient, already under the influence of a deep acting chronic remedy, suffers from an acute ailment, for which relief

Management of the Case

must be given, the "acute" of that chronic remedy will help without disturbing the main remedy. Some examples are : The chronic of Acon. is *Sulph*; of *Bell*, is *Calc*; of *Ars.* are *Verat.*, *Thuja*, *Nat-s.*; of *Bry.*, are *Alum.*, *Phos.*, *Nat-m.*, *Kali-c.*; of *Colo.*, is *Caust.*; of *Ign.*, are *Nat-m.*, *Sep.*; of *Ipec.* are *Cupr.*, *Ant-t.*, *Nat-s.*; of *Lach.* is *Lyc.*; of *Merc.* are *Syph.*, *Thuja*, *Aurum.*; of *Nit-ac.* are *Sulph.*; of *Nux-v.*, are *Sulph.*, *Lyc.*, *Sep.*, *Kali-c*. (According to Roger Schmidt in *Hahnemannian Gleanings*, April, 1978). Some more, according to Elizabeth Hubbard are, again putting the acutes first : Coloc. — *Staph.*; Bacill — *Calc. ph.*; Hepar-s. — *Silicea* ; Puls. — *Silicea*.

60. **Inimical or incompatible relationship.** If the patient's condition worsens, when a remedy is given before or after certain other remedy, we know that the two remedies are incompatible or inimical to each other. The list of remedies shown as inimical in the book on relationships has grown out of such bitter experiences of master prescribers. We shall cite a few examples given by Dr. S.P. Koppikar in his article on "Relationship" (Journal of Hom. Medicine, 3/1/1963):

(i) Acetic acid and vinegar, usually employed to antitode anaesthetics, opium and tobacco, will increase the sufferings if used against some others like *Bell.* and *Arnica*.

(ii) Coffee is a fairly common antidote to mány drugs. Yet it increases the excitement and frenzy produced by *Cantharis*. It complicates cases of *Colchicum*. *Coffea* and *Cham.* upset the effects of one another.

(iii) China given for the debility produced by *Ledum* is very injurious.

(iv) A case of cholera which improved by one dose of *Veratrum* 200 relapsed when *China* was given to remove the residual debility. Luckily, another dose of *Veratrum* 200 stopped the trouble, and later, *Acid-phos*. acted as a good pick-me-up.

(v) Gladwin found that it took a long time to undo the trouble caused after *Phos*. was given to a patient for severe frequent colds when he was under the influence of *Causticum*.

(vi) *Mercury* and *Silicea* have a number of common spheres of action and are needed in abscesses, boils, bone troubles, glandular diseases, ear troubles, sweating, etc. Farrington says, "These remedies, so inimical, are perplexingly similar in modalities." We are therefore advised to interpolate *Hepar-sulph.* in case it is necessary to give them one after the other. *Hepar.* is an antidote and a complementary to *Mercurius.*

61. The explanation for such inimical relationship, muses Koppikar, lies in their extensive similarity. Just as a remedy produces aggravation when it is similar-most to the natural disease, because the patient is very sensitive to the stimuli, when a person is already under the influence of one remedy, he is very sensitive to a further stimuli of the same nature. "Oversensitiveness, Allergy and Anaphylaxis are all similar reactions but differing in degrees of intensity." He, therefore, advises that if the remedy is still acting, we should wait and give time for the hypersensitive period to pass off; or give an intervening complementary which breaks through the reactions of the previous remedy. (Compare this with the remarks on "Timing of Remedies" under heading "Complementary Relationship.")

62. **Antidotal relationship.** This was apparently the first relationship which Hahnemann had to discover and make use of, since antidotal drugs had to be urgently identified and applied whenever the provers' sufferings caused by the violent action of the remedies had to be cut short. What is the basis for the antidotal action of remedies? Basing himself on the law of similars, Hahnemann argued that if a natural disease could be removed by a similar artificial disease (drug effects), there was no reason why one artificial disease produced during provings, could not be removed or alleviated by another similar aritificial disease. The antidotal relations are, therefore, based on symptom similarity. It has been observed during their practice by master prescribers, that when severe aggravations have resulted from a high potency, the aggravation is made milder by one or two doses of a low potency of the same medicine.

63. Low potency users sometimes have to contend with aggravation arising from the low potency repeated frequently over long periods. Such aggravation can be relieved by the action of the high and very high potencies of the same medicine. Stuart Close has said : "It is a fact that high potency of a drug is sometimes the best antidote for the effects of the crude drug."

Management of the Case

64. Coffea, Camphor, Nux-vomica, etc. are considered to have antidotal power in respect of a large number of remedies. Yet in view of the fact that this power derives from symptom similarity, it appears to be good practice to choose a remedy which can counter the troublesome symptoms on the basis of maximum possible symptom similaity rather than as a "general antidote." This point of view appears to get support from a case treated by Dr. Younan. An old opium-eater found that he had high blood sugar. He was also extremely constipated with balls of hard stool. Plumbum 200 cured him soon both of the diabetes and constipation. Few books except Knerr's "Drug Relationship" mention Plumbum as an antidote to Opium, while Hubbard's "Brief Study Course" mentions it as a complementary to *Opium*. It would thus seem that there is a thin line dividing antidotal and complementary relationship. May be the "timing" of administration makes a similar remedy antidotal or complementary. On the whole, symptoms similarity holds the key even in this matter, as in all others.

65. **Obstacles to cure.** In the management of the case towards a cure, different types of obstacles play no small part. Hahnemann has not overlooked to emphasize in the *Organon*, that the removal of causes of disease is a prerequisite for cure. Among the various obstacles may be listed :

(i) Conditions calling for mechanical/surgical interference.

(ii) Unbalanced diet or wrong habits of eating.

(iii) Bad habits which contribute to ill-health, such as excessive smoking or drinking alcoholic beverages; late sleeping; irregular food; sexual vices or excesses.

(iv) Want of sufficient rest or exercise.

(v) Unhealthy environment, such as ill-ventilated workplace, air pollution, living in damp and dirty place, etc.

(vi) Occupational causes, such as inhalation of poisonous fumes, extreme physical strain and fatigue, high humidity, travelling in the hot sun, etc.

(vii) Unhelpful or unsympathetic emotional atmosphere at home or at work.

(viii) After effects of the powerful modern drugs such as Chloromycetin, Cortisone, etc. and last, but by no means the least.

(ix) Chronic constitutional diathesis calling for one or more anti-miasmatic remedies.

We shall take up for consideration only some of these factors which call for a little more detailed elucidation, the rest of the items being more or less self-explanatory.

66. **Surgical cases.** While taking the case the physician owes it to himself as well as to the patient to satisfy himself that the condition does not call for surgical intervention. Failure to do so, especially in life endangering situations, would be inexcusable. Acute appendicitis, tumours in vital parts, fractures needing immobilisation, and even the giving of an enema in intractable constipation or catheterisation in dysuria would come under this head as would the giving of Intravenous Glucose in a case of Dehydration.

67. **Diet.** Besides the diet being generally balanced, care has to be taken to see that the diet is appropriate to the type of disease the patient is suffering from. The diabetic, the nephrotic, the cardiac and the hepatic patients will each need a separate diet chart, and the physician's advice to the patient should not be wanting in this respect. The importance of blood-chemistry should not be overlooked or under-rated, and proper diet has a vital role in its making. We remember a case of inveterate eczema treated with ill success for about a year under the expert homoeopathic care of Dr. Grimmer (reported in the Journal of American Institute of Homoeopathy), till laboratory tests revealed that the patient was suffering from Hypoproteinanaemia. When the patient was put under proper diet, the eczema gradually receded of its own accord.

68. Another point which needs consideration is, what items of food should be avoided while under homoeopathic treatment? There is widespread misunderstanding on this score and it may be as well for us to dispel some wrong notions, such as that coffee, onion, garlic, etc. are taboo.

69. Dr. J.N. Kanjilal emphasises in his article "Homoeopathic Regimen" (*Hahn. Gleanings*, Feb. 1976) that since ho-

moeopathy treats the individual patient, taking into account his peculiar constitution, desires, aversions, etc., we cannot be blind to the real requirements of the soul or personality of the individual patient, in taking a decision with respect to the regimen for him. From the theoretical point of view, pathological diagnosis may dictate a particular type of food and drink as being essential, but if it goes against the taste and desire of the patient, it is likely to do him little good, rather it may cause harm. Vice versa, from theoretical consideration, a particular item of food or drink may appear harmful to the patient, but if he has a strong craving for the same, you cannot totally prohibit it without causing any harm. For example, in a case of dropsy total prohibition of drinking water may cause harm if the patient has strong thirst. On the other hand, with disease having perverted his desires, a patient may strongly demand such an item of food or drink which is likely to be very harmful to him. A rational physician cannot blindly abide by such desires and aversions; rather, he has to critically assess the real nature of those desires. Yet, he can never totally ignore the desires and aversions. Judicious prescription of diet and regimen is far easier in acute cases when the desires, etc. are so glaring, than in chronic cases. What applies to diet holds true for all other aspects of the regimen such as the patient's preference for cold or warm environment, covering, bath, rest, sexual act, etc.

70. It has been the general observation of a number of physicians like Kanjilal, Sankaran, etc. that we need not impose abrupt stoppage of long accustomed habits and addictions like tea, coffee, tobacco, liquors, etc. though we must advice them to gradually reduce them. However, where the morbid affection can be traced directly to a particular addiction, *e.g.*, excessive smoking in cases of chronic pharyngitis, tobacco chewing or excessive intake of tea or coffee in case of gastritis, liquors in cases of cirrhosis of the liver, we have to insist on quick control and ultimate abandonment of those maintaining causes.

71. One more point about restrictions on diet has to be considered. Hahnemann and Kent have unequivocally stressed that when a patient is under the influence of a certain remedy, the items of food or drink which cause the trouble and thus call for that remedy should be avoided. If this is not done, the action of the remedy will be hindered. In fact Hahnemann has expressed himself against the indiscriminate restrictions which needlessly increase the difficulty of patients. Kent, in his *Lec-*

tures on *Materia Medica* and Mrs. J.T. Kent in an article have advised us to caution patients who are under the influence of certain remedies, to avoid the use of certain foods, lest the action of the remedies be upset, and the patients fail to get their benefit. Some examples of remedies and their aggravating foods are given in the table that follows.

72. It goes without saying that after he is cured, the patient can eat those very things with impunity.

Remedy	Food to be avoided	Remedy	Food to be avoided
Bryonia	Sauer-Kraut, vegetable salad, chicken salad.	Pulsatilla, Carb-veg., China.	Fats(Ghee, Oils) Butter, Fruits, (in indigestion)
Lycopodium Thuja	Oysters	Bryonia, Lycopodium, Petroleum.	Cabbage
Chamomilla Nux-vomica, Causticum	Coffee	Arsenicum, Nux-vomica, Lyco, Rhus-tox,Puls.	Cold and frozen foods.
Calc-c. Nitric-ac., Sepia	Milk	Argent-nit., Ignatia.	Candy, Sweets.
		Kali-bich. Nux-vomica.	Beer
Antim-crud.	Sour things, vinegar and sour wine.	China, Ignatia, Nux-vom., Puls.	See "Food agg." in Repertory
Graphites, Puls.	Pork		Tobacco
Cantharis, Nux-vomica, Sepia	Drinking cold water.	Puls.,Colch., China ars.	Eggs.

Management of the Case

73. In regimen too, individuality is the keynote. A cold wash or ice bag is contra-indicated in the case of an *Antim-crud.* patient, who is made worse by it. A *Ledum* patient of rheumatism feels worse by hot applications, though the joints are inflamed and swollen. A *Tabacum* patient of heart troubles feels worse in lying position; a *Gelsemium* patient of Anginal pain cannot stay in bed, as he feels better by movement. A *Psorinum* patient of Asthma feels better when lying on back with limbs wide apart, while a *Medorrhinum* patient of Asthma feels better when in knee-chest position.

74. It may be noted here that cooking in aluminium vessels has deleterious effects on health, and this point should be enquired into when case-taking. *Cadmium-oxide* in potency is reputed to be the most rapid antidote to the bad effects of eating food cooked in aluminium vessels.

75. **Air pollution.** In all large industrial towns, industrial fumes and smoke are vitiating the atmosphere. The *Sulphur dioxide* which is said to be one of the chief ingredients of the "air pollution", is said to be responsible for certain respiratory diseases like Bronchitis, Bronchial asthma and Emphysema. The provings of *Sulphurous acid* which Dr. Grimmer conducted and subsequent clinical applications have shown that this remedy in the 30th potency is most effective in meeting these respiratory conditions caused by air pollution.

76. **Emotional environment.** Persons who are completely free from anxieties, fears, irritations and frustrations of one type or another are indeed rare. It is a strong conviction with homoeopaths that most of the ills that man is heir to have their origin in these mental conditions, and no wonder that strong mental symptoms play a vital role in the selection of the remedy. Not only does the homoeopath unearth the peculiar twists of mind to guide him in the selection of the remedy, but this very process casts him in the ideal role of a counsellor, nay, a psychiatrist. Whenever he finds an emotionally chronic patient, it is in fact his duty, and should be his pleasure, to use his authority to advise those looking after or attending on the patient to assure congenial, sympathetic and hope inspiring atmosphere without which medicine alone would fail of its purpose. In this connection the following major needs of each person, if he is to be at peace with himself and those around him, must be kept in mind ·

(i) The first major need is the physical need of food, shelter and safety.

(ii) The second need is that he achieves or succeeds in a given area that seems important to him.

(iii) The need to avoid failure — he does not have the capacity to face, much less to learn from failure.

iv) Ability to master an area, to be superior in one thing.

(v) Need to receive recognition and approval of those who, he feels, are important in his life.

(vi) Need for sympathy and affection.

(vii) Need for security — in job, in finance, in the love of one's family.

(viii) Craving for something new, something different, a chance to be creative, to try a new adventure — for a free outlet or expression of his creative energies.

(ix) Need for physical sexuality and love, the satisfaction of biological need — unless the person finds complete absorption in a mission (like a Monk or a Scientist) more satisfying.

77. When a patient comes to the doctor, he is in a crisis, he comes with a cry for help. At this juncture the homoeopathic doctor is able not only to listen to him, relieve his tension, give him a catharsis, and give him the right type of advice, but also, in the process, to find the curative medicinal agent and thus help the patient to an equilibrium of functioning. Above all, the patient's hope of recovery should never be given a blow even under the most difficult conditions, but on the contrary he should be doubly reassured of ultimate recovery.

78. **Drug effects — Tautopathy.** Patients take all kinds of drugs, either from doctors or by self-medication, in their anxiety to get rid of their diseases. Not all the drugs are innocuous, and many of them leave strong after effects, which act as obstacles to cure. This was so even in Hahnemann's time, and it has been the practice of many homoeopaths to antidote these effects with a first prescription of *Nux-vomica*. But such antidotes are obvi-

ously powerless in the face of the modern powerful drugs. The curative action of homoeopathic remedies is achieved not by their chemical action but through dynamic action which stimulates and strengthens the vital force i.e., the natural defence mechanism, to overcome the disease. But, "it has been noted that antibiotics unfavourably influence the defence mechanism in the human body, a fact which has been confirmed also by animal experiments. It was found that the administration of Penicillin to healthy individuals causes a decrease in the leucocyte count'. ("Gainslen and Lehmann). Again, "Antibiotics in the usual dosage do not effect complete destruction of the micro-organism, because they act mainly as bacteriostatics. The final destruction of the germs is, therefore, left to the body's own defences, e.g., Phagocytosis, antibody formation, bactericidal activity of the serum, etc." (Thalhammer, Replot, Chemsuz, Vogt, Gunther). Allergic shocks are many on records during antibiotic treatment, not to mention various side-effects. "Peptic ulcer and migration of prostatic cancer to the breast are known side-effects of therapeutic hormones. Metastasis to the breast may occur when estrogen is given for prostatic carcinoma." Dr. L.G. Cope, Physician at the Post-Graduate Medical School of London has said : "Cortisone and Corticotrophin do not cure, they merely suppress some manifestation of disease." Further, patients are known to become resistant to drugs.

79. When the natural defence mechanism of the body is thus thrown out of gear, it is small wonder that even the highest potencies of homoeopathic remedies fail to penetrate the barrier. Fortunately, the law of similars and the law of least action can together rescue us from this situation. (The law of least action, formulated by Maupertius, the French mathematician, and known to homoeopaths as the law of quantity and dose reads : The quantity of action necessary to effect any change in nature is the least possible ; the decisive amount is always a minimum, an infinitesimal). According to this law, which is better known an Arndt-Schultz law, "Small doses stimulate, medium doses paralyze and large doses kill." More concretely : A toxic substance (drug) which has become fixed in the system can be liberated and eliminated from the system by an infinitesimal dilution of the same substance; in other words, the effect of crude drugs on a living organism can be antidoted by the minimal dose of the same drug. Mr. D.W. Everitt. a pharmacist of England, named this method as tautopathy, and in our own country Dr. Ramanlal P. Patel has done much to popularise it.

Sulphathiazole, Penicillin, Chloromycetin, Streptococcin, Staphylococcin, Cortisone, etc. run up to potencies of 6th, 30th or above are now available.

80. Before administering any tautopathic potency we have to find out from the patient or the previous physician what medicines were given. We then have to give the same medicine in potentised form in 6th to 30th potency. Dr. Patel writes, "After waiting for four days or a week, we are amazed to see how it clears up the case. Sometimes I have noted that there is no need of prescribing any other homoeopathic drug as, in such cases, patients recover completely . . . If we cannot wait long, we may, after giving the tautopathic drug in 30 or higher, prescribe the homoeopathic drug in low potency as an alternating or intercurrent medicine . . . as different potencies have different planes of action." Dr. Sankaran has reported (Journal of Homoeopathic Medicine, December 1966) a case with difficulty in articulating speech after a history of typhoid for which the patient was given Chloromycetin. Causticum, the indicated remedy failed in different potencies. He was thereupon put on *Chloromycetin* 30, three doses a day for three days and later on *Causticum* 1M and "there was an immediate and very satisfactory improvement and within a month he was arguing in the court." Dr. N.P. Sukerkar reports a case of chronic stomatitis, irregular menses and attacks of tachycardia in a patient with a history of two attacks of paratyphoid within two years when she was treated with large doses of *Chloromycetin*. She felt better within four days of receiving two doses of *Chloromycetin* 200. In another two weeks she received two doses of *Chloromycetin* 1M. After a month "she was a new person . . . . better in every way." She was then given a dose of *Typhoidinum* 1M" as I have invariably followed these cases with *Typhoidinum* 200 or 1M." (J.H.M. Sept. 1963).

81. These examples show the advisability of taking advantage of tautopathic drugs whenever a patient comes with a past history of heavy or prolonged drugging with modern medicines, before we can hope for the indicated homoeopathic remedy to be effective.

SELF-TEST

1. What is the significance of Hering's Laws of Cure? Explain how they help us to decide whether a remedy is acting curatively or not. (Para 2)

Management of the Case

2. What are the five factors which govern the time taken for positive action of a remedy to show itself? Is the time taken in acute diseases long or short? (Page 7)

3. What course should we follow as regards repetition of dose, in order to obtain positive action in continued fevers? (Para 10). How does it differ from chronic cases? (Para 11)

4. How can we avoid aggravation of symptoms which is likely to arise after giving of a remedy? (Para 29)

5. What are the circumstances in which we are justified in repeating the same remedy, but in lower potency? (Para 38). How do they contrast with the circumstance in which we can repeat the same remedy, but in higher potencies? (Para 37)

6. When would it be necessary to administer an entirely new remedy? What type of symptom is the best guide in the selection of the new remedy? (Para 41)

7. Why do we, sometimes, have to give one remedy after another? Is it advisable to do so, and why? (Para 42)

8. What are the circumstances in which we should refrain from repeating the dose, but must wait and watch? What is the harm in repetition in such cases? (Para 46)

9. Explain what is meant by the statement : "There is a thin line dividing the antidotal and complementary relationship." What part does the "timing of administration" play in changing the nature of reaction to antidotal or complementary? (Para 55-58)

10. In diet and regimen too, individuality is the keynote. Explain with examples, how this principle is applied in practice. (Para 63-67)

LESSON 9

THE CHRONIC MIASMS AND NOSODES

1. The discovery and development of the theory of the chronic miasms on the part of Hahnemann can truly be said to be yet another epoch-making event in the history of curative medicine. As we have noted earlier, finding that even the best selected remedies acted only as temporary palliatives in chronic cases, Hahnemann delved deeply into the past personal and family histories of a large number of such cases and it is only after twelve long years of such close study and verifications of his tentative conclusions, that he announced to the world the full details of his discovery. He propounded that the true natural chronic diseases are those which owe their origin to a chronic parasitic miasm or germs (or chronic micro-organisms, as we would call them now-a-days), and this, fifty years before Koch and Pasteur discovered micro-organisms as the cause of illnesses. He called them chronic because they constantly extend their tentacles and, notwithstanding the most carefully regulated mental and bodily habits, diet or a robust constitution, they never cease to torment their victim with constantly renewed suffering to the end of life. Then again, "All chronic diseases are so inveterate immediately after they have become developed in the system, that unless they are thoroughly cured by the (homoeopathic) art, they continue to increase in intensity until the moment of death."

2. Dr. Bach used to say, "How did Hahnemann know that infection was instantaneous? It took us three months at U.C.H. to demonstrate this during the war ... If you scarify a rabbit, and take two dabs one in each hand, of streptococcus and of iodine, and dab on iodine as fast as you can after the other (streptococcus) you are too late to prevent infection."

3. Hahnemann further tells us that "the least remains of a germ may eventually repoduce the full disease" and hence the treatment must go on till the cure is complete.

4. Yet another characteristic of the chronic disease is that they do not merely end with the individual patient's life but the taint is passed on from generation to generation.

5. It thus became Hahnemann's aim, in his study, to take into consideration these deeper conditions from which sprang the acute diseases. And it was his aim to find a remedy which would meet the acute condition, and the presumably hidden underlying chronic condition as well at the same time.

6. As a result of his long study Hahnemann traced the sources of chronic diseases to three types of infections, the *Psoric*, the *Syphilitic* and the Sycotic; he called them "Miasms" which we may better understand to mean "stigmata" or "taint," arising from the respective intractable poisons. As for the two venereal miasms of *Syphilis* and *Sycosis* (gonorrhoeal), there was no doubt even in his time and his dicta about them are now amply confirmed.

7. About the *Psoric* miasm, however, there has been much controversy because Hahnemann attributed it to the stubborn skin eruptions, the acarus of the itch mite, leprosy, etc. He described *Psora* as the hydra-headed "mother of all diseases" and asserted that there was a traceable relationship between many chronic ailments enumerated in pathological works under distinct names on the one hand, and the various types of skin and glandular manifestations, nutritional disturbances and acute as well as infectious diseases on the other. He found that various forms of disease were first made manifest on the skin attended with considerable itching, as skin was the natural place where *Psora* thrives and did least harm. But when suppressed by many forms of treatment such as ointments, removal of organs, etc. this constitutional state becomes more manifest in a train of distressing symptoms in any part of the body, so long as the skin manifestation is quiescent.

8. While conflicting opinions have been expressed about how far the *Psora* theory is scientific or not, Margaret Tyler, who is perhaps one of the few prescribers who achieved many magical cures because of her unique mastery of the miasmatic approach, says "Some day someone among the pathologists will

demonstrate his perspicacity in regard to *Psora* also, by proving that the acarus is the intermediate host of some microorganism responsible for one or more chronic diseases of manifold manifestations. For, Hahnemann gives numerous instances, from many writers, of itch cured by outward applications, having been followed by chest troubles — Asthma, epilepsy, gastric ulcer, dropsy, albuminuria, even eye troubles and cataract." In support of this statement Tyler says that "It is possible to cure itch by internal treatment" and cites the case of a boy who got nothing but the *Psorinum* CM. (Oil of Lavendar being too costly for local application) and was found to have been cured by it.

9. **Suppressions.** Since time immemorial it has been the first and primary object of physicians to remove any morbid state on the skin or mucous membrane, and regard such removal by whatever means as a "cure". They had little regard for the fact that such manifestations on the skin are but an effort on the part of the vital force to protect the more vital parts of the organism, and that in the exercise of this protective function, the lesions are removed or thrown out to tissues and parts where the morbid disease force can do least harm to the life. Therefore, the homoeopathic system has always frowned upon such forcing back of the poisons into the interior by strong local treatment, as it works detrimentally to a radical cure. The readiness with which skin diseases are treated or the discharges from mucous surfaces dried up exclusively by local measures, this readiness and anxiety has been responsible to no small extent for driving the *Psoric, Syphilitic* or *Sycotic* poisons within, to attack the more vital organs and regions. This has resulted in the great increase of incurable chronic maladies that affect mankind.

10. But it is not only the external applications that suppress disease. All medication which is not homoeopathic is suppressive in nature and effect, So long as we depend on the diagnosis of the "disease" and treat the disease and not the patient, so long will the treatment be suppressive. A "mere constipation" will be neglected or palliated till there is an enlargement of liver or an intestinal disorder as a concrete manifestation of "disease". A "mere cold, or tendency to constant colds" will be regarded as of no consequence or just palliated, till he develops bronchitis, asthma or phthisis. Chronic diseases have their progression from childhood, and if the vital force is not given aid in the right direction (which only homoeopathic potencies

can do), instead of the normal formation of tissues and normal functions of organs, we shall be confronted with a steady evolution of various "new" diseases each time an "old" one is "cured", until we get frank abnormalities like tumours asthma, emphysema, Bright's disease, and so on. All this only means that what is diagnosed as "disease" today is really no "disease", but its "effect". A true homoeopath, therefore, does not go by a particular "disease" in any particular part of the body, but he understands that the whole man is sick. He does not limit his attention to the present illness alone, in a chronic case, but takes the man as one entity in the entire time phase since childhood, and even going back into his ancestry. If the man's physical organs like liver, heart, lungs or kidney are sick today, it only means that the man was sick long before these expressions of diseases came. The homoeopath who has mastered the nature of the chronic miasms will not find it difficult to decide what are the miasms which the child has inherited and what course they will take in future, or have already taken in the past in the case of a grown-up man. It is this knowledge alone which enables a homoeopath to do his best work, by undoing the suppressions and putting the man on the road to recovery. If, however, there is advanced pathology, cure may not be possible and one will have to be satisfied with palliation. These remarks are not mere theory, but have been born out of the concrete experience of hundreds and thousands of masters of the homoeopathic art.

11. **Miasms and totality.** Why is it necessary for us to know about the chronic miasms? Is it not sufficient if we follow the totality of symptoms and select the most similar medicine possible for curing our cases? J.H. Allen answers, "The fact is, we cannot select the most similar remedy unless we understand the phenomena of the acting and the basic miasms; for, the true similia is always based on the existing basic miasms, whether we be conscious of the fact or not."

12. If we have no knowledge of Psora, Syphilis and Sycosis, it would mean we have no knowledge of the characters and habits of the enemy. The work of these miasms is often hidden for years; so latent and pent-up are these forces in the organism. If we base our prescription only on the totality of the symptoms that are entirely nervous or reflex, in reality we would not have considered the more important and basic values in the totality. The reflexes are always secondary, while the primary

and basic symptoms (values) are directly of miasmatic origin. The nervous phenomena may be palliated by such a procedure, but it returns, and time is lost in the experiment; but the physician skilled in anti-miasmatic prescribing overlooks the foamings upon the surface, dips deeper into the case looking for *prima causa morbi*, and applies a remedial agent that has a deeper and closer relationship with the perverted life force. The nature and character of disease (perverted life force) depends wholly upon the form of the miasm and the character of its bond with the life force. Therefore, our study of disease should become a study into the nature of the miasm present and the degree of its activity. The life force manufactures any pathological formation depending upon the existing or acting miasm. If the miasm be psoric we have psoric manifestations. If sycotic, we have sycotic pathology; if syphilitic, we have the polymorphic pathological presentations of that miasm.

13. **Fragmentary presentation of diseases.** The reason why diseases continue to reappear, though in ever varying or modified forms, is because they do not constitute the disease in toto, and the ostensible disease is a mere fragment of a much more deep-seated evil that has taken possession of the whole organism. Therefore, we ought not to treat them as separate and completely developed maladies in local parts only, since there is something within the whole organism that is at variance with the life in general.

14. **Symptoms guiding us to the miasmatic background.** Hahnemann, therefore, advised that our prescription should be based on those symptoms that are centralised upon the existing, active chronic miasms. How can we do this? Again, J.H. Allen exhorts, "By the study of the Organon of Medicine and the Chronic Disease. How shall we learn the symptoms of the miasms? By a study of each of the chronic miasms, Psora, Syphilis and Sycosis, in all their stages and in all their blendings." The Materia Medica is but the reflected image of the disease that are to be cured. You can see Psora in *Sulphur* and in *Lycopodium*, in *Arsenicum* and *Psorinum*; you can see Syphilis in the *Mercuries*, in the *Iodides* and in *Nitric acid*; you can see Sycosis in *Rhus*, in *Thuja, Kali-sulph., Capsicum, Medorrhinum* and a host of others. A study of the whole range of derangements of health, and the types of derangements — from the simple physiological to the gross pathological — which each remedy can cause (and, therefore, can cure) would be amply rewarding.

15. As the other side of the coin, the constitution of each patient should be carefully studied, for the various diseases he has suffered from will be found to be dependent upon some miasmatic basis. The physician who cannot detect the presence of Sycosis in his patient, without a history of gonorrhoea, says J.H. Allen, "has very little knowledge of the miasmatics. But with such knowledge he can head off Phthisis in its incipiency, before an abscess forms in the lung tissue, as he would be familiar with the phenomena".

16. Among the remedies having the same symptoms as to the external form, the one corresponding to the active, basic miasm ranks higher. Therefore, in selecting the remedy we should arrange the symptoms according to their value, giving preference to those last appearing, for they are the symptoms of the active miasm, and classifying the remainder as belonging to the latent grouping. If these should continue after the active symptoms have disappeared, it may be necessary to study them for a new selection.

17. In our study of miasms it is worth remembering that often times a single persistent symptom may guide us to the discovery of some one of the chronic miasms which we were searching for, for an indefinite time, during the treatment of a case. For example, the severe itching or the plethora of subjective symptoms of Psora; the ulcerative processes, aggravation at night or tendency to constantly wash the hands of Syphilitic miasm. The day-light aggravation, chronic pelvic disorders of women or sleeping in knee-chest position of the Sycotic miasm.

18. **Some characteristic differences between the three miasms.** We shall now mention a few of the most important characteristic differences between the three miasms, which when they are driven in, become latent and begin to attack the vital organs, although it may not be correct to draw a hard and fast line between them. Knowledge of these differences will help us to classify the symptomatology of each case at a given occasion and to find the corresponding similimum.

19. It is well to bear in mind that when we are dealing with a case with mixed miasms, we always find one miasm uppermost as revealed by symptoms as compared with the others, and naturally that uppermost miasm should claim our

prior attention in selecting the remedy. When that is removed, the next prominent miasm must be carried for taking the totality of symptoms present, until the patient is freed from the inheritance of generations. Yet. Sycosis, if present in any form, or in any stage, usually takes precedence of the three miasms.

20. For a detailed exposition, in Schematic form, of the comparative characteristics of the three Miasms, including Pseudo-Psora, the Tubercular taint, the reader is strongly urged to study the small, but valuable work "A Comparison of the Chronic Miasms" by Phyllis Speight. However, a few important differentiating characteristics of these Miasms are given in the Appendices 'F', 'G' and 'H'.

21. **Acute primary infections**. We have not dealt with the acute primary action of the *Syphilitic* or *Gonorrhoeal* infections, such as the Chancre of Syphilis or the muco-purulent urethral discharge of Gonorrhoea after the prodromal period of 12 to 15 days and of 8 to 12 days respectively. These acute phases are easily curable by the remedies that conform to the nature of the discharge provided they are not complicated with the third chronic miasm Psora. It is when they have been suppressed and driven in that they are a dozen times more grievous than when in the primary stage.

22. There is one point worth noting in this connection. When a man who has gone through the primary manifestations of one of the contagions marries, his wife too takes the contagion, but she does not go through the primary manifestations. The disease is transferred from husband to wife in the stage in which it then exists at the time of their marriage, and from thence goes on in a progressive way. When we give anti-sycotic or anti-syphilitic treatment to such people, they will bring back only that stage which they began with. It will not bring out a discharge or a chancre. She can get well without its return. The reverse order in her case only means the reverse order of those symptoms she has had. The same holds true of the infant with syphilitic or sycotic parents.

23. It is good for the physician to know the miasmatic history of the patient. If a patient has gone through a serious acute illness, he will remain semi-quiescent instead of making for

The Chronic Miasms and Nosodes

speedy recovery. But when, at this time, he is given an anti-syphilitic or anti-sycotic or anti-psoric remedy as the case may be, he will then begin to rally fast. If this is not known to the physician, many patients will gradually sink for want of vitality to convalesce.

24. Deep-acting remedies are miasmatic. A list of remedies having anti-psoric, anti-syphilitic and anti-sycotic action, as given in Kent's Repertory, is given in Appendices J., K., L., M. A list showing the depth of action of remedies given in the editorial of *Hahn. Gleanings* (May, 1978) has also been given in Appendix 'I'.

25. It will be seen that as a rule all the deep-acting remedies belong to one or more miasms. This fact simplifies our task very much since, if we select the similimum from one of the deep-acting remedies, all of which are fully represented in the Repertories, the selection will automatically cover the miasm concerned also. Yet, a more conscious effort to identify the miasmatic background of the patient and also to check up if the remedy selected does meet that miasm, would be advisable. This exercise on the part of the physician will develop his mastery of this aspect of chronic prescribing. This ability will also give him the power to forestall and prevent the development of destructive processes of many chronic diseases, right from childhood or youth. In fact, treatment commencing at the antinatal period is the special field of homoeopathy which gives the hard-working physician the most brilliant results in the eradication of chronic diseases and hereditary taints. As one grows older and pathology develops, the road is paved with incurability.

NOSODES — AN EXTENSION OF PSORA

26. In an excellent paper on "Nosodes" (*Hom. Heritage* Jan. 1979) Dr. Guy Buckley Stearns, M.D., remarked about influenzinum that "If we were to add another chronic miasm to those already suggested, influenza should be placed at the head of the list. It is vicious, hydra-headed and ubiquitous. Its ramifications are so extensive that a full description calls for the rich vocabulary that Hahnemann applied to psora". On reading this we wondered how many miasms we are going to have. We got the answer in Dr. Koppikar's lecture delivered at the International Homoeopathic Congress, 1980 (*Hom. Heritage*, Dec. 1989), in the course of which he has drawn pointed attention to Margaret

Tyler's pregnant remarks : "One cannot doubt that were Hahnemann alive today, the chronic parasitic non-venereal disease psora would have long ago sorted itself out into not one but a dozen such," Ever since Hahnemann developed Psorinum, homoeopaths have followed on with quite a number of preparations of disease products for the cure and prevention of diseases. To which class do all these preparations belong? We are inclined to think that they all belong to Psora which Hahnemann with such great vision, described as "hydra-headed", "mother of all diseases". As Tyler aptly says, "Psora has been sorting itself out into not one but a dozen such". All the non-venereal nosodes we have, are but the hydra-heads of Psora, which Kent describes is a susceptibility to disease, being the effect of man's evil thoughts.

27. It is to Dr. Swan that we are indebted for many of agents, known as Nosodes, and to his indomitable perseverance in the face of the most strenuous opposition to his advocacy of them by his oft-repeated generalisation, "Morbific matter will cure the disease which produced it, if given in a high potency, even to the person from whom it was obtained." The law of homoeopathy is that a drug or poison which can produce a symptom, or a group of symptoms in a healthy person, will cure the similar symptom, or group of symptoms when occuring in the sick. Now, it is well known that the poison which causes a sickness or disease, inheres in the products of such sickness or disease. Thus, the saliva of rabies, or mercurial salivation, of measles, scarlet fever, diphtheria, contain the poison that produced the disease. Potentise the saliva and you capture the poison in all cases. To the charge that this was "Isopathy" he replied that the application of the crude poison to effect a cure is Isopathy (like vaccination for small-pox), but the potentisation of the isopathic product makes it homoeopathic to the disease which produced it, and it cannot have any curative action on that disease till potentised.

28. As for proving them on healthy persons, Swan pointed out that Morbilin, Scarletinin, Diphtheritinum, Variolinum, Pyrogenium, Psorinum, Syphilinum, Medorrhinum — all these are the fullest proved poisons in existence; they have been proving for hundreds of years by tens of thousands of persons, old and young, male and female. Carefully collect all the symptoms produced by them on healthy people, and you have their pathogenetic effects, to guide you in curing people suffering from

similar diseases. Nevertheless, Swan himself proved a number of Nosodes. H.C. Allen's *The Materia Medica of the Nosodes* today represents the most complete work on the symptomatology of the Nosodes.

29. When Hahnemann postulated the theory of the Miasms as being the cause of chronic diseases, he sought to reach the underlying taints which caused the innumerable morbid aberrations. The fundamental aim of the real physician is to remove those taints. As the Nosodes have been found of incalculable service in reaching constitutional dyscrasia beyond the sphere of our ordinary, even miasmatic remedies, Allen's work is invaluable to every prescriber desiring to get at the characteristics of the Nosodes and the various diseases to which they are specifically related.

30. It is beyond the scope of this book to mention even briefly the numerous cases in which one Nosode or another has opened way to magical cures of intractable and baffling diseases, but one thing becomes clear from them that the more immunity is studied, the more obvious it becomes that every disease due to a poison of any kind needs an exactly prescribed anti-poison. The individual variations in the case of any constitutional taint are thus met by precise indications derived from the study of the Nosodes. As Dr. Koppikar says in his editorial of *Homoeopathic Heritage* (July, 1989), "The Psoric condition" may be one, but the psoric `infections' are quite a few. Even viruses can cause Psora. Malaria can become Psoric. That is why we find Nosodes like Influenzin, Diphtherinum, Pneumococcin, Bacillinum, Pyrogen, Morbillin, Streptococcin etc. extremely powerful and most valuable remedies in the treatment of chronic and even acute diseases."

31. **The Duncan Method.** Nosodes can be prepared from diseased tissues and secretions or from bacterial cultures. Occasionally, excellent results have followed the use of potencies of the culture made from a local infection of the patient himself. H.C. Duncan of New York has given his name to an autogenous treatment wherein he takes any disease exudate from a patient, puts it through a Berkfeld filter and injects the filtrate. He claims excellent results. Undoubtedly this would work just as well if potentised and given by mouth.

32. **Will Nosodes Complete the Cure?** Opinion is divided as to whether the Nosodes can complete the cure or whether

they improve the patient upto a point only and thereafter the constitutional remedy, anti-psoric, anti-syphilitic or anti-sycotic as the case may be is necessary to complete the cure. Stearns, Pulford and Farrington held the opinion that the Nosodes did good work when the "apparently indicated" remedies did not help, but after sometime you have to follow them up with some other indicated remedy. Thus, the role of the Nosode and the constitutional remedy becomes complementary in tackling difficult cases. No progress can be made by dependence on any one of these alone. There is another school of thought: Nosodes can cure cases independently, on the basis of their characteristic symptoms, just like other remedies. A glance through H. C. Allen's book on Nosodes confirms this view.

33. **Magical Cures with Nosodes.** We shall now give in very brief outline only, some of the magical cures effected by the Nosodes. These concrete instances will not only enlighten us about the potencies to be used, the question of repetitions, and whether they can cure alone without the aid of other remedies.

34. **Tuberculinum :**

(i) At a get-together of doctors in a restaurant, the waiter, a tall, thin German who had been in the war, asked the doctor what he should do for a painful boil on the nape of his neck. Dr. James Krichbaum looked at him and, before anyone else had a chance to think, said : "That man is fighting tuberculosis. He needs a dose of *Tuberculinum.*" A powder of the 10M was given and brought relief at once and the condition was cured within three days.

(ii) A teacher had developed severe pain in her right hip, diagnosed as sciatica. Most careful prescription failed. For the acute inflammation of hip joint, the leg was placed in an extension apparatus, but the pain continued. One day, at their wit's end, Drs. Rabe and Stearns applied the rule that, where an apparently indicated remedy fails, one should study the Nosodes. *Tuberculinum-bovine* 10M was given with prompt relief. Two repetitions in higher potencies carried her through but she was left with an ankylosed hip joint. Too much time had been lost at the start. (Stearns)

(iii) Another case with the same character of symptoms, but with a red streak down the middle of her tongue, which led to *Chamomilla* had great relief from it; but within fortyeight hours, it ceased to help and a dose of *Tuberculinum-bovine* 10M took up the cure and she recovered without the use of an extension splint and without any resulting lameness. By the way, *Tuberculinum* has "red streak in the centre of the tongue". (G.B. Stearns)

35. **Psorinum.** I remember the case of a boy who had the Itch badly. I did not want to give him *Sulphur* because I had recently seen a much sulphured boy with repulsive and horrible pustular mix up. I gave him *Psorinum* C.M. and when he again appeared, was found to have been cured. (Tyler)

36. **Variolinum :**

(i) What about the illness of persons who have had small-pox-even forty or fifty years previously — which are astonishingly amenable to infrequent doses of Variolinum? One remembers a very neurotic patient, everybody's despair, who was found to have once had smallpox. She returned to comparative normality after Variolinum was administered (Tyler)

(ii) A lady 39 years old had small pox badly at 9 years old and was badly pitted. She got *Variolinum* 200, 1 dose. After a month, less deeply pitted. *Variol.* 200, 1 dose. After four months : She says, "I am very much better." Since then, at intervals, for various ailments, she has been given a dose of *Variol.* which has helped her. Now, at a short distance, one would not notice that she had smallpox. (Tyler)

(iii) A patient now 56 years with cataract and glycosuria. Had small pox as a 3 years old, was given several doses of *Variol.* at long intervals. The sugar varies; but a report a few months later reads : "Wonderfully well; no thirst or hunger. Eyes clearer; good colour; less pitting". (Tyler)

(iv) Another out-patient for gastric troubles, retching, etc., had for years been to different doctors. Had small pox when 7 years old; now 55. Got *Variol.* 200, 1 dose in March, July and September, says "The medicine worked like magic on me."

(v) A case of abscesses in both nostrils which prevented her for years breathing through nose, till *Variol.* which not only improved the unsightly deformity, but enabled her to breathe again through nostrils. (Tyler)

37. Pneumococcin. What about sicknesses that occur after Pneumonia? . . . A case of *Chorea* in a child, with a temperature and heart affected. The child had Pneumonia twice, and Broncho-pneumonia twice. One single dose of *Pneumococcin* 30 promptly cured the Chorea and put the heart right. (Tyler)

38. Medorrhinum :

(i) Scald head in an infant three weeks old. The child cries day and night, cannot be quietened even by being carried about. It drives the patient wild . . . Having treated the father several years ago for gonorrhoea and knowing his outs. I at once prescribed *Medorrhinum* 200, which, to my great surprise, gave decided relief. I followed this with *Calc-sulph.* 30 as an intercurrent remedy with good success. (L. Guthers)

(ii) Another child, screams day and night. It cries itself to sleep and awakens crying; cannot be pacified at all; hands clenched and striking against its head. After nursing throws up milk which is sour and curdled. Both father and mother had been subjects of gonorrhoea. After *Medor.* 200 the child was quietened at once and my faith in it was much stronger. (L. Guthers)

(iii) During the war we had cases of severe Gonorrhoeal rheumatism among the sailors, which responded excellently to *Medorrhinum.* (Tyler)

(iv) In one case, the disease having been contracted 9 years previously there was high temperature, profuse sweating, several joints affected — swollen, very painful and full of fluid; besides which there was grave iritis and conjunctivitis. The patient was a disgusting spectacle; unable to sleep for pain and jerking of limbs, and could not see even to feed himself. After a few doses of *Medorrhinum* 30, he rapidly improved. Joints less swollen; sleeping without the jerks and starts. For fluctuations, the medicine was repeated, 30, 200, 1M at longish intervals. He was soon able to read large print than small. A corneal ulcer appeared, and rapidly disappeared. And he went out practically well, and able to read ordinary print. (Hahnemann says that the cure of venereal diseases is only difficult and tedious when they are complicated with psora). (Tyler)

(v) A delicate case of a girl, 9 years old, came for soreness and discharge, vulva. Swab showed gonococci. *Medorrh.* 10M, one dose. Next month, better herself, better colour. "Some days hardly any discharge which is now watery. No irritation now." *Med.* CM. After two months, "Discharge was gone." Child has grown Swab — "no gonococci." (Tyler)

39. Pyrogen :

Pyrogenium is a wonderful remedy because of its wide range of usefulness : (P.C. Majumdar). Dr. Sankaran called it "Homoeopathic broad-spectrum antibiotic". According to Majumdar, it is in the true type of enteric fever that its efficacy is so marked . . . Also in ptomaine poisoning. The following case of Dr. Majumdar illustrates its use :

A robust middle aged man had to sit for a long time near a putrefactive dead body. From the next day he developed pain over the whole body as if bruised, utter prostration, high fever, purging and vomiting. Pulse full, yet very frequent. Temperature 105°F. Tympanitic distension of abdomen. *Pyrogen* 6th, one dose every six hours. After two doses temperature fell to 99 F., pains subsided as well as purging. Next day owing to indiscretion in food purging and fever returned. *Pyrogen* 200, one dose. Patient was cured.

40. Diphtherinum.

Envisage the possibility that even diphtheria or mumps, in a generation back, may possibly prove an indication for such a remedy as *Diphtherinum* or *Parotidinum*, which may be found to influence the case, whatever its nature. We say of "whatever nature" advisedly because, in the most amazing case we ever came across, "diphtheria, badly, at years of age, and never well since", led to the administration of *Diphth-*

erinum 200, to end, within a fortnight, twelve years of great pain in the eye, in a monstrosity one cannot otherwise describe of a girl of eighteen. When first seen she had an enormous head, bulging forehead, big right eye displaced downwards on to the cheek. "Multiple tumours of brain" : sight and hearing affected; wasting of one-half of the tongue; paralysis of one side of throat. Much pain and lachrymation in the displaced right eye. That a few doses of potentised *Diphtherinum* could have terminated, once and for all, twelve years of pain that morphia had only lulled to temporary unconsciousness . . . affords a striking example of what the advanced homoeopathy of Hahnemann's later researches, when still further extended to embrace other chronic conditions based on early acute infectious disease, can accomplish. (Tyler)

41. We could go on giving many, many more cases of this type cured by such "advanced homoeopathy" not only in the West, but even by many homoeopaths in India, but space forbids. We feel tempted to report Tyler's cure of Carcinoma of head of pancreas with *Parotidinum* 200, three doses six hourly, on her past history of Measles and the hint : "Mumps affects the pancreas" ; she had then to be given *Morbill* for history of Measles. Another case of a 66 years old patient nearly blind in both eyes; glaucoma on left eye; much pain; "too old for surgery; arteries hard and tortous". And *Pneumococcin* 200 a few doses (on history of pleurisy and double pneumonia) improved his sight amazingly; haemorrhage nearly gone. Dr. Sarabhai Kapadia's case of severe burns, not improving inspite of indicated remedies, till *Syphilinum* was given on the basis of history of syphilis in the father. Long standing Leucorrhoea cured by *Tuberculinum* on the father's history of tuberculosis — are a few more cases.

42. **Bowel Nosodes**. The Nosodes developed by Dr. John Paterson after nearly forty years of research — numbering only eight — have also been giving excellent results in practice. This little book *Bowel Nosodes* by J. Paterson deserves to be studied and put into practice.

43. **Conclusion**. We have travelled far after Hahnemann first lighted the torch. The early pioneers and masters had to work enormously hard, wading through pages and pages of the Materia Medica Pura, to understand the genius of the remedies and apply them in practice. Through their labours, they have illumined the path more brightly than they found it, and have

The Chronic Miasms and Nosodes

left their valuable experiences in the form of clinical confirmations of a vast number of symptoms; exposition of the highlights and Key-notes of the remedies; Repertories and detailed records of how they treated the cases together with the lessons they learnt from them as regards the problems of selection of remedy, potency, repetition, etc. By proving many new remedies, including Nosodes, they have enriched the Materia Medica which is capable of standing us in good stead in treating even most difficult cases provided we are prepared to study the case deeply and search through the Materia Medica, with the help of the Repertory or otherwise, for the curative remedy. It is all up to us make the best use of this rich legacy, nay, even to carry it forward and advance it with our own contribution to its growth.

44. Just at present every one is anxious to simplify, standardise and speed up the process of selection of the remedy. Going rapidly with his mind's eye over the entire course of lessons given in this book, the writer strongly feels that the law of similars will ever remain unchallenged as it is founded on the immutable truth of Nature; and the totality of symptoms is a natural corollary of the diversity of individual vital force and susceptibility; and there are a few components of the totality which are more important than others in the selection of the remedy. They are Mentals, Physical Generals, i.e., symptoms pertaining to the patient as a whole, such as cravings and aversions, appetite, thirst, sexual function and impulse, sleep and dreams, including general modalities of time, weather, temperature and other circumstances. Also peculiar uncommon characteristics. Then again, if we are not able to get marked mentals, we are left with the modalities. Modalities are nothing but etiology. Understood this way, our task becomes considerably simple. Etiology can be subdivided further into several branches, and if we catch hold of the most important etiology, our task seems to become simplicity itself.

(i) If we examine the patient closely and deeply, with a "High Index of Suspicion" about Miasm, as A. Neiswander urges us to do (because patients do not reveal everything),an anti-psoric, an anti-syphiliticor anti-sycotic remedy may straightway open the case and make it easy for the constitutional remedies to follow and act positively.

(ii) Perhaps the etiology is physical trauma, for which we have wonderful remedies in the Materia Medica.

(iii) In case it is mental trauma, such as fright, disappointment, shock, grief, then too our search gets limited to a small number of remedies which are prominent in this field.

(iv) If the patient has suffered at any time in the past from any disease such as Measles, Small pox, Mumps, Diphtheria, Influenza, Typhoid, Pneumonia, or other septic fevers, the cases treated by Margaret Tyler and others have shown us what amazing results can be achieved by the administration of the appropriate Nosodes even in seemingly incurable cases.

(v) Similarly, the use of tautopathic remedies can counter the adverse effects left behind by the massive dosage of such drugs as *Chloromycetin, Cortisone* etc.

(vi) Lastly, in those cases where we have no clear-cut etiology as referred to in the preceding five factors, we can take it for granted that none of those obvious obstacles to cure exists, and proceed to find the constitutional remedy on the basis of the totality of symptoms under the heads of Mentals, Physical Generals, Peculiar uncommon symptoms, Concomitants and Qualified Particulars with the help of the Repertory. Making etiology the fulcrum on which the whole question of selection turns, appears to hold the greatest promise of helping a larger number of our patients towards smooth and speedy cure. But even etiology is not as easy to come by as would appear at first sight; it is only with the cultivation of the art of searching interrogation with a "high index of suspicion" and "letting our imagination play" as Burnett used to say that we can become masters of this art, and, when we do so, we can rest assured that the Law of Similars will not fail us.

SELF-TEST

1. Why do we consider treatment which suppresses skin conditions or secretions like leucorrhoea by local measures, instead of by oral medicines, harmful? (Para 9-10)

2. What are Nosodes and what is the secret of their magical cures? Mention a few Nosodes with cures effected by them. (Para 34-41)

Study in Depth

Chronic Disease, Its Cause and Cure — P.N. Banerjee.

A Comparison of the Chronic Miasms — Phyllis Speight.

LESSON 10

How to Study the Materia Medica

1. We have so far emphasised the need for repertorisation for finding the remedy. However, there are times when this method fails. This happens for a number of reasons. It is possible that we have not taken the case in full and have missed some important characteristic symptoms. May be, we have not interpreted the symptoms correctly and have selected the wrong rubric. Then again, as Kent says, "It is quite possible for a remedy not having the highest marking in the anamnesis to be the most similar in image, as seen in the Materia Medica." It may also happen that we have attached too much importance to the face-totality rather than to the fundamental cause which is not so obvious; and so on. In these circumstances, a sound knowledge of Materia Medica can be of great help.

2. **Ability to differentiate between Remedies, A Must** : Thorough knowledge of Materia Medica also becomes essential as we aim at higher and higher levels of efficiency as prescribers. Dr. John Clarke has said in his *Prescriber* that the best Repertory is one that is carried in our mind". He obviously meant thereby that if one knew the Materia Medica well (i.e., all the characteristic features of each remedy), that itself constituted the best Repertory. A thorough knowledge of the Materia Medica involves the ability to differentiate one remedy from other similar looking remedies. This task is facilitated if the practitioner has as a basis for comparison some knowledge of the individuality of the remedy; something that is peculiar, uncommon or sufficiently characteristic in the confirmed pathogenesis of a remedy. It is only with such knowledge in respect of many remedies that it becomes easy for him to differentiate (and eliminate) one unsuitable remedy after another mentally (as we

How to Study the Materia Medica

do in a repertorial chart), and arrive at the remedy in a flash, almost intuitively.

3. Knowledge of differential characteristics of remedies also helps us in case-taking because "what the mind does not know, the eyes do not see." Lack of knowledge of the characteristics of a remedy will prevent us from checking up with the patient whether he has them. For example, if we do not know that *Medorrhinum* or a craving for oranges, or *Phos-ac.* has craving for refreshing or juicy things, we will miss this point even if the patient mentions them.

4. How to study the Materia Medica, therefore, boils down to finding a method for mastering the characteristics of at least the polychrests to begin with. A close observation of able practitioners of this art, and analysis of their thought process, and its evolution over a period of time, has led the writer to the conclusion that there are no short-cuts to master these differential characteristics of remedies. However, the process of learning can be made simple, methodical and effective. Even if we read one remedy from one, two or three books at a time, all the really important characteristics will not be uniformly impressed on our minds. Therefore, the writer would suggest a better way of studying them.

5. **An effective method of studying Materia Medica** : Carefully go through the specimen study of *Arsenicum-alb.* given at the end of this lesson. You will find that the study is divided into five broad headings, *viz.* (1) Mentals, (2) Strange, rare and peculiar symptoms, (3) Physical Generals, (4) Qualified Particulars and (5) Cases. The Section "Physical Generals" in turn is divided into subsections (a) to (k). Now take a note-book & divide it into these Sections and sub-sections, leaving sufficient space to enter symptoms as they are found by you in various books.

6. Start entering in the notebook from Nash's *Leaders*, say *Nux-vomica.* Continue these entries for *Nux-vomica* from Allen's *Key-notes*; after that from Tyler's *Drug Pictures*. After this study you will find that you have made a fairly good study of *Nux-vomica.* Now refer to Kent's Repertory (preferably Vols. I and II of *Synthetic Repertory*) and enter under the relative headings those rubrics against which *Nux-vom.* is given.

Note : Against each entry mention the source, *viz.* "N" for Nash, "A" for Allen, "T" for Tyler, "KR" for Kent's Repertory and

"SR" for *Synthetic Repertory*. The grade of the remedy given in the repertories should also be shown, viz. *Nux-vom.* 3 or *Nux-vom.* 2.

7. After completing these entries for Mentals, Peculiars and Physical Generals, take up making entries in Section (4), *viz*, Qualified Particulars, by referring to Kent's Repertory from Vertigo to Skin. As this part of study involves much work, it can be done last, at your convenience.

8. **Study Case Reports** : In Section (5) you note down case reports (briefly) which you may read in journals, or hear as narrated by other practitioners where the remedy has helped. Don't fail to note down the guiding symptoms of the case, the potency and repetition, the prescriber's name and the source of information. A number of cases studied this way will furnish you with the most characteristic symptoms which have guided prescribers to the remedy very often. For example, *Puls.* has been mild, gentle yielding nature, tearful disposition, *Amel.* by consolation, better in open air (worse in closed stuffy rooms), wandering pains, aversion to fats, worse from eggs, etc.

9. To cap all this effort, study the remedy from Kent's *Lectures on Materia Medica.* The drug picture of *Nux-vom.* on your mind will be complete more or less, and now, you have only to learn to observe patient and perceive the remedy in their symptomatology.

10. It need hardly be stressed that since the work of taking notes as above involves checking and cross-checking to see that similar entries are not already made, and since the entries are being made after due thinking, in your own mind, they will leave an indelible mark on your memory.

11. The above effort will give the student a fairly good grasp of the essential features of the remedies he has studied. However, he has yet to acquire the most important skill of translating this knowledge into practice. This involves the ability to differentiate one remedy from another. Many remedies are similar to one another in one or more respects. They are also different in one way or another. Unless we know the technique of differentiating remedies, and casting out those which do not meet our requirements, we shall not be masters of the art. We shall now turn our attention to the method by which we can acquire this art.

12. **From Science to Art in Prescribing**: The artistic method enables us to reach still higher levels of efficiency. Kent's advice in this behalf deserves close attention. He says in his booklet *How to use the Repertory*, "As homoeopathy includes both science and art, Repertory study must consist of science and art. The scientific method is the mechanical method, taking all the symptoms and writing out all the associated remedies with grading, making a summary with grades marked at the end" (i.e. repertorisation). "There is an artistic method that omits the mechanical, and is better . . . the artistic prescriber sees much in the proving that cannot be retained in the Repertory, where everything must be sacrificed for the alphabetical system. The artistic prescriber must study Materia Medica long and earnestly to enable him to fix in his mind sick images . . . sick personalities of human beings . . . . I have known such intuitive (artistic) prescribers" who cannot explain how they achieved marvellous cures . . . but if this artistic healing "is carried too far, it becomes a fatal mistake, and must, therefore, be corrected by repertory work done in even the most mechanical manner."

13. **Take The Most Peculiar Symptoms First** : Quoting Kent further : "The artistic method demands that after taking the case most carefully, the symptoms must be judged as to their value as characteristics in relation to the patient . . . to determine those which are strange, rare amd peculiar. Symptoms most peculiar to the patient must be taken first, then those less and less peculiar until the symptoms that are common and not peculiar are reached, in order, from first to last . . . The task of taking symptoms is often a most difficult one. It is sometimes possible to abbreviate the anamnesis by selecting one symptom that is very peculiar, containing the key to the case. A young man cannot often detect this peculiarity, and he should seldom attempt it. It is often convenient to abbreviate by taking a group of three or four essentials in a given case, making a summary of these, and eliminating all remedies not found in all the essential symptoms. A man with considerable experience may cut short the work in this way."

14. We have quoted Kent to stress how important it is to use the Repertory as well as to know the Materia Medica well, and also to bring out sharply that the crux of the artistic method seems to lie in the choice of peculiar and characteristic symptoms for selecting the remedy. Kent also said that three or four essentials that hold the key to the case can guide to similimum.

15. **The three legged stool** : Hering said much the same thing to Dr. Boyce who was consulting him for his wife. He said to Boyce, "Let us apply the triangular test, and if we find three important characteristic symptoms, pointing to one remedy, let me assure you that we can prescribe it with utmost certainty. I have tested its application in hundreds of cases, and when clearly defined, it seldom fails to fulfil its mission." (*H.H.* Sept. 1979).

16. Now let us turn to Dr. H. V. Miller (*H.H.* July 1979) : "The suitable remedy must generally contain several characteristics. A good prescription is said to be based upon at least two or three characteristics, but four or five of them will amount to almost absolute certainty . . . We individualise a remedy when we become familiar with its peculiar combination of characteristics. For instance, circumscribed heat of the vertex is said to be a characteristic of *Sulphur*. It is a symptom common to several other remedies, i.e. *Calc.* and *Graph.* If we find this vertex heat accompanied by cold, sweaty feet, and vertigo on going upstairs, *Calc.* is indicated. If it is accompanied by profuse leucorrhoea and a very fleshy lady, *Graph.* is the remedy. Many times we shall find it accompanied by other indications for *Sulph.*, such as a *Sulphur* diarrhoea, a Sulphur appetite, etc . . . . Generally, when some peculiar symptom of a case corresponds with a charateristic symptom of a remedy, we have good reason to conclude that the balance of the case will also correspond more or less with the remaining characteristic of the remedy.

17. **Minimum Syndrome of Maximum Value**. It is obviously this same idea which has been expressed by Sir John Weir, Dr. Paschero and Dr. Eugenio F. Candegabe as the "minimum syndrome of the maximum value". They say that the essence or vital orientation of a drug always manifests in a small and typical group of symptoms, the tout ensemble, the minimum syndrome. The small group that determines the drug leads to the understanding of its essence. If this group of symptoms comprises different classes of symptoms, viz. a mental, a physical general, a strange, rare and peculiar and, where possible, a qualified particular, we can be assured of the total correctness of the remedy, based on the totality of symptoms.

18. It is the common experience of many prescribers that they are able to spot the remedy even while taking the case, based on their repeated observation of a certain group or combination of symptoms leading to a particular remedy. This is an

How to Study the Materia Medica

ability acquired through experience. However, it may not be amiss if we present to the readers a tentative list of characteristic symptoms of a few remedies, to give them an idea of how through the "minimum syndrome of maximum value" we could understand the genius or essence of remedies. This list is at Appendix "K". A word about the limitation of these groupings : Dr. Miller has already shown how these groupings can vary and lead to different remedies. It is, therefore, not possible nor advisable to name a cut and dried group. These groupings can only "make us think" of the remedy, and we have to examine for further indications of the drug. It must also be understood that all the symptoms given cannot be found in one case, but if at least four or five of them are found together in a patient and further examination confirms, we may be reason-ably certain that the remedy covers the balance of the symptoms. Yet, as Kent has warned, and we repeat, "if this artistic healing is carried too far, it becomes a fatal mistake, and must be corrected by repertory work done in even the most mechanical manner."

19. Using a Characteristic as a Pivotal Point : (to differentiate between remedies). Learning the group of characteristic symptoms of remedies does not end our problem of matching this group with the symptoms of the patient, because the combination can vary from patient to patient even for the same remedy. H.C. Allen has shown us how to solve this problem in the preface to his *Keynotes*. He says : "The student must differentiate the apparently similar symptoms of two or more medicinal agents in order to select the similimum. To enable him to do this correctly and rapidly, he must have as a basis for comparison some knowledge of the individuality of the remedy; something that is peculiar, uncommon or sufficiently characteristic in the confirmed pathogenesis of the polychrest remedy that may be used as a pivotal point for comparison. It may be a so-called *Keynote*, a characteristic, "red strand of the rope", and central modality or principle — as the aggravation from motion or *Bryonia* . . . or the apathetic indifference of *phos acid* some familiar landmark around which the symptoms may be arranged in the mind for comparison" (and differentiation).

20. We draw attention to Allen's advice to use "a keynote or a characteristic as a pivotal point . . . as a landmark around which the symptoms may be arranged." This broad hint actually

gives us a technique for comparison and differentiation. Let us see, through a couple of examples, how we can develop this technique to arrive at the similimum.

21. **Case No. 1** : Mr. P. aged 32 complained of (1) Urticaria since several years, so much that he (2) lost hope of recovery. The urticarial eruptions came on (3) exposure to sun, or (4) eating fruits, (5) vegetables, or (6) sour things (7) he had diarrhoea from milk.

In this case we may take "diarrhoea from milk" as the pivotal point, for which Kent's Repertory (p. 614) gives CALC., Kali-ar., Kali-c., Lyc., Mag-c., Mag-m., Nat-a., Nat-c., Nic c., Nux-m., Sep., Sil., Sulph. Obviously, one of these will be the similimum. Now, if we take the remedies against "agg. from exposure to sun" (we must know at least the more prominent of them - or else refer to Kent's Repertory (p. 1404), all these remedies, on comparison, will be eliminated except calc., mag-m., nat-c., and Sulph. If we take one more symptom "Fruit agg." (p. 1363 with calc., mag-m. and Nat-c.), we will find that Nat-c. is strongly indicated. The rest of the symptoms are covered by Nat-c. This example shows how simple, rational and dependable the technique is.

22. In the preamble to Materia Medica Pura (Vol. I, Pp. 20-23), Hahnemann describes this method in detail, the method of casting out unsuitable remedies to arrive at the similimum : He gives two cases, of Bryonia and Pulsatilla. The only difference is that Hahnemann has referred to the symptom numbers in the Materia Medica Pura, whereas we find it more convenient to refer to the rubrics in the Repertory. Readers are advised to study Hahnemann's examples.

23. **Case No. 2** : A male 60 years complained of sudden, frequent and ineffectual urging to urinate; also of great sleepiness all the time. He has lost his 30 year's business partner recently (Grief), and on account of his ailment he had become totally indifferent to his business though his sons needed him badly. He had an aversion to work, and even to think. Was sleepy all the while. He had no appetite for food and the only things he liked were fruits and fruit juices. He had lost weight considerably in the last six months.

Which remedy represents this combination of symptoms? If we take "Thinking, aversion to" (87) as the pivotal point, we will

How to Study the Materia Medica

find that the only one competing remedy, *Phos.*, has no "ailments from grief" nor has it the desire for fruit and juices, whereas *Phos-ac.* covers the whole case, including the chief complaints of urination and sleepiness.

24. This discussion shows that the more we equip our minds with a knowledge of the characteristic combination (grouping) of symptoms of a number of remedies, the more efficient we can become as prescribers.

25. **Seek Confirmation from Materia Medica** : Despite all care in selecting the remedy by repertorisation or a knowledge of the peculiar, uncommon characteristics, it is advisable to refer to the Materia Medica as a Court of Appeal. For this purpose *Hering's Guiding Symptoms* or Clarke's *Dictionary* may be used. What does such a reference consist of? If it is a throat case, we refer to the heading "Throat" in the schema; if it is Stomach, that part of the schema is referred to. In addition, we may verify if the remedy has the mentals, modalities and concomitants.

26. **Referring cases to Materia Medica.** When we refer to the Materia Medica it is important to remember that no case can possibly have all or most of the symptoms belonging to the remedy which is the similar-most. The Materia Medica is a collection of the symptoms produced by a number of provers, not of one prover. Each individual has his own peculiar susceptibilities and weak points and his sufferings are limited to them. The stool under *Nux-vomica* shows constipation as well as diarrhoea, and the Nux patient who has constipation will not have diarrhoea. Absence of any symptoms in a case does not contraindicate the remedy, whereas the presence of a symptom, even if it is in two words, would indicate it. Only the outstanding characteristics of a remedy are an exception to this rule, such as aggravation from heat of *Pulsatilla*, aggravation from motion of *Bryonia*, etc.

27. **A System to Remain Abrast and Ever Ready.** Knowledge which is not constantly used gets rusted. A homoeopath should constantly recharge his batteries of Materia Medica knowledge by :

(i) Constant reading of literature on the subject.

(ii) Subscribing to homoeopathic journals which bring to

him old classics as well as the experience of his professional brethren.

(iii) Participating in periodical meetings of the profession where experiences are exchanged.

All these methods keep him fresh in thought and up-to-date in knowledge.

28. How can the physician make sure that the various nuggets of gold he picks here and there, while reading and talking or hearing, can be recalled at will, at a moment's notice? Be assured, we cannot rely on our memory for this, however good it may be today. This problem can and must be solved if we are to be able to place our hands on the gold biscuits whenever needed, it can be solved only if we follow a system. "Red streak in the middle of the tongue" we learnt a little while ago, is found in *Chamomilla* and *Tuberculin*. Shall we enter it under these remedies in Boericke's Materia Medica? No, this will not help. It amounts to begging the question. When do we need this information again? Obviously, when we see another tongue with a "red streak in the middle". Therefore, the best way to get the remedies when needed is to enter them against a suitable rubric under "Tongue" in the Repertory. This method should be followed in respect of every bit of new information we get, provided of course it is reliable. For this purpose, we should paste two or four blank pages at the beginning of every small or big section in the Repertory and enter the information in these pages immediately we come by it. In case pasting of such pages in the Repertory is considered inconvenient, we should have a note-book divided into as many sections as in the Repertory, so that the new information can be straightway entered in the relevant page of the note-book. When we refer to the Repertory we should make it a habit to look into this note-book as well. This way, not a bit of new knowledge will be "lost" or "misplaced" in due course.

29. **Materia Medica to Repertory**. Then there is yet another way of keeping our mind (knowledge) sharp, so that it has a clear grasp of what we see in a patient or read in the Materia Medica; and on the other hand, keeping our main instrument, our main source of "instant knowledge", *viz.* the Repertory, ever sharp and well stocked with all variety of parts required in the construction of the Curative Engine, the similimum. This

method is no other, but that of learning the Repertory from the Materia Medica, and the Materia Medica from the Repertory. How do we do this? Whenever we read any Materia Medica, we should check up if the symptoms are included in the Repertory against a suitable rubric. This exercise has three advantages : One, we develop confidence in the Repertory when we find that most of the symptoms, even obscure symptoms, are in the Repertory; secondly, the true meaning of the rubric and its depth becomes clearer to us when it is read in conjunction with the descriptive text; and thirdly, in case the remedy is not found in the appropriate rubric, we can add it and make the Repertory a more efficient instrument.

30. **Repertory to Materia Medica.** The habit of thumbing through the Repertory during our spare or idle moments pays good dividends, and removes many of our pet misconceptions, and sometimes reveals to us the remedy for a difficult case, which we had been hunting for long. One acquires a new slant on old remedies; or we find a remedy to have a high rank in respect of a symptom which we had never thought of. For example, it has been dinned into our ears that *Lachesis* is left sided and *Lycopodium* right sided; but Boger-Boenninghausen's Repertory reveals that under "lower extremities" *Lach.* and *Lyco.* have the highest grading on the right and left sides respectively. Again, *Oxalic Acid* is better known to be worse "Thinking of his disease", but Boger-Boenninghausen's Repertory reveals under "Conditions of Aggr. etc." that Nitric Acid is the only remedy which carries four marks against this rubric, with a few more remedies having three marks. (This fact helped us greatly in a case of Psoriasis). Then again, *Lac-caninum* is well known as if it is the only remedy having action on "alternating sides" of the body; here again, the same Repertory reveals that *Cocculus* is equally prominent in this peculiarity. We could discover similar gems by thumbing through the Kent's Repertory at will. Often a repertorial analysis brings before us a small group of remedies with unsuspected light thrown on them, which had never struck us while reading the Materia Medica.

31. After all, a deep knowledge of our remedies is our basic stock-in-trade and we should leave no opportunity unutilised to keep our granary full, taking care to see at the same time that the store room is well arranged (in a Repertory) so that we can place our hands on the articles we need at a moment's notice.

SELF-TEST

1. Why is it that lectures and talks on Materia Medica impress the individuality of remedies on our mind, better than the formal schema-wise text? (Para 2)

2. What is the best plan to follow for learning the essential features of the most commonly used remedies?

3. Absence of any symptom of a remedy in a patient does not contra-indicate the remedy" Explain.

4. Give an example or two as to how we can apply the "three legged stool" approach in practice?

5. What method should we follow to make sure that any important symptom of a remedy, which comes to our notice, becomes available to us at a moment's notice, whenever required?

6. What are the advantages of checking up that the more important or peculiar symptoms of remedies given in the Materia Medica are, in fact, represented in the Repertory?

7. What is Allen's advice for differentiating one remedy from another, while they are apparently similar in some respects?

ARSENICUM ALBUM — A STUDY

I. **STRANGE, RARE** and **PECULIARS** (General) : Burning pains like fire, amel. by heat, hot drinks, hot applications (except piles and headache which are better cold applications). Cannot bear sight or smell of food (Colch. Sep.). Gastric derangement from watery fruits, cold fruits, ice cream. Great remedy for food poisoning. Vomiting and purging at the same time. A.F. venomous stings, septic conditions. Skin symptoms alternate with internal affections. Great prostration out of proportion to the illness, and rapid sinking.

II. **MENTALS** : Oversensitive, fastidious, fault-finding. Restless, but too weak to move. Anxious, fearful. Agonising fear of death, fear of financial loss; wants company. Suspicious; fixed ideas; hallucinations.

III. PHYSICAL GENERALS :

a. Thermal : Cold air, cold and damp

b. Periodicity: 1 to 2 p.m. or 12 to 2 a.m. Agg. Night
Acute : Every other or every 3rd, or 4th day;
Chronic : 7th day or every 2 weeks according to chronicity or Annually (Lach.)

c. Appetite: Less of A. with thirst; with nausea (hunger with nausea: (Verat.). Eats seldom and much. (Rev. Sulph.)

d. Thirst: Burning thirst; drinks little and often. Craves ice-cold water which distresses the stomach and is vomited immediately.

e. Cravings : Ice-cold water, milk, acids, coffee, sour things.

f. Aversions : Sweets, butter, fats, meat.

g. Others : Modalities : Agg. Exertion, Sea shore.
Modalities : Amel. Hot applications (Dry); hot food and drinks; warm wraps. motion; walking about; lying with head elevated; Company; Open air.

h. Causation: Eating ices, fruits, esp. watery, tobacco chewing; sea bathing; alcoholism, bad meat and food. Eruptions undeveloped or suppressed. Care, grief, fright.

i. Sexual - Male :
Female : Increased sexual desire during menses. Stitching in rectum during menses.

j. Sleep & Dreams: Anxious, restless. Starts from S. Dreams: care, sorrow and fear. Talks in sleep.

k. Sweat: with great thirst.

Lesson 11

Different Ways of Selecting the Remedy

1. We have so far seen that Hahnemann has laid down clear guidelines in his *Organon* for the selection of the remedy by stressing the importance of "peculiar, rare, strange and characteristic symptoms", "mental symptoms" and the "totality of symptoms". However, different masters of homoeopathic practice have, through the exigencies of their practice and exercising considerable originality, but without departing from the law of Similars, evolved and successfully followed different methods of selecting the remedy to suit different types of cases, the primacy of importance being given to different aspects of the totality depending on the nature of the case. Experience led them to these different approaches as follows :

(i) Specifics.

(ii) Certain remedies act as Prophylactics.

(iii) Certain key-notes lead more quickly and effortlessly to the curative remedy.

(iv) Causation of illness immediate or remote, leads to a single or a small group of remedies.

(v) Organopathic remedies have given remarkable results when pathological conditions have to be treated without the necessary symptoms being available.

(vi) A knowledge of the relationship of remedies helps in selecting the appropriate remedy to follow another which has ceased to act after a partial effect. (see Paras 55-64 of Lesson 8).

(vii) In some cases unless tautopathic remedies (to antidote the effects of allopathic overdosage of antibiotics, cortisone, etc.) are exhibited, no progress towards cure is possible. (See Paras 79-81 of Lesson 8).

(viii) The miasmatic approach (deep rooted morbid effects) and the use of nosodes and the appropriate antipsoric), anti-sycotic or anti-syphilitic remedies opens up the case and makes the patient more responsive to the indicated remedy. (See Lesson 9).

2. We shall now take up the first five of the above-mentioned strategies, one by one, for consideration.

3. For much of material that follows we are indebted to *Principles of Prescribing* in which Dr. K. N. Mathur, M.B.B.S., M.F. Hom. (Lond.), an experienced and learned homoeopath, has presented different ways of prescribing, quoting clinical experiences of pioneers of homoeopathy.

4. **Specifics.** Truly speaking, there is no drug or medicinal formula of any kind which is universally curative either in a general sense or in a particular disease. Every homoeopath knows this. How, then, can we speak of "specifics in Homoeopathy? The truth is that while no remedy is or ever can be 100 per cent accurate in all cases of a particular disease or condition, in a few diseases or conditions the disease symptoms so accurately fit a known drug picture that it is only in a small percentage of cases that we require to go past this remedy. It is little wonder, then, that the disease and the remedy get so intimately associated in the mind of the physician that he is apt to think of the remedy as specific. In Appendix "B" are given remedies together with the conditions in which they have proved to be "Near-specific" in a majority of cases.

5. **Prophylactics.** Hahnemann had noted that remedies can act as prophylactic medicines when the homoeopathic remedy in its provings brings out symptoms similar to the particular disease. He found that Belladonna acts as prophylactic against Scarlet fever; Pulsatilla against Measles; Drosera against Whooping cough; Baryta-carb. against Quinsy; Graphites against Erysipelas, etc. Genus Epidemicus, the word coined by Hahnemann, denotes the homoeopathic remedy that is similar

to the totality of symptoms found in the majority of patients suffering in an epidemic disease, and which if given to the patients before the onset of the disease, prevents the epidemic disease or, when given during the disease cures the patient. Some of the remedies which have proved efficacious as prophylactics are given in Appendix "C".

6. **Key-note Prescribing.** Guided no doubt by Hahnemann's dictum in Paragraph 153 of the *Organon* that in the selection of the remedy "the more striking, singular, uncommon and peculiar characteristic" signs and symptoms of the case should chiefly and almost solely be kept in view, Dr. Henry N. Guernsey coined the expression "Key-notes to the Materia Medica" and drew the attention of homoeopaths to their importance. Dr. H.C. Allen's *Key-notes and Characteristics* and Dr. E.B. Nash's *Leaders in Homoeopathic Therapeutics* owe their popularity among generations of homoeopaths to the value of Key-notes in "aiding the student to master that which is guiding and characteristic in the individuality of each remedy and thus utilise more readily the symptomatology of the homoeopathic Materia Medica." Dr. Nash has shown in his book *The Testimony of the Clinic* how remedies selected on the basis of Key-note characteristic symptoms have given wonderful results especially in acute cases. In his work on obstetrics, Dr. Guernsey has given the key-notes of remedies, "such only as had been in my experience and that of others, tried, proven and chosen', so that the mind might be directed at once in the true direction, the choice to be confirmed by the totality of symptoms; so that (as in music) the key-note being struck, all the other tones would be harmonised with it. Guernsey says, "I again repeat that the key-note system does not in any way interfere with the doctrine of "totality"; it is the guide to its being properly and practically carried out." Guernsey explains what is a key-note; "In instituting comparisons between medicines, by taking all the symptoms and comparing them carefully, we will find that each one presents, besides the fundamental similarity to all the others, peculiar differences from all the others; and these invariable points of peculiar difference are the "key-notes". For example, "There is something within the pathogenesis of *Aconite* which is indicative of *Aconite* alone; embodying its one characteristic, unfailing, predominant, effect, which makes it to differ from all other drugs, and which pervades all its other effects with more or less predominance. These symptoms or conditions form the key-notes of *Aconite* as a medicine, and furnish the key to its indication in disease." The

key-note simply suggests to the mind (by the shortest, surest and most practical method) the medicine . . . and if there has been no error in viewing the key-note of the disease, there will be found in the Materia Medica under that remedy the remaining features and symptoms of the patient, or in other words the "totality". Through this system the complex and difficult text of the Materia Medica is rendered pure and clear — and every shadow uplifted from its pages . . . The practitioner is thus enabled to individualise his case and find the similar remedy having the totality of the case, and be able to cure it. Some clinical experiences are given below:

Abscess on face. Purplish, mottled, great burning, bloody, thin excoriating, foul smelling discharge — Tarentula 12x — J.T. Kent.

Painful Micturition :

(i) Cannot pass urine sitting; must stand always, or will not start — Sarsaparilla CM — J.T. Kent.

(ii) Unable to urinate without standing with feet wide apart and body inclined forward (stones in bladder) — *Chimaphila umbellata.*

(iii) Great urging and straining to urinate; pains go down thighs during effort to urinate. Can emit urine only when he goes on his knees, pressing head firmly against floor, (Renal colic, etc.) — *Pareira brava.*

Bright's disease. Ear complications with kidney disease. Right eye, profuse lachrymation, sacular under-lid. Face puffed, worse right side. Thirstless and agg. warmth. Is it *Apis* or *Ars.*? Not with these modalities. Now the mother of the child says : "Her water smells strong, like that of a horse." And *Nitric acid* 1000th cured the case. (J.T. Kent).

Phosphorus. Obstinate dysentery in a child. Several remedies failed utterly. While the mother was changing the diaper, chanced to notice that the anus was wide open. I could have inserted my little finger to the depth of two inches without touching the bloody mucus-lined walls. The tenesmus was continuous. Three days after *Phosphorus* was given, nothing remained of the trouble except the resulting weakness. (E.B. Nash).

Kali Bichromicum. Chronic rheumatism. Wandering pains; they occupy small spots that could be covered with the point of a finger. (Champlin).

Pyrogenium. Typhoid; Koch's abdomen? Lack of relation between pulse and temperature (temperature 102.4 and pulse 180 p.m.). Two days after *Pyrogen* 1000 was given in water half-hourly, temperature came down to 100, pulse 138 with respiration 28. Temperature normal after four days — in all seven days since the start. (Dr. S.R. Wadia).

Arum Triphyllum. Constant picking at the nose and lips until they bleed.

Apis. Habitual abortion at the end of the fourth month, from an "incompetent os" (analagous to its involuntary stool from every motion as though the anus was wide open').

Argentum Nitricum. Diarrhoea from apprehension, when ready to "go to church or opera"; anticipations aggravate.

Borax. Dread of downward motion in nearly all complaints.

China. Ailments from loss of vital fluids. (*Phos-ac.*)

Phosphoric Acid. It is listless, apathetic; indifferent to the affairs of life. Has no will to retaliate even if slapped.

Baptisia. Painless sore throat, (Painful : *Phosphorus*).

Conium. Bad effects of suppressed sexual desire, or suppressed menses. Urinary flow intermits, and hence great difficulty in voiding urine (useful in prostatic or uterine affections).

Chamomilla. Child exceedingly irritable, fretful; will be quiet only when carried about. Child is cross, cannot endure any one near him; will even order his mother out of the room; averse to talking.

Lachesis. Diseases begin on the left and go to the right side. (They go from right to left side : *Lycopodium*).

Lac Caninum. Symptoms change from one side to the other every few hours or days.

Different Ways of Selecting the Remedy

Kali Carbonicum. Bag-like swelling between the upper eyelids and eyebrows. (Bag-like swelling, puffy, under the eyes: *Apis*).

Lycopodium. Affects principally the right side, or pain goes from right to left. Aggravation of complaints at 4 p.m. or 8 p.m. Amelioration after midnight.

These examples are sufficient to illustrate how key-notes can guide us to the remedy and make our search easier provided there are no Generals to contra-indicate, and the Materia Medica confirms that it has the other symptoms of the patient.

7. Causation. During the provings of remedies Hahnemann noticed that some drugs showed symptoms belonging to causations. For example, *Aconite* and *Opium* have symptoms pertaining to the effects of fear; *Colocynthis* and *Nux-vomica* have symptoms pertaining to the effects of anger (also *Chamomilla* and *Staphysagria*); *Ignatia* and *Natrum-mur*, have symptoms pertaining to the effects of grief; Arnica, Bellis-per., *Ruta* and *Symphytum* have symptoms pertaining to trauma; *Cantharis, Arsenic-alb.* and *Causticum* have symptoms pertaining to the effects of burns, and so on. Hahnemann and other pioneers made good use of sensations "as if" caused by, or "aggravated from" to arrive at "caused by". As pointed out by Dr. S.P. Koppikar (the present editor of *Homoeopathic Heritage*), the early homoeopaths would have prescribed the remedies on the symptoms, but as they took care to note down the etiology in such cases, in course of time these clinical rubrics have become available to us.

8. The second type of causation is when suppression took place. The cure of a case of "hardness of hearing" (without any modality) solely on the basis of history of suppression of eczema of scalp (corresponding to *Mezereum*), by *Mezereum* by the brilliant intuition of Dr. Caroll Dunham belongs to this category. Another case is the cure by Dr. Boger of a left sided salpingitis with swelling and high fever after the suppression of profuse leucorrhoea, with one dose of *Pulsatilla* MM. A case of chronic otorrhoea following suppressed menses has been cured by *Pulsatilla* 1 M at the Subodh Mehta Medical Centre. Paralytic weakness of lower extremities in a boy of 11, following "healing" (suppression) of a septic wound was cured by Dr. Sarabhai M. Kapadia with *Cocculus* 1M in water at four hourly intervals.

9. There is a third type of causation, which may be described as "Never well since . . .". These are remote causes, and Allen gives a number of them under different remedies in his *Key-notes and Characteristics*. Another description of these causes is, "Bad effects of . . ." Dr. S.P. Koppikar will bear extensive quotation on this point : "Early in my practice, I discovered that if I treated the cause (especially in acute diseases), 90% of the trouble would be knocked off. Take for example, a fever like "Flu". Just find out how the illness started, or what was the exciting cause. If it followed a drenching, especially when overheated, *Rhus-tox*, cut it short; if after infected food or drink, etc., *Arsenicum-alb*. or *Pyrogen*; if after exposure to summer heat, or dry cold, *Aconite*; drinking ice water on a hot summer day, *Bellis* or *Bryonia*; after swimming, *Antim-c*. and so on. Thus I realised that if I had, ready on hand, about forty or fifty etiologically useful remedies, I could tackle most of the acute diseases straightaway. I had to prescribe for about 50 to 80 patients in two hours (in Sri Ramakrishna Math Dispensary) and it was a surprise to me that every time I prescribed on etiological ground the case got well much quicker.

10. "I mugged up the etiological keynotes of remedies like *Aconite, Arnica, Ant.-c., Bell., Bryonia, Carbo-veg., Rhus-tox., Pulsatilla, Sulphur*, etc., in Allen where the remedy starts with "complaints from . . ." Luckily the list was not long. I also added a few important remedies from the chapter on "Causation" in Clarke's *Clinical Repertory*. Later a few Nosodes. I made it a rule to ask every time "How did you get it?" or "What were you doing out of ordinary the previous 24 hours?" The patients too liked my work. There was no aggravation, "perhaps I thought, the etiologically indicated remedy does not cover exactly the presenting symptoms".

11. "Next, to my surprise, I discovered that the same technique could be used in real chronic cases. I found that many a patient had gone through definite "traumatic" of life-changing" illnesses, which had perhaps brought about the present picture. I simply administered the remedies etiologically one after another (preferably) in the reverse order of the development of the case. Say four or five remedies might come up, one or two nosodes perhaps. The whole prescription — to follow in a certain order — was thought of and written down at the first sitting. I must say it has done immense good to a large number of patients.

Different Ways of Selecting the Remedy

12. "Of course, I have not become a one track, etiological fadist, please. Every case might and does "indicate" a homoeopathic (similar) remedy, based on location, sensation, modality, mental or bodily characteristics." (*Hom. Heritage*, Oct. 1979).

13. Application of art (etiology) in everyday practice. Dr. Koppikar elaborates this point in his *Clinical Verifications and Reflections*: It is one thing to admire great art, quite another to use it . . . Let me remind you that an artistic prescription is one where the given picture of the case is almost not the indication for the prescription and also, the selected remedy may not contain the present trouble of the patient prominently, so far as is known. For example, *Medorrh.* was not known to have produced severe diarrhoea. Yet a case of infantile diarrhoea not improving despite careful prescribing, was cured by *Medorrhinum*, given because the doctor remembered treating the baby's father for gonorrhoea years ago.

14. "Rev. Cannon Upcher's famous case of a uterine "fibroid" (as recorded in Clarke's *Prescriber*) cured by Bacillinum (for family history of T.B.), *Thuja* (re-vaccination, and never well since) and *Bellis-perennis* (history of a bad fall on to her stomach), each prescription based solely on the causes one after another, *viz.* tubercular history, vaccination and fall, is a typical example of art.

15. "So, now, can this not be done by every one of us every day? I think 90% of my best cures were based on this technique. The remedy or remedies were selected purely on etiology without much bothering whether the remedy covered the present symptoms or not. To apply the technique of this art in our daily practice, two things are necessary, *viz.*: (i) Implicit faith in the capacity of any remedy to cure any case . . . The range of curative powers cannot be guessed easily. The right remedy can cover any condition, including pathology. (ii) To follow Hahnemann strictly in case-taking. His most important advice, further emphasised by his great disciple Von Boenninghausen, is to complete each symptom especially with regard to its modalities. I suggest one extra thing; for every trouble mentioned by the patient, ask when it started (exact date, time of day, season, occasion, etc.) and how (cause) it started. You will then get the chronological development of his or her troubles one after the other. Some have just come and gone; others have almost changed the life and personality of the patient. These latter are

the most valuable ones. Insist that the patient should think over and recapitulate what might have brought on these important changes. A single cause will call for a single etiological remedy in high potency. Where we have three or four separate causes, all we have to do is to follow the wall-breaking method of Rev. Cannon Upcher (quoted above), starting with the remedy covering the latest etiological factor and programming on the first day itself to follow it up with the other etiologically indicated remedies in the reverse chronological order. Follow the plan giving the remedies at intervals of 10 to 30 days."

16. A list of etiological conditions with their corresponding remedies is given in Appendix "D".

17. **Organopathic remedies.** It is a well-known fact since the time of Paracelsus, that certain remedies have specific action on specific organs of the body. This fact has been taken advantage of by medical men since time immemorial. Even the homoeopathic system of medicine has found it advantageous and necessary to utilize this factor as is borne out by the fact that "location" of complaints is one of the important aspects to be taken into account in selecting the remedy. Homoeopathy can, therefore, be said to have "swallowed up" organopathy, though homoeopathy is something else besides, because the "elective affinity" of remedies have to be "similar" in other respects too, i.e. to the diseased patient. When a large number of remedies have "elective affinity" (organopathic attraction) to particular organs, how can we choose one among them with certainity of its curative action ? This can be done when the requisite characteristic features of the patient and the remedy are available. In one sided cases, where such symptoms are not available in a patient, we have to resort to the principle of prescribing on the basis of organotherapy. Drs. Clarke, Burnett, R.T. Cooper and C. M. Boger have, in their writings given their experiences about the usefulness of this approach when other guiding symptoms, such as causations, modalities and miasms were wanting.

A brief list of such organopathic remedies is given in Appendix "E".

Self-Test

1. What are the advantages of key-note symptoms and what are the precautions we should observe in using them?

Different Ways of Selecting the Remedy

2. What is the relationship between "causation" and "aggravation from"? What is Dr. Koppikar's advice when prescribing etiological remedies in chronic cases?

3. What are the circumstances under which we have to resort to organopathic remedies?

Lesson 12

Role of Therapeutic Hints

1. We believe that in the lessons that have gone before, we have given sufficient guidance as to how to find the remedy in a given case, whether acute or chronic. To recapitulate : We have to take the case properly and fully eliciting especially the symptoms that characterise the individual patient (apart from the common ones which pertain to the disease), evaluate the symptoms in their classifications of Modalities (including Causations both fundamental and exciting), Mentals, Locations, Sensations and Concomitants; refer these totality of symptoms to the Repertory and make a repertorial analysis, and finally check up by reference to the Materia Medica and make sure that the characteristic symptoms of the remedy or remedies, emerging from the repertorial analysis, do indeed match the characteristic symptoms of the patient. This procedure will become more and more speedy and intuitive as the physician gains experience and, through experience, acquires an uncanny grasp of the genius of each remedy and its application in practice.

2. **Therapeutic Hints.** Inspite of the method clearly outlined above, and also the assertion made throughout the past lessons that in homoeo-therapeutics, individualisation of the remedy is of supreme importance, and that diagnostic labels are more apt to mislead than help us, there is an insistent demand from new students for "at least a group of remedies which are known to have acted curatively in different ailments." It is probably to meet this demand and also probably because the authors felt it necessary and in the interests of the science, that many leading practitioners have left a record of their experiences of remedies which have proved their curative powers in different conditions. They have handed down their experiences sometimes in journals (later incorporated in books) or in complete book form. We shall mention a few of such leading books on "Therapeutics" for the information of the readers, leaving it to them to select any

one or two of them which they may like to possess for constant reference.

3. **Clinical Therapeutics.** By Temple S. Hoyne. As Dr. Jugal Kishore writes in his foreward to the Indian Edition, "this is truly a text-book of applied Materia Medica. Under each remedy Dr. Hoyne has given cardinal symptoms under the regional headings with emphasis on the application of the Materia Medica in clinical conditions. He has quoted extensively the records of eminent authorities on the use of a particular drug in certain clinical conditions." The author drew freely upon the current and past homoeopathic journals during the period of 1840 to 1880 and made the Materia Medica a living subject. Dr. Jugal Kishore calls it a "Text Book of Applied Materia Medica." (First published in 1880, pp. 1250, Reprinted by : B. Jain Publishers (P) Ltd., New Delhi).

4. **The Prescriber.** A Dictionary of the new therapeutics : By Dr. John H. Clarke, M.D. (pp. 352, including a valuable essay on "How to Practice Homoeopathy"). First published in 1885, this book has gone through many editions. All kinds of complaints one commonly meets with are taken up in alphabetical order and the remedies found useful for them with the potency recommended are given. These features are of much practical use. Dr. Clarke writes in his Introduction : The *Prescriber* is a ready instrument by means of which the practitioner can put the precepts of homoeopathy to the test. With this book at his elbow he will be able to find, in a case of any disease, the remedies that are most generally appropriate, with their differential indications . . . it will sometimes happen that the differential symptoms named in the *Prescriber* are not sufficient to enable a choice to be made with due certainty. In that case, if reference is made to the Materia Medica, the actual symptoms of the different remedies can be studied in full and compared with each other". Further, Dr. Clarke adds : "it is the glory of Hahnemann that he liberated medical practice from its bondage to the names of diseases. Every case of disease is a problem in itself . . . Clinical Repertories form one out of many of the means of fitting the remedy to the case." . . . "The use of repertories is in itself an art which the homoeopathist must diligently cultivate."

5. **Homoeopathic Therapeutics.** By Samuel Lilienthal, M.D. (third edition published by the author in 1890, pp. 1154). This grand old work has been aptly described as "an un-

abridged dictionary of homoeopathic therapeutics". The value of this work can be gauged from the author's preface to the third edition : "Take this third edition as the old man's testament to his many students and younger colleagues, for your success rejuvenates your old teachers. Though three years, faithful work was necessary to collate and critically examine every symptom, still it can only be considered as an aid in studying up a case. Perfection is impossible . . . . It is for the physicians to give us clinical reports and verifications, and it is the duty of the reviewer to sift them carefully, whether he can accept the grain of wheat, or throw it aside among the chaff. Let every man and every woman do his and her duty, and our Materia Medica will be a pura, . . . so that gradually a work can be issued worthy to be named homoeopathic therapeutics." This magnum opus covers a large number of remedies and each one of them in considerable detail, under a variety of complaints, and can be said to be the last word in homoeopathic therapeutics.

6. **Essentials of Homoeopathic Therapeutics.** It is a Quiz Compend : By Dr. W.A. Dewey. M.D. (First published in 1894, pp. 285 including a useful complaint-wise index, giving names of remedies dealt with under each complaint). This book in the form of questions and answers gives a group of remedies most commonly called for in various conditions with their comparative, differentiating symptoms, and is ideal for new students.

7. **Practical Homoeopathic Therapeutics** : By Dr. W.A. Dewey, M.D. (First published in 1900, a few years after the *Essentials* just described, pp. 475 including a useful index). This is an enlarged version of the *Essentials* by Dr. Dewey. The author has included many more remedies with comparisons. In the words of Dr. Dewey, "The work has been undertaken to supply the practitioner of homoeopathic medicine with reliable, practical and condensed indications for the more important remedies in diseases . . . The periodical literature of our school, as well as the works of all standard authorities have been carefully examined and the practical points contained therein have been included in this volume. No attempt has been made to give indications for all the remedies that may be indicated in the various affections. This would be but a repetition of what already has been well and faithfully done by our great authors on therapeutics. The object has been to restrict rather than to elaborate, to give the practical indications for a few of the most prominent remedies rather than to dwell on the elaborated

possibilities of many." The indications for the remedies given are those "born of the experience of the foremost prescribers — the successful men — of the homoeopathic school of medicine and, may, therefore, be considered as trustworthy".

8. **Pointers to the Common Remedies.** By Dr. Margaret Tyler (pp. 337). That an ardent follower of Kent, a strong advocate of repertorisation and one who had a deep insight into the genius of the remedies in the Materia Medica should have thought it necessary or advisable to give "pointers to remedies" found commonly necessary in a variety of clinical conditions is significant. It is not known how she yielded to the temptation to write down "Therapeutic Notes," when her preceptor, J.T. Kent, did not. Perhaps she intended to be of help to physicians less gifted than herself, or to the beginners ! If we take, just for comparison, the section on "Dysentery", Lilienthal gives sixty-two remedies whereas Tyler mentions twenty-one. Dewey's *Practical Therapeutics* contains twenty-two while Bishambar Das's *Select Your Remedy* (to be next described) contains twenty-two some of which are rare, such as *Streptococcin, Staphylocin, Septicaemin, Chaparro Amargossa,* and *Trombidium.* Tyler's presentation of the indications for each remedy seems to be more pointed and clear, containing more of the true guides and less of the chaff; all of them coming undoubtedly from her keen observation and rich experience.

9. **Select Your Remedy** : By Rai Bahadur Bishambar Das (First published in 1953 it has already gone into a number of editions duly revised and enlarged, pp. 592). This book represents "all the knowledge and experience" which the author gathered "during 35 years of practice and study". The arrangement adopted follows the anatomical schema and the diseases, as are commonly named, are given in the appropriate chapters together with the medicines to be used on the basis of symptoms shown against each. The author further adds, "Medicine is such a vast subject that it cannot be expected to be covered in a publication of this kind, but I am confident that with the aid of this book a practitioner will be able to cure 90% of the cases that he may be called upon to treat."

10. **How to get the best out of the Therapeutic Guides**. The therapeutic guides have their limitations as well as advantages. We shall now discuss both these aspects and try to show how we can overcome the limitations and at the same time take advantage of their good points.

11. **Limitations of Therapeutics.** Therapeutic hints, in Homoeopathy, suffer from serious limitations, especially from the point of view of a physician whose aim is, or ought be, to enhance his expertise and to learn from every case to fulfil his aim. Therapeutic hints may serve a layman who "tries remedies" without the sense of responsibility which a regular physician has. If a layman succeeds, well and good, and if he fails he has the ready excuse of lack of knowledge and training. But this is not the case with a professional homoeopathic physician. He too may sometimes succeed with the hints, but if he fails it is his duty to find out why he failed. One who merely follows the therapeutic hints will have no means of knowing why he failed.

12. The reason for most failures in homoeopathy is failure to individualise the remedy, which involves the entire process referred to in the first paragraph of this lesson. As stressed by Dr. C.M. Boger in his foreword to his *Synoptic Key of the Materia Medica*, "the prescriber has to keep in mind the fact that the actual differentiating factor may belong to any rubric whatsoever" (Boger's emphasis) from the five classes of symptoms, to which the Objective symptoms must be added as the sixth class. It is obvious that it is out of the question for any master of the art to provide a variety of symptoms under all these six classes for each remedy given in the hints. This is the first reason why therapeutic hints, howsoever comprehensive, are apt to fail us.

13. It is well known that certain remedies occupy a high rank in respect of certain symptoms; and they are shown in capital or bold letters in Boger-Boenninghausen's Repertory or in bold letters and italics in Kent's. They have been assigned these high ranks because they have proved themselves repeatedly curative of the symptoms in question. Now, it is important that a high grade complaint in a patient must be met by an equally high grade remedy in the Materia Medica. The therapeutic hints do not show the grades of the remedies in respect of the symptoms concerned, and in the absence of this knowledge the physician will not be able to select the appropriate remedy. This is one more reason why therapeutic hints may not provide a very dependable guide in the selection of the remedy.

14. There is yet another reason why therapeutic hints are apt to mislead us. As is already known to readers, homoeopathy does not treat any individual disease but the patient as a whole.

Role of Therapeutic Hints

For example, a patient comes with headache with the associated complaint of pain in throat while swallowing. Another case of headache may have some digestive complaint as a concomitant. It becomes difficult to refer to these different complaints in the therapeutic hints and find the one remedy that covers both complaints in addition to the modalities, etc. We give only two examples to prove the point. A case of skin eruptions was only palliated with the indicated remedies, but when he developed severe coryza, *Arsenicum* prescribed for it helped his skin eruptions too, quite fast. This was because it was found later that his skin eruptions generally alternated with the flare up of coryza, and a remedy which covered both equally strongly alone could cure. Another case of inveterate warts which had resisted not only allopathic and Ayurvedic but even homoeopathic medicines over the years, yielded readily to *Arsenic Iodatum* which was prescribed for hectic fever, severe cough and night-sweating, on the basis that he was a phthisical patient. These examples emphasise the importance of totality of symptoms including the miasmatic etiology. Therapeutic hints could not have helped in these cases. The same holds true for most of the cases coming to a homoeopath for treatment.

15. Then again, going through the various remedies covering a particular condition and weighing their relative applicability to a given case does take some time, which can as well be utilised to refer to a Repertory which will give us both the advantage of individualisation and matching the remedy in the same rank as the symptoms of the patient, and that too irrespective of the "Diagnosis".

16. **Taking advantage of Therapeutic Hints.** Therapeutic hints do have a value, however. For one thing, we can know a group of remedies which different authors have found to be most commonly useful in specific conditions. This helps us to study those remedies well and store their depth of action as well as differentiating points well in mind. Such hints also give us additional guidelines, such as, if *Colocynth* fails *Stannum* or *Kali-carb.* will help; or in Amenorrhoea if Natrum-mur though indicated, fails, *Kali-carb.* will help; or that in rheumatic conditions *Calcarea. Fluor* will complete the action of *Rhus-tox.*, and so on.

17. Therapeutic hints sometimes will give us rarely used remedies which we could try when the remedy indicated

through repertorisation or a study of the usual remedies in the Materia Medica fails; for example, *Chaparro Amargose* for "Chronic or acute dysentery or diarrhoea when everything else has failed" mentioned at p. 342 of *Select Your Remedy*, or "Wyethia — an excellent remedy for chronic pharyngitis and laryngitis where there is constant desire to clear the throat for dintinct utterance. Give in 30 dilution."

18. Such hints also sometimes reveal "little-known" uses of well-known remedies, that is, well-known, or very much associated in our minds with "other uses." For example, *Select your Remedy* recommends *Sabal Serrulata* for laryngeal phthisis, which is omitted even in Lilienthal's much larger work, whereas this remedy is usually associated in our minds with complaints in the genito-urinary sphere, such as prostatic enlargement undeveloped or shrivelled mammae, etc.

19. We have referred to the need for a comparative study of remedies given in the hints in respect of each condition and the storing of essential differentiations in mind. The same procedure could be extended in a more systematic manner, so that the results of such study would be available to us at a glance or at a moment's notice. Lilienthal's *Homoeo. Therapeutics* gives, under many sections, the key-notes of remedies in bold letters. These key-notes could be added as a special section in the Repertory for ready reference, apart from the "rare remedies" and the "little-known uses" of well-known remedies mentioned above.

20. As an example, we give below the remedies where keynotes in bold letters are given by Lilienthal on *Asthma Spasmodicum* :

Ambra : Asthma senile at siccum; also children.
Angustura : Neurosis of the Vagus.
Apis-mel : He does not know how he can get another breath.
Argentum-nit : Pure, nervous asthma; craves the cold wind blowing in his face and lungs.
Arsenicum-alb : Periodical asthma.
Arsenicum-iod : Occasional asthmatic attacks in phthisical and psoric patients.
Asclepias tub : Humid asthma.
Baptisia : Dyspnoea from want of power in lungs, not constriction, all due to nervous depression.

Role of Therapeutic Hints 241

Baryta-carb : Asthma senile (after Ant.-tart.). Asthma of scrofulous children, with enlargement of tonsils and cervical glands.
Bromium : Asthma of sailors as soon as they go ashore.
Cannabis sat : Humid asthma.
Capsicum : Catarrhal asthma, with red face and well-marked sibilant rales.
Carbo-veg : (Lyc.) asthma from abdominal irritation, with marked flatulence, asthma of old or debilitated people; during the fit they look as if they would die, so oppressed are they for breath.
Carduus-mar : Nervous asthma of miners; cachexia of tunnel labourers.

While treating a case of asthma, much time could be saved by going through these brief notes, and selecting a few remedies for further study.

21. Similar "notes" can be taken in respect of the complaints which the physician has to treat often, and they will not only form a good study of Materia Medica through therapeutics and for therapeutics, but such study will be of ready assistance at any time in future when needed.

These notes could be taken as a part of the Repertory thus enriching or enlarging the scope of the rubrics. Whenever any of these remedies are confirmed by clinical experience, we should underline them. When we have a remedy with three such underlinings (or confirmations), its rank should be raised to capitals.

22. **The Art of Selecting the Remedy.** We thus come to the definite conclusion that there is no short-cut to the correct remedy, except that basing it on the totality of the case. All other methods, by whatever name described, can at best be palliative. On the other hand, a remedy selected on the basis of totality of the characteristic symptoms, in which etiology or peculiar symptoms play a prominent role, is capable of bringing forth a magical response.

23. Let us not forget that homoeopathy is a science. The law of similars is a very jealous one. As Margaret Tyler never tires of asserting, there is a stop-spot of every remedy, even *Tuberculinum*, and it will only act in its field, and fail to do any work in a field which does not belong to it. "Only the remedy that has

evoked the exact conditions of the individual patient will cure the patient; that is, not merely palliate while he recovers, but cure." It is obvious that "totality" can also be expressed as a "several legged bench" if we may express it that way. We get the best results when all the legs of the bench touch the ground firmly. Reconciliation of these several factors cannot ordinarily be done except through repertorisation. But Repertorisation is also an art. How can we master this art?

24. Art, in my humble opinion, consists in translating the various principles of homoeopathy into practice. This translation into practice is a matter of technique, which can be developed with practice. The Oxford Concise Dictonary defines "technique" as "the part of the artistic work that is reducible to formula." The writer believes firmly that the practice of homoeopathy can be reduced to a formula, at least as far as the common ailments are concerned — i.e., a technique which any one can follow to get the desired result.

25. Now, a technician needs tools. The best of technicians will not be satisfied with tools which are second-grade. The Materia Medica alone was the tool available to the old masters. We are fortunate that the results of their arduous studies and clinical experience have been handed down to us in their various works. Besides, their own needs in day-to-day practice led them to compile Repertories as an aid to comparison as well as differentiation of remedies. The Repertories thus, are our most valuable heritage. Pierre Schmidt, one of the most eminent homoeopaths of the present day, says that he consults the Repertory at least fifty times a day, and he has been doing this over a long period of practice. Does not his example show that if we too make it a habit to use this tool, higher levels of success — and that more often at the first shot — are not beyond our reach? For this, we must firstly, master the principles and philosophy of this science, and through study and critical learning from each experience, gradually develop the art of evaluating the most important symptoms in a case which holds the key to the remedy. Secondly, we must equip ourselves with the best of tool or tools, and keep them very sharp. Thirdly, we must master the technique of handling the tools, which is not so hard after all. Given these three requisites — Principles, Tools and Techniques — success and satisfaction in our efforts in every curable case will be within our easy grasp. While we are mastering these techniques, in the initial stages, we may take some

longer time on each case, but as we gather more and more experience, the time taken by each case will get shorter and shorter. In addition, we will develop an inexplicable insight into the genius of remedies. That is the lesson of experience from the masters of this art. Let us follow their examples for the glory of the science, for our own success as healers, as well as the satisfaction of our patients.

SELF-TEST

1. What are the features which distinguish Hoyne's *Clinical Therapeutics* from other books on Therapeutics? (Para 3)

2. What is the advice of Dr. Clarke in a case when the differential symptoms named in the *Prescriber* (or any other work in therapeutics) are not sufficient to enable a choice to be made with due certainty? (Para 4)

3. According to Dr. Lilienthal, what type of work is worthy of being named "homoeopathic therapeutics"? What is the description given to his own work on the subject? (Para 5)

4. What are the advantages of *Practical Homoeo. Therapeutics* of Dr. Dewey, from the viewpoint of a busy practitioner? (Para 7)

5. What are the limitations of therapeutic hints in homoeopathic practice? (Para 11, 12, 13)

6. How can we turn therapeutic hints to our advantage inspite of their limitations ? (Para 17, 18, 19)

7. What is the reason for most failures in homoeopathy? How can we make sure of selecting the similimum? (Para 12, 22, 25)

Books mentioned above are available with M/s. B. Jain Publishers (P) Ltd., Post Box - 5775 , New Delhi - 55.

Lesson 13

Literature on Homoeopathy

(Books recommended for essential reading and reference.)

1. One has to be choosy in regard to his reading, and this is especially so in the present day when we are flooded with literature; yes, even on homoeopathy. Some wise man has said that "some books deserve not more than a glance, some need to be read carefully, studied not once but again and again, and some others should be constantly referred to whenever in doubt." Books acquire importance according to the stage of our learning. What is important in the early stage becomes superfluous in the advanced stage. As for the books of reference, we have to cultivate a sort of friendship, a familiarity of high degree, if we are to get from them the direction or information we need without much of hunting, that is, almost at a glance.

2. Bearing these points in mind we shall recommend a few important books for those who are absolutely new to this subject. For this purpose, we shall divide the students of homoeopathy into three classes or stages :

(i) Elementary stage.

(ii) Middle stage.

(iii) Advanced stage.

We could also categorise them as equivalent to "School level", "Graduate level" and "Post-Graduate level" respectively. Of course, this is an arbitrary division which is made only for the sake of convenience. Depending upon the depth of interest of the student and his speed of learning, he could first glance through the books in a library and then decide on those he would like to buy for his constant reference, irrespective of the "stages" assigned to them here.

ELEMENTARY (BEGINNER'S) STAGE

Principles and Philosophy

1. **Brief Study Course in Homoeopathy** — by Elizabeth Hubbard. As the name implies, this is a very good introduction to homoeopathy for beginners, written by one who was a master of the art of prescribing. The author covers all important aspects of Homoeopathy — principles and practice — in a nutshell. This book provides a good stepping stone to higher levels of knowledge.

Homoeopathy — Principles and Practice. This small booklet by Douglass Borland who, in his time, reared a generation of young homoeopaths in England, covers the principles and practice of homoeopathy and makes it very easy for beginners to know the subject, before they go on to study more detailed books.

2. **On the Comparative Value of Symptoms** — This essay by Gibson Miller has deservedly become popular for its masterly exposition of this important aspect of homoeopathic philosophy and its application in practice. A close study of this booklet even repeated at intervals, is a must for any serious minded student of homoeopathy.

3. **How not to do it** — By Margaret Tyler. In this small booklet the reputed author cautions those untrained in the fundamental doctrines of homoeopathy against some common but serious errors, such as prescribing for the disease, too frequent repetition, how to minimise labour in repertorising, hasty prescribing, prescribing during amelioration, the danger attending on the use of high potencies in advanced cases of pathology and the supreme importance of not interfering with the action of a well considered prescription. Tyler's forceful words, born out of her bitter experiences, have a highly educative never-to-be forgotten effect.

Materia Medica

4. **Leaders in Homoeopathic Therapeutics** — by E.B. Nash. His style of presentation creates an immediate interest in the subject and makes it easy for the beginner to follow up later with the study of more detailed works on the subject. Please also read Para 11 (i) of Lesson 3.

5. **Key-notes and Characteristics of the Materia Medica with Nosodes** — by H.C. Allen. This book is the result of years of study by the author, as student, practitioner and teacher in Hering Medical College. It was written at the earnest solicitation of many alumni of the college, with the object of aiding the student to master that which is guiding and characteristic in the individuality of each remedy and to place the mastery of the characteristics within the reach of everyone in the profession. The undimmed popularity of this book is a testimony to its practical usefulness.

6. **Key to Materia Medica** — by Pulford. A full description of this work has been given in para 10 of Lesson 8. The reader learns from this book not only the most characteristic symptoms of each remedy, but it also has the advantage of the symptoms presented in the schema (anatomical sections from head downwards).

7. **Pocket Manual of Homoeopathic Materia Medica** — by William Boericke. This valuable book can almost be described as indispensable to every homoeopathic practitioner. For more details please see para 13 of Lesson 8.

Repertories

8. **Therapeutic Pocket Book** — by Boenninghausen. This was the first ever Repertory, the plan of which was approved by Hahnemann himself. This work had served the profession for nearly a century, till it was overshadowed by Kent's and later by its own enlarged and revised edition brought out by C.M. Boger. To those who know how to use it, its usefulness is not yet dimmed by other repertories. It contains rubrics not found even in the other repertories. In our opinion, this book is worth its price for the preface by Boenninghausen and the brilliant introduction by H.A. Roberts.

9. **A Synoptic Key of the Materia Medica** — by C.M. Boger. This useful work has been fully described in para 11 of Lesson 8.

Therapeutics

10. **Beginner's Guide to Homoeopathy** — by T.S. Iyer. This book is a good introduction to homoeopathy for beginners, as it covers not only philosophy, but detailed advice on practice.

Various diseases are described with their etiology, course and prognosis together with the homoeopathic remedies that are likely to be found useful. All these, coming from an Indian author, born of his experiences, make this work a useful addition to the library shelf of the beginner.

11. **The Prescriber** — by John H. Clarke. Various complaints are taken up in alphabetical order in this book and their treatment with several remedies is given together with the dosage. Besides the therapeutic guidance it gives, the "Introduction" is worthy of careful study.

12. **Pointers to Common Remedies** — by Margaret Tyler. The therapeutic hints given by this master prescriber, giving detailed symptoms of each remedy for a given clinical condition, are highly useful and deserve close study.

13. **Miscellaneous**. The following Essays, Papers or Tracts, being low-priced, should not be missed by the new student, as they provide us with the experiences and views of different authors of note. The title of each book is self-explanatory, and hence detailed comments are not considered necessary.

14. **Different Ways of Finding the Remedy** — by Margaret Tyler (p. 16)

15. **Difficulties in Homoeopathic Prescribing** — by Sir John Weir (p. 28)

16. **Clinical Verifications and Reflections** — by S.P. Koppikar.

17. **Practical Homoeopathic Prescribing** — by P.G. Quinton (p. 18)

18. **Acute Conditions, Injuries, etc. (Special Indications of 36 Outstanding Remedies)** — by Tyler and Sir John Weir (p. 43)

19. **The Significance of Past History in Homoeopathic Prescribing** — by D.M. Foubister (p. 20)

20. **Stories of Conversion to Homoeopathy** — Compiled by P. Sankaran. (p. 42)

21. **Fifty Reasons for being a Homoeopath** — by J. Compton Burnett (p. 72).

22. **"The Homoeopathic Heritage"** — (Editor: Dr. S.P. Koppikar). B. Jain Publishers, 1921, Chuna Mandi, New Delhi-110055. (Annual Subscription — 1984 : Rs. 40/-).

Middle (Graduate) Stage

Principles and Philosophy :

23. **Lectures on Homoeopathic Philosophy** — by James Tyler Kent (p. 276). These lectures were delivered by Kent in the Post-Graduate School of Homoeopathy and are regarded by the profession as the ablest and most authoritative commentary on the various doctrines propounded in the *Organon of Medicine*. Kent says that "To safely practise the art of curing sick people, the homoeopathic physician must know the science", and any one who is anxious to master this science cannot do so without a careful study of these lectures.

24. **Organon of Medicine** — by Samuel Christian Hahnemann. A number of authors have translated this work in English (from the original in German); and there are also a number of "easy presentations". These smaller works no doubt serve the limited purpose of acquainting the reader with the doctrines of this science. However, this work with commentary by Dr. B.K. Sarkar helps us to understand the Master's ideas on all points of theory and practice. All the pioneers like Hering, Lippe, Kent, Stuart Close, H.A. Roberts, etc. used always to turn to the aphorisms in this basic text on the theory and practice of this system left to us by the founder. As such, to practise homoeopathy correctly, every homoeopath must study this work thoroughly.

Materia Medica

25. **Kent's Lectures on Homoeopathic Materia Medica**. Kent was a giant in his knowledge of remedies, in his application of them in practice based on philosophy, as well as in his ability to build unforgettable word pictures of the remedies. Hence, any one who wants to master the Materia Medica should lose no time in taking up this for study.

26. Homoeopathic Drug Pictures — by Margaret Tyler. This is a unique work which compels attention by its style and at the same time instructs as well as inspires the reader.

27. Hering's Condensed Materia Medica — Hering says in his preface to this work : "The most complete works on Materia Medica present by their size great obstacles to the rapid acquirement of a practical knowledge of the genius of each remedy. The real object in preparing this work has been to give in a condensed form such absolutely necessary material as would enable the student, in a comparatively short time, to gain knowledge of such important leading symptoms and conditions as are characteristic of each remedy — knowledge which is imperatively necessary for everyday practice."

28. Dictionary of Practical Materia Medica — by Dr. John H. Clarke (Three Volumes). Homoeopathic science owes not a little to the patient and untiring labours of Dr. Clarke in collecting information about the curative powers of all types of remedies and presenting it in his volumes. In compiling this work Dr. Clarke decided to include all the remedies of which definite use had been recorded in homoeopathic literature. "If some are inclined to object that I have included too many", he says in his preface, "I reply that my work is a Dictionary, and I have never yet found a Dictionary that explained too many words." The plan of the book has been conceived and executed with an eye to practical usefulness. Each remedy is described under several headings: First comes the source and manner of preparation of the remedy; next is given an alphabetical list of the disease in which it has manifested some curative power. The next featue, "characteristics" describes the leading features of the drug, including the key-notes, modalities and sensations. This condensed presentation of the true genius of each remedy is remarkably educative. Then follows the schematic symptoms from head downwards, which tell us the exact symptoms produced or cured by a drug . Again, when a prescriber has found his correspondence in some leading symptoms, he may wish to test the correspondence in other particulars. For these purposes nothing short of a detailed list of symptoms in each section of the schema is of service. The paragraphs of "Relationships" and "Causations" further enhance the value of this work.

29. Physiological Materia Medica. *(Containing all that is known of the physiological action of our Remedies together with* *their characteristic indications and pharmacology)* — by W.H. Burt, M.D., pp. 992. There can be no serious practitioner of homoeo. therapeutics who will not find this work to be of much practical value. The author has taken enormous pains to collect the material from various sources, and asserts in his preface that the subject matter of each drug has been attested by competent authorities, and hence is made up of solid practical facts, that can be relied upon at the bed-side with positive certainty. The most valuable feature of this work is a special study of the physiological action of each drug, for says the author, drug pathology is quite as necessary to the scientific physician as disease pathology. The first thing to learn about a drug is its physiological and pathological action upon the healthy human organism. To know what tissues it acts upon and just how it affects them, leads directly to its curative action; one drug acts upon the nerves of motion, another upon the nerves of sensations; one relaxes, another contracts; one acts upon the mucous membranes, another upon the bones — each one producing certain pathological conditions in localised parts. The knowledge of this localised action gives us the key to its therapeutics. The second important feature, *viz.*, therapeutic key-notes given in the schema (head to foot) culled from well-known practitioners, complements the first part.

No wonder that the first large edition was sold out in ninety days and the second within a year, necessitating a third edition within sixteen months.

The entire approach of the book will be found to be not only an eye opener, but also of great practical use to graduates in modern medicine, who may find the description of physiological action and tissue affinity of the drugs to be more instructive than symptomatology alone.

Repertories

30. **Boenninghausen's Repertory with Characteristics** — by Dr. C.M. Boger. The special features of this Repertory and their usefulness even for beginners, have been dealt with in Lesson 5, Para 8.

31. **How to find the Similimum with Boger-Boenninghausen's Repertory** — by Dr. Bhanu D. Desai. As the title indicates, this small book provides valuable guidance for using the Boger-Boenninghausen's Repertory. The book repre-

sents the extended experience of the author over 35 years of practice, during which he has used the Repertory almost exclusively. Its value as a guide to easy repertorisation is enhanced by the actual working out of 25 cases of different prescribers, and fifty more cases given as an exercise in repertorisation. One who works out these exercises will have no difficulty to quickly develop mastery in using this Repertory to find the remedy in any type of case.

32. A Concise Repertory of Homoeopathic Medicines — by S.R. Phatak. Unlike other repertories, this one presents all the rubrics in alphabetical order. This unique feature together with the fact that the author has drawn largely from Boger's *Synoptic Key* and has also made a number of his own additions, makes this Repertory a quick and useful bed-side reference tool. It contains many rubrics not found in Kent's.

33. The Comparison of the Chronic Miasms — by Phyllis Speight. The author presents in an easily understandable form of charts a comparison of the characteristic symptoms of Psora, Pseudo-Psora, Syphilis and Sycosis, under the heads of Head, Mind, Eyes, etc. These she has culled from Hahnemann's *Chronic Diseases*", J.H. Allen's *Chronic Miasms* and H.A. Robert's *Principles and Art of Cure by Homoeopathy*. An extremely useful book of reference on Miasms, which deserves careful study.

Therapeutics

34. Practical Homoeopathic Therapeutics — by W.A. Dewey. This work has been dealt with in Lesson 9 in detail.

35. Select Your Remedy — by Bishamber Das. This treatise contains the practical experience of 45 years of medical practice by the author. A very useful book, it describes the salient symptoms of a number of remedies which may be called for in a given condition. No book on therapeutics can individualise the remedy, but from the group of drugs which it provides us with, we can go to the next stage of individualisation. This book has also been dealt with in Para 9 of Lesson 9.

36. Graphic Drug Pictures with Clinical Comments — by Pulford. While outlining the characteristic symptoms of each remedy, the author has given the various clinical conditions in which the remedy has proved or is likely to prove useful. This admixture of Materia Medica with therapeutic comments is very useful both for beginners and veterans alike. Not very detailed, and for that reason very useful.

37. **Potency Problem** — by P. Sankaran. This is a very instructive compilation of the views and experiences of a large number of practitioners and may be read with profit by those who would like to widen their horizon on this important aspect of prescribing.

38. **Selection of the Similimum and Management of the Patient** — by P. Sankaran. This was the last booklet written by the author during his final illness. It deals with the most important and the central point of homoeopathic practice, i.e. the selection of the similimum. The secrets of the art are revealed in the simplest way by one who used it sucessfully in treating thousands of cases.

ADVANCED (POST-GRADUATE) STAGE

Principles and Philosophy

39. **Principles of Prescribing** — by Dr. K.N. Mathur (pp. 671). The main purpose of this book, according to the author himself is to collect all the prescribing principles based on the truth of illustrated cases and can be verified by other homoeopaths. These principles of prescribing are collected from old and new homoeopathic journals and books, so that they are available in the form of a book for all times, as the journals and old literature may not be available always. They will be useful for the coming generations of homoeopaths. The author has succeeded in his aim admirably, and the compilation of typical cases from a large number of practitioners, foreign and Indian, repays careful study.

Materia Medica

40. **A Study of Materia Medica** — by Dr. N.M. Choudhury. These are lectures on the lines of Kent's *Lecturer*, by an Indian prescriber and teacher of note; can be read with much benefit.

41. **Clinical Materia Medica** — by E.A. Farrington (pp. 826). Homoeopathic literature has been greatly enriched by the pen of this master-mind whom Hering recognised as well fitted to a place in the highest rank among the expounders of the

most intricate aspects of our Materia Medica. These lectures on clinical application of remedies, giving comparisons of several remedies for a given condition, by this brilliant teacher have guided many homoeopaths.

42. **Key-notes and Red-line Symptoms** — by Adolph Lippe. Lippe is held in high esteem as a prescriber of unique ability wherever homoeopathy is practised. This book contains not only the key-notes which Dr. Lippe had found useful; but the key-notes brought to the notice of the profession by many other authors as well. As such, it is a very useful book of reference and study.

43. **Master-key to Homoeopathic Materia Medica** — by Dr. K. C. Bhanja, B.A., H.D. (National Homoeo Laboratory, Calcutta-700014), pp. 488. In this book the author, who was a master prescriber, has presented the homoeopathic remedies in a novel method which is at once arresting and practical. The remedies are described not in the usual Hahnemannian schema but in quite a different pattern, *viz.* :

(i) Introductory with the ground key-notes.

(ii) General guiding symptoms which are sub-divided into :

    (a) Adaptability (*i.e.* suitable for).

    (b) Mentals.

    (c) Physical Generals.

    (d) Aggravations and ameliorations in general.

    (e) Aggravation and ameliorations relating to particulars.

    (f) Marked features, which vary according to the genius of each remedy — *e.g.*; for *Eup.-per.* the heading of marked features are : Sore bruised feeling, vommiting and biliousness and anomalous character; for *Pulsatilla* they are : Ever changing, alternating. thirstlessness. Thick bland, yellowish green discharges, erratic, one-sidedness, chilliness, bitterness, suddenness and metastasis.

(g) Other leading indications, i.e., various complaints in which the remedy is found useful.

(h) Relationship.

(i) Comparisons.

(j) Potency

(k) Lastly a useful chapter on antidotal relationship.

The author has immeasurably enhanced the value of this book narrating his own as well as other's experiences at appropriate places. Even more important, he has obviously correlated the entire text with his own observations in practice. These facts make this one of the most practical and "must be studied and constantly referred to" books on Materia Medica.

44. **Materia Medica of the Nosodes** — by H.C. Allen (pp. 576). This treatise on the Nosodes has no equal in homoeopathic literature. It was completed by the distinguished author a short time before his death and represents the result of years of study, experience and of proving and confirming the symptomatology. In view of the important, nay, key-role played by nosodes in homoeopathic treatment, no serious student can dispense with a constant study and mastery of the nosodes.

45. **Chronic-Miasms** — by J.H. Allen. No one can claim to have mastered the art of homoeopathic prescribing without a thorough knowledge of the chronic miasms. This book is a great help in acquiring such knowledge. Dr. Allen says in the preface that the demands of his students, and requests from the profession at large induced him to put his knowledge of these subjects into book form. He further states that each miasm has its own peculiar history, its physiological expressions, its mental phenomena, its aggravations of time and circumstances, its secondary and tertiary manifestations upon mucous surfaces or upon the skin. All these characteristics of Psora, Pseudo Psora (Tubercular), Sycosis and Syphilis are fully explained in this work. The peculiar features of each miasmatic remedy are also given.

46. **Guiding Symptoms of our Materia Medica** — by Dr. Constantine Hering. The unique importance of this work comprising ten volumes has been explained in Lesson 3.

47. Chronic Diseases by Hahnemann. In this Hahnemann's original work on the chronic miasms, he explains how he unravelled the nature of these hidden stigmatae (poisons) in the human body and the nature of havoc they cause. The first volume deals with the philosophy of chronic miasms and the second delineates the characteristics of the various anti-miasmatic remedies. A study of these volumes from the master's pen is necessary to round out one's mastery of the chronic miasms.

Repertories

48. Kent's Repertory. This is an essential tool of every homoeopath and its usefulness has been explained in Lesson 5 (Para 9).

49. A Study of Kent's Repertory — by Margaret Tyler. This little booklet explains how to use Kent's Repertory.

50. Repertory of Hering's Guiding Symptoms — by Dr. Calvin B. Knerr. Voluminous as the *Guiding Symptoms* are (in ten volumes), this Repertory based on the *Guiding Symptoms* could be likened to the key which unlocks the door to the hidden wealth. The Repertory is in the usual schema form (Mind, Head, Eyes, etc.) and unlike Kent's or Boger-Boenninghausen's Repertories, attempt is made to give each rubric as a complete symptom, i.e., with location, sensation and modality. For example, "Vertex, heaviness : pain, like a weight, better pressing, worse sounds, hearing, talking or from strong light, *Cact.*" (p. 157). As in other repertories, the remedies have marks : 4, 3, 2 or 1. The author says in the preface : "Although the Repertory is a faithful reproduction of the *Guiding Symptoms*, its contents, classified and indexed, as a matter of course, in no way can it take the place of the larger work. This Repertory many times helps when the others fail."

51. Kishore Cards — by Dr. Jugal Kishore. Card Repertories save us a lot of time and labour, as all that we have to do with such a Repertory for getting the remedy, is to pick out the relevant rubric cards and place them one upon another. The punched hole we see through all the cards represents the remedy. This card Repertory prepared by Dr. Jugal Kishore, is reported to contain a large number of rubrics and to have proved more useful than other card Repertories.

Therapeutics

52. Homoeopathic Therapeutics — by S. Lilienthal. This is a stupendous collection of remedies which have been found useful in varying types of diseases, and is bound to help any one who hunts through it for the remedy. (See Lesson 9).

53. Clinical Therapeutics — by Temple S. Hoyne. Please see Para 3 of Lesson 9.

54. Therapeutics of Fever — by Dr. H.C. Allen. Running into 571 pages, including a repertorial section, this is an extremely useful work from the pen of one who possessed rare powers of observation and insight into the various remedies of the homoeopathic Materia Medica. The author says in his preface: "Experience has conclusively verified the teachings of Hahnemann, that the most obstinate and intractable cases occur chiefly in psoric or tubercular patients, and the more deep the dyscrasia the more protracted the fever. Hahnemann's lesson in the *Chronic Diseases* on the treatment of acute syphilis must be applied to fevers of all types and acute diseases of every name and every kind, irrespective of habitat . . . . The same law of cure, the same rule of practice applies to each patient. It is the patient not the fever that is chiefly and especially to be considered. It is the individual with his or her peculiar idiosyncracies and constitutional inheritances with which we have to deal. As a rule, the family history is much more suggestive of the curative remedy than the rapid pulse and high temperature, and should be carefully studied. When discovered, the constitutional miasm — psora, sycosis, syphilis, tuberculosis — should be especially noted, for here will often be found the key with which to unlock the secret of the severity of the attack or the relapsing tendency of the fever." D. Allen continues, "It is the experience of the author that if the remedy be selected from the totality of the objective, subjective and miasmatic symptoms, the patient may be cured in any stage of the fever. It is not necessary for any fever to "run its course." These remarks of the author are sufficient to reveal the stamp of authority backed by experience which the detailed description of the characteristics of various remedies given herein bears.

55. Diarrhoea — by James Bell. This is yet another classic work on a single disease condition, *viz.* diarrhoea and dysentery, which no homoeopathic physician should be without.

56. **Pneumonia** — by Douglas Borland. This is one more classic from the pen of an experienced artist in homoeopathic practice. Even though modern medicine has taken the dread out of pneumonia, the author shows how with homoeopathy we can do better.

57. **Accoucher's Emergency Manual** — by Yingling. This small booklet is worth its weight in gold (even at the dizzy rates prevailing today). Is not easy and safe parturition and the ushering of healthy babies in this world worth the low price of this booklet?

58. **Some Emergencies of General Practice** — by Douglas M. Borland. This masterly lecture of the famous physician is particularly useful because the success in handling emergencies may make or mar the reputation of the physician. This lecture will infuse into homoeopaths a new enlightenment, confidence and courage in handling such cases.

Journals

59. **Homoeopathic Heritage**, B. Jain Publishers, 1921 Chuna Mandi, Paharganj, New Delhi- 110055.

60. **Indian Journal of Homoeopathic Medicine** — (Quarterly) — Society Road, Irla, Vile Parle, Bombay - 400056.

61. **Quarterly Homoeopathic Digest**, Dr. K.S. Srinivasan, 1253, 66th Street, Korattur, Madras - 600080.

Books mentioned above are available with M/s. B. Jain Publishers (P) Ltd., Post Box - 5775 , New Delhi - 55.

Appendix "A"

Questionnaire For Taking The Case

Please indicate a normal condition of health by writing "N". (1) A moderately experienced pain, by putting one plus (+); a severe one by two pluses (++); and a very severe one by three pluses (+++). (2) Where two opposite conditions are given together (*e.g.* tall/short), strike off the one which is not applicable. (3) Put a cross (x) against questions not applicable to the patient.

Date : _____

Name : _____

Sex : M/F.   Occupation : _____

Address : _____

Married/Unmarried : _____

Height : Tall/Medium/Short : _____

Build : Thin/Normal/Obese.   Age : _____

(1) (a) Please state briefly the serious complaints the patient has suffered from since childhood.

| Nature of complaint. | Year of occurrence. | How long did it last. | Any recurrence thereafter. |

(b) Any history of Asthma, T.B., Cancer, Psoriasis, Insanity & c. in close relations? _____

Appendix "A" 259

2. Present (Chief) Complaints : Please state all the disorders patient has latterly suffered from — even if he considers any of them unimportant, or not related to his main complaint.

Part of body   Sensations and   Modalities   Probable
* affected.   complaints.   Agg. or Amel. by   Cause.*
(Right/left side)

(For a list of sensations please refer to Q. No. 16; and for a list of modalities, refer to Q. No. 14).

3. a. Any disorder of senses of Taste/Smell/Hearing/Vision/ Touch : _____

   b. Appetite/Hunger : Is it normal : _____ Excessive? _____ Deficient _____ Capricious (at unusual times)? _____ (Wanting).

   Does he feel filled up after a few morsels of food _____ Abdomen bloated _____ Flatulence (gas)? _____ Heartburn? _____ Eructations? _____

   c. Food items for which patient has a craving or aversion and which disagree with him.

Food Items	Craving	Aversions	Disagree
Sweets	—	—	—
Salty things	—	—	—
Sour things	—	—	—
Milk	—	—	—
Eggs	—	—	—
Meat/fish	—	—	—
Butter	—	—	—
Spices (Condiments)	—	—	—
Potatoes/Starchy foods	—	—	—
Fried things	—	—	—
Drinks, Warm/Cold	—	—	—
Drinks, ice cold	—	—	—
Onion/garlic	—	—	—
Lime, chalk, undigestible	—	—	—
Raw vegetables	—	—	—
Juicy, refreshing things	—	—	—
Alcoholic liquors	—	—	—
Any other	—	—	—

Thirst : Please indicate the intensity of his thirst with suitable ticks.
Thirsty (drinks a lot in a day).
Thirstless (drinks comparatively little in a day).
Quantity and Frequency : Thirst for large/small quantity and at long/short intervals.

4. **Stools** : Please indicate severity with plus marks :

Nature of Stools	Soft	Hard	Bloody	Slimy	With Urging	Must Strain	No. of Stools
Normal	—	—	—	—	—	—	—
Constipated	—	—	—	—	—	—	—
Loose	—	—	—	—	—	—	—
Dysenteric	—	—	—	—	—	—	—

Piles :

Bleeding : _____ Blind : _____ Protruding : _____
Itching : _____ Burning : _____ Fissures : _____
Painful : _____ Fistula : _____
Aggravated by : _____ Ameliorated by : _____

5. **Urine** :

Profuse/scanty : _____ Frequent : _____
Dribbling : _____ Burning : _____
Involuntary _____ Day/Night : _____ Colour : _____
Odour : _____ Painful : _____ Deposits : _____
Sugar : _____ Stones (Kidney/Bladder) : _____
Position in which urine passed easily : _____

6. **Breathing** :

Any complaints : _____
Bronchitis : _____ Asthma _____ Rapid _____
Oppressed : _____ Rattling : _____ Wheezing : _____
Difficult Expiration/Inspiration : _____

Cough :

Hollow _____ Harassing _____ Tickling _____
Spasmodic _____

Appendix "A"

Expectoration :

Taste : _____ Odour _____
Copious/Little : _____
Watery : _____ Tenacious : _____

7. Sexual (a) Male :

Desire : Strong/Weak : _____ Erection, Strong/Weak _____
Emissions : In sleep : _____ During stool : _____
Too early _____
Coition, any complaints during : _____ or after : _____
History of Venereal diseases, if any (give details) :

(b) Female :

Age at first menstruation : _____

Menses :
Profuse/Scanty : Too early/Too late.

Flow

| Nature of complaints in relation to menses. | Red Before Menses. | Dark During Menses. | Pitch-like After Menses. | Smell Fetid |

Leucorrhoea :

Watery : _____ Thick/tenacious : _____
Fetid smell : _____ Acrid/excoriating : _____
Causes itching : _____
Abortion, if any : _____ during which month of pregnancy.
Coition : Aversion to : _____ Desire, Strong/Weak : _____
Number of children : _____ Sterility : _____

8. Sides of Body Affected :

(Please name the anatomical region, also stating right or left side of body).

Complaints first appeared in _____ Right/Left side.
Complaints then extended to _____ R/L from _____

Complaints wander or shift from one place to another (no fixed place) _____
Complaints appear in a spot : (Where) _____
Complaints radiate to different parts _____ R/L.
Direction of pains : go up _____ go down _____ diagonal _____

9. Cold or Hot (Burning) Sensations :

Cold/Hot (Burning in : Vertex _____ Eyes : _____
Ears _____ Face _____ Stomach : _____ Abdomen : _____
Back : _____ Palms : _____ Soles : _____)

10. Sweat if excessive :

(a) Where _____
(b) When : (State time and circumstances) : _____
(c) Odour of sweat : _____
(d) Does it stain clothes : Yellow : _____

Very little sweat (dry skin) : _____
Partial sweat on : Head/feet/soles _____

11. Skin, Glands and Bones :

Nature of disorder   Where   Dry   Oozing   Itching

Moist Watery Viscid Bloody Pus Burning

12. Sleep :

Normal, sound : _____ Disturbed, _____ Difficult, after walking : _____ .
Too sleepy (even day-time) : _____ Sleeplessness : _____
Unrefreshing : _____

Position in Sleep :

Lies on back : _____ on Right/Left side.
Lies on abdomen : _____ Head raised (high pillows) : _____
Dreams : Pleasant : _____ Unpleasant : _____
Nightmare : _____ Snoring : _____

Appendix "A" 263

13. **Constitutional Tendencies** :

Does the patient

(i) Catch cold easily with sneezing/blocked nose, often : _____

(ii) Get stomach/abdominal complaints frequently : _____

(iii) Have throat complaints often : _____
(iv) Suffer often from cough with/without phlegm : _____

(v) Any disorder of respiration : _____
(vi) Get urinary complaints often : _____
(vii) Find that wounds take long to heal : _____
(viii) Bleed easily, from any part (urine/stool/nose/mouth : _____

(ix) Feel fatigued/tired easily : _____,
(x) Any Addiction to : Alcoholic liquors/tobacco/drugs, etc : _____

14. **Modalities** (General) :

Please indicate by plus marks (or exact statement) the time, the temperature (weather) and the circumstances when the patient's sufferings are markedly increased (aggravated) or very much relieved, i.e., ameliorated. (Please state the exact time, if so observed : e.g., 10 a.m., 12 noon, or 5 p.m., or 9 p.m. or 12 midnight, and so on).

Time :	Morning	Forenoon	Noon	Afternoon	Whole Day (Sunrise to sunset)
Agg.	—	—	—	—	—
Amel.	—	—	—	—	—

	Evening	Before Midnight	After Midnight		Whole Night (Sunset to sunrise)
Agg.	—	—	—	—	—
Amel.	—	—	—	—	—

Aggravation during *full moon* — ; *new moon* — ;
Other fixed intervals —

Modifying Conditions	Agg.	Amel.
Temperature		
Dry Heat/Summer	—	—
Dry Cold/Winter	—	—
Wet Cold/Rainy Season	—	—
Cool Open Air	—	—
Wind/Fan/Draft	—	—
Sun Exposure to	—	—
Change of Weather	—	—
Bathing/Washing	—	—
Drinks, Cold/Warm	—	—
Uncovering	—	—
Circumstances		
Darkness/Light	—	—
Eating : Before/During/After	—	—
Raising/hanging down, of limbs	—	—
Exertion, mental	—	—
Exertion, physical	—	—
Loss of vital fluids (Blood, semen & c.)	—	—
Rubbing/message	—	—
Standing	—	—
Sleep before	—	—
Sleep during	—	—
Sleep after	—	—
Supressions (Eruptions, Coryza, Menses & c)	—	—
Fasting — delay in eating	—	—
Company, Society	—	—
Looking up/down	—	—
Looking sideways/intently	—	—
Lying down	—	—
Lying on back	—	—
Lying on right/left side	—	—
Lying on painful/painless side	—	—
Motion, movement	—	—
Motion, beginning of	—	—
Motion, continued	—	—
Motion slow, gentle	—	—
Odours, strong	—	—
Over-eating	—	—

Appendix "A"

Temperature	Agg.	Amel.
Over-lifting	—	—
Noises, sensitiveness to	—	—
Pressure	—	—
Pressure of clothes or neck-tie	—	—
Riding in car/ship/plane	—	—
Sitting	—	—
Stooping	—	—
Stool, before	—	—
Stool, during	—	—
Stool, after	—	—
Suppressed emotions	—	—
Turning over in bed	—	—
Touch	—	—
Urination : Before/During/After	—	—

15. **Patient's emotional make-up.** Self-assessment by the patient of this aspect is difficult, as one can rarely be objective with regard to one's own emotions and temperament. So, please have this assessment made by a friend or relation, showing the intensity by one, two or three ticks — i.e., in addition to patient's own assessment. The physician, for his part, should elicit various instances in the life of the patient which can throw significant light on his mental-emotional state.

Emotional State	Intensity	Conditions which agg.
Anger, easy to — expresses	—	—
Anger, easy to — Supresses	—	—
Broods over insult	—	—
Careful/scrupulous/fastidious	—	—
Fears of all kinds	—	—
Fear of darkness	—	—
Fear of evil/misfortune	—	—
Fear of ordeals/exams	—	—
Fear of being along	—	—
Obstinate/headstrong	—	—
Sensitive/takes offence easily	—	—
Gentle, can be persuaded	—	—
Grief-stricken	—	—
Timid/Cowardly	—	—

Emotional State	Intensity	Conditions which agg.
Loquacious	—	—
Suspicious	—	—
Restless	—	—
Jealous	—	—
Anxiety	—	—
Delusions/Fantasies	—	—
Despair	—	—
Disappointed in love	—	—
Depressed/sad/melancholy	—	—
Fault/finding	—	—
Hurried/impatient	—	—
Anxieties/anxious	—	—
Indifferent to loved ones (family)	—	—
Likes/Dislikes — Sympathy	—	—
Moods, very changeable	—	—
Memory Weak/lost	—	—
Proud arrogant	—	—
Sex, constant thinking of	—	—
Tired of life/suicidal	—	—
Weeps easily	—	—
Sex, suppressed desire	—	—

16. **Sensations, pains and complaints** (General and Particular) : A list of the more commonly felt sensations is given below by way of suggestion only. If any of these pertain to the patient, please put a plus (+) against them, and also write down the region of body where it is felt. Sensations not found here may be added.

Emotional State	Intensity	Aggr. by amel. by
Ball or Plug	—	—
Burning/Heat	—	—
Benumbing	—	—
Bruised	—	—
Bursting/Splitting	—	—
Chilly	—	—
Cramps	—	—
Constricting (like bandage)	—	—
Contracting (as if too short)	—	—
Crawling (insect-like)	—	—
Dizziness/Vertigo	—	—
Emptiness	—	—
Fullness/heaviness	—	—

Appendix "B"

Emotional State	Intensity	Aggr. by amel. by
Fatigued/exhausted	—	—
Tickling (itching internally)	—	—
Tingling	—	—
Whirling	—	—
Lethargy/indolence	—	—
Itching/scratching	—	—
Hammering	—	—
Neuralgic/spasmodic	—	—
Labour-like/bearing down	—	—
Numbness	—	—
Pounding/hammering	—	—
Restlessness (mind/body)	—	—
Scraping	—	—
Sinking/falling	—	—
Jerking/twitching	—	—
Stitching/sticking	—	—
Stiffness/rigidity	—	—
Stinging/prickling	—	—
Sprained/dislocated	—	—
Throbbing/pulsating	—	—
Trembling/quivering	—	—
Tightness/tension	—	—
Paroxysmal/recurrent	—	—

Appendix "B"

Near-Specifics

Strictly speaking, there are no 'specifics, in homoeopathy; the remedy which meets the totality of symptoms in a case is the specific for the individual. Yet, certain remedies have repeatedly proved useful in certain conditions and this knowledge could prove useful the physician, to start with at least. Therefore, before administering any of the remedies recommended in the notes that follow under "Near-Specifics", "Prophylactics" "Causations", "Suppressions" or "Organopathic Remedies" it is most essential to make sure, by reference to the Materia Medica, that it suits the patient. Only thus can one be sure of getting satisfactory results. The potencies, where given, are suggestive rather than mandatory.

Indications	Remedies
Acne of young girls	Calc. phos. (of boys : Calc-picrata)
Angina pectoris	Latrodectus — 200
Angina pectoris worse from slightest motion.	Bryonia — Q-30
Angioneurotic oedema	Antipyrine — 2x
Aphthous stomatitis	Mercurius solubilis — 200
Appendicitis, worse slightest touch.	Belladonna — 30,200
Appendicitis; pain in ileocaecal region, with vomiting of green bile; deathly sensation in epigastrium.	Iris Tenax — 3 to 30x, 30th
Asphyxia, neonatorum	Antimonium-tartaricum— 6-30
Asthma, better from lying in knee-chest position.	Medorr. — 1M and 10M.
Atheromatous arteries	Cactus grand
Blepharo — spasm — first remedy to be thought of.	Agaricus — 30, 200
Blindness, after a lightning stroke. Sees green halo around candle light.	Phosphorus — 200 to 10M
Blood pressure, to lower	Allium-sat. — Q 20-40 drops.
Boils and Ulcers with great sensitiveness to touch, bloody pus.	Hepar-sulph. — 200, 1M, 10M.

Appendix "B"

Indications	Remedies
Bone affections, exostosis, osteo-sarcoma.	Hecla-lawa — 3x to 6x.
Brain fag of students	Picric-ac. or Anac.
Bronchitis in the aged where suffocation from excessive secretion is present.	Hippozaenium — 30
Burns of first and second degree with burning sensation.	Cantharis — Q diluted locally and 30-200 internally.
Carbuncles, or Gangrene with burning pains.	Anthracinum — 30 or 200.
Cardiac dropsy	Adonis Vernalis — Q 5-10 drops.
Cervical nerves, last five, affections of.	Gelsemium — 30, 200.
Chancre of syphilis, primary	Syphilinum 1M one dose daily every night for a month.
Colic of infants, from incarcerated wind.	Senna — low potency.
Colic, recurrent attacks, relieved temporarily by *Colocynth*.	Kali-carb. cures permanently 30, 200.
Constipation of new born infants.	Alumina, Bryonia — 30.
Convulsions from concussion of brain, opisthotonos.	Cicuta-visrosa 6 to 200.
Convulsions, puerperal, continue after delivery.	Cicuta-virosa 6 to 200.

Indications	Remedies
Cyanosia in new born — Asphyxia neonatorum.	Laurocerasus, Q to 3c.
Cystitis	Canth 200 — Sars, Dulc.
Dengue fever, with aching in bones and soreness of flesh.	Eupat. perf. — 6, 30, 200.
Diabetes with rheumatic pains.	Lactic acid — 6x, 30, 200.
Diarrhoea, from apprehension when ready for church or opera.	Argentum-nit. — 30 or 200 (also Gelsemium).
Diphtheria, alternating sides with shining membrane.	Lac-caninum — 200 or higher.
Diphtheria, nasal	Nitric acid — 200, 1M.
Diphtheria, nasal or laryngeal.	Kali-bich. — 200
Diphtheria, nose-bleeding, persistent, during detatchment of membrane.	Phosphorus.
Diphtheria — Diphtheric paralysis.	Diphtherinum — 30, 200.
Diphtheria — great oedema, stinging pains when swallowing, stupor — almost a specific for true diphtheria.	*Apis* — 200 to 10M
Dropsy, after typhoid.	Apis-mel. — 6, 30 or 200.
Dysentery, bloody, with tenesmus before, during and after stools.	Mercurius cor. — 30, 200.
Emphysema, with intense dyspnoea, must sit up.	Mercurius-sulph — 30, 200.

Indications	Remedies
Exertion, physical — bad effects of; Overlifting — inordinate exertion of muscles; sore bruised pain all over.	Rhus-tox. — 30, 200, 1M.
Eye — Haemorrhage into anterior chamber, after Iridectomy.	Ledum-pal — 30, 200.
Eye, traumatic injuries, after a blow from an obtuse body.	Symphytum — 30-Q for external application.
Fevers, septic or puerperal — when the best selected remedy fails.	Pyrogenium — 200, 10M.
Furuncles, small	Picric acid — 30.
Gall stones	Cholesterinum 3x to 200.
Gall stones colic — Oxaluria.	Berberi-vul. — Q 30, Cholesterinum, 200-1M (attacks come and go suddenly).
Goitre, hard — after Iodum failed.	Bromium 30-200
Gonorrhoea, chronic.	Fluoric acid — 6, 30.
Grief, shock — bad effects of (insomnia, suppressed menses, etc.)	Ignatia — 200-1M.
Gummata	Kali-iodatum — 30, 200.
Headache, bursting, from exposure to sun (Sunstroke) :	Glonoine — 30-200.
Headache, begins at sunrise, worse at noon, and declines by sunset.	Spigelia — 30, 200.

Indications	Remedies
Haemoptysis	Acalypha indica — 6 or 30.
Haemorrhage, postpartem.	Cinnamonum — Q 3 drops in sugar.
Haemorrhage, bright red — Profuse menses.	Ficus-religiosa — Q 5 to 10 drops; or 30.
Haemorrhoids, most sensitive to touch; even a sheet of toilet paper is painful.	Muriatic acid — 3, 30. (Cf. Hypericum).
Heart, dilatation, with debility.	Crataegus oxy. — Q 10 to 20 drops.
Heart disease with scanty urine; albuminuria.	Eel-serum — 12, 30, 200.
Hiccough during pregnancy.	Cyclamen — 30.
Hoarseness of singers, as soon as they begin to sing.	Selenium — 30th.
Hysteria; ailments with dry mouth and sleepiness; great flatulence; Globus hystericus.	Nux-mos. — 6, 30.
Impetigo contagiosa.	Antimonium-tart. — CM. single dose (Pulford).
Infantile liver and spleen.	Calcarea — 3x.
Injury to head — chronic effects; epilepsy, forgetfulness etc.	Natrum-sulph. 30, 200, 1M.
Injuries to nerves — bunions, corns, when pain is excruciating. Pain after laparotomy or after dental extraction.	Hypericum — Q to 200, 1M.

Appendix "B"

Indications	Remedies
Jaundice.	Chelidonium — 1x, Myrica. — Q, 3, 200. Carduus Marianus.
Jaundice, malignant — haemorrhagic diathesis.	Crotalus-hor. — 30, 200.
Jaundice, obstructive — Liver disorders.	Chelidonium-maj. — 1x, 6, 30.
Kidney diseases — organopathic remedy; swollen feet. Bright's disease. Albumen, blood and mucous in urine.	Solidago — Q or 3.
Ligaments, torn	Hamamelis — 6x, 30 (after Arn. and Rhus-tox. failed).
Liver and spleen enlarged : with fever : without fever :	Ferr-ars — 3x Ferr-iod. — 3x
Mastitis — breast tumours : breasts inflamed, stony hard, painful.	Phytolacca — 30, 200 (Cf. Bryonia).
Mastoiditis	Capsicum — 30, 200.
Milk, allergy to — milk passes undigested in nursing children.	Magnesia-carb. — 200.
Milk in nursing women, to increase.	Lactuca-virosa — Q.
Miscarriage, habitual — as a uterine tonic.	Viburnum-pruni — Q teaspoonful thrice a day — even 30th.
Mumps — produces perspiration, reduces temperature in high fevers with dry skin.	Pilocarpus — 30 along with indicated remedy.

Indications	Remedies
Neuralgia, intercostal	Ranunculus bulb. — 30, 200.
Night terrors in children	Kali-brom. — 30, 200.
Oedema from Kidney disease with albuminuria	Plumbum-met. — 30, 1M.
Ophthalmia, purulent	Argentum-nit. 1M, a priceless remedy, with an occasional dose of Pulsatilla 200 to favour action of Arg-nit.
Ophthalmia neonatorum	Argentum-nit. — 30 to 200.
Otitis media	Belladonna, one of the best remedies.
Paralysis, Bell's	Causticum — 30, 200, 1000.
Perforation of septum; punched out ulcers — Pain in spots which can be covered by a finger.	Kali-bich. — 30, 1M.
Piles, bleeding with heart symptoms.	Collinsonia — 30, 200.
Placenta preavia	Erigeron 1x.
Prolapse of rectum	Ruta. 30.
Prostate, senile hypertrophy	Ferr. pic. — 6x, 30.
Reynaud's disease — formication under the skin; dry gangrene especially of extremities like toes etc.	Secale-cor. — 30, 200.
Rheumatism of joints	Collinsonia — Q a few drops in a tumbler of water, a teaspoonful every two hours.

Appendix "B"   275

Indications	Remedies
Rheumatic pains, after gonorrhoea.	Sarsaparilla — first to 6th or 30th.
Rheumatic pain in legs and loss of walking power.	Berberis-vul. — Q or 30.
Ringworm, ring shaped lesions and patches of eczema.	Tellurium, 6th or higher. (Nat carb., Nat. mur., Sep., Bacill).
Sciatica, with alternation of numbness and pain.	Gnaphalium — 30, 200.
Sexual weakness with too early ejaculation of semen in coitus.	Titanium 30.
Shingles	Ranunculus-bulb. 10M — 3 doses (Pulford), *Variolinum*, 200
Spleen enlarged, malarial	Ceanothus — Q or 30.
Stammering in children	Bovista. 30.
Stammering in children; has to exert himself a long time before he can utter a word; makes great effort to speak; distorts the face (Bov., Ign., Spig.).	Stramonium 200.
Stammering; repeats first syllable three or four times.	Spigelia — 30, 200.
Teethig diarrhoea in irritable children.	Chamomilla — 30, 200.
Testicles, atrophy (or undescended) in boys.	Aurum-met. — 30, 200.
Tonsillitis, right sided	Mercuriusiod. flavus — 30, 200.

Indications	Remedies
Tonsillitis, left sided	Merc. iod. Ruber — 30, 200.
Traumatic soreness, of soft tissues — Railway spine. Tumours after a blow.	Bellis per. — Q 3, 30, 200.
Tumours, uterine	Aurum muriaticum — 6 or 30.
Tuberculosis of bones, glands, larynx and lungs. Hoarseness of tubercular patients.	Drosera 30, 200, 1M.
Tuberculosis, pulmonary.	Arsenicum-iod. — 3x along with the constitutional remedy.
Ulcers, carbuncles of purplish colour; great burning, stinging pains.	Tarentula cub. — 200.
Urine, retention of, after labour or injury with blunt weapons.	Arnica — 30, 200.
Urine, scanty — with cardiac or renal dropsy with thirst.	Apocynum-cann. — Q 10 drops t.d.s.
Urticaria, chronic.	Bovista — 30.
Voice, total loss of — of professional singers.	Argentum-met.
Vomiting with diarrhoea; excessive exhaustion from least exertion; frequent thirst for small quantities of cool water.	Arsenicum-album — 30, 200 or 1M.
Whooping cough.	Drosera — 6, 30, 200 or 1M.
Worms — inveterate cases, after Cina, Spigelia, Sabadilla, Teucreum fail.	Scirrhinum — 200 or 1M.

Appendix "B"

Indications	Remedies
Wounds — punctured :	Ledum.
Wounds — lacerated :	Calendula Q locally as well as internally — 30, 200.
Clean-cut, surgical :	Staphisagria.
Sentient nerves; shooting pains travel up along nerves :	Hypericum — 200, 1M.
Wounds — of periosteum : of bones : (fractures) :	Ruta 20. Calc.-ph., Symphytum; Pyrogen (septic); Thyroidinum (to speed up healing).
ecchymosis, from :	Arnica — 200, 1M to CM.
Yellow fever	Crotalus Horridus — 30, 200.

Appendix "C"

Prophylactics

"Homoeopathic prophylaxis never causes anaphylaxis or shock, never results in secondary infection, never leaves in its wake serum or vaccine disease or any other severe reaction; it simply protects surely and gently. I generally give a dose of the 10M in most cases and the reaction is good at least for the epidemic". — Dr. A.H. Grimmer.

Indications	Remedies
Air-sickness	Borax; Cocculus 1M.
Bronchitis, capillary of children (mucous rales, bluish face, sweating)	Ant. t. 1M works wonders.
Car sickness	Cocculus, Tabacum.
Chicken-pox	Antim-tart., Puls., Variol.
Cholera	Camphora or Lach. or Sulph. 200th, 3 doses daily.
Croup	Phosphorus 10M (Guernsey).
Diphtheria	Diphtherinum 10M. Merc-cynapium 10M.
Dysentery	Mercurius dulcis (Bacillary). Ars.-alb. (Amoebic).
Emotional diarrhoea	Gels. or Arg-nit. 10M.
Erysipelas	Graphites 1M.
Convulsions, puerperal, immediately after delivery.	Amyl-nit.

Appendix "C" 279

Indications	Remedies
Convulsions, before, during and after delivery.	Cicuta.
Convulsions, during and after delivery.	Hyos.
Placenta, adherent — to prevent	Hydrastis 30
Soreness of parts after labour, to prevent.	Arnica 200.
Abortion, tendency to (Habitual) Any month	Viburnum-prun. 30.
Early months	Apis, Vib-op. 30.
First month	Croc., Vib-op.
Second month	Kali-c., 1M.
Third month	Sabina, Apis, Cimi. Croc., Kali-c., Kreo., Sec., Thu.
Blood black	Kreosotum
Fourth month	Apis 10M.
Fifth to seventh month	Sep.
Seventh month	Sep. 1M., Ruta.
First half of pregnancy	Nitric-ac.
Os, incompetent due to	Apis 10M.
Still-born births (of dead child), to prevent.	Cimic. 1M.
Harelip in children	Calc. sulph. 12x — give to mother, twice a day from 3rd to 7th month of pregnancy.

Indications	Remedies
Haemorrhage, post-partum after hard labour	Millef, 30, given before confinement
Heat stroke	Glonoin 10M
Herpes, recurrent	Hepar-sulph. 10M
Hydrophobia	Bell., Canth., Hyos., Lyssin., Stramonium.
Influenza	Influenzinum 200, 3 doses 8 hourly.
Malaria	Nat-m. 200, weekly one dose for 6 weeks before going to malarial area. Ars. 200 weekly one dose for one month. If malarial symptoms appear while on Ars. then, China-off. 200 one dose for 3 days. If symptoms persist, higher potency of Natrum-mur. once a week will eradicate the disease in most cases (Benj. Goldberg).
Measles	Morbillinum M. Pulsatilla M.
Mumps	Parotidinum 30.
Pus infection	Arnica; Psorinum; Pyrogen 200 to 10M.
Quinsy	Bar-c., Hepar-s., (Painful); Psorinum; (eradicates predisposition).
Rickets	Calc-phos. (failing it, SIL.).
Scarlet fever	Bell. or Scarlet. M.

Appendix "C"

Indications	Remedies
Sea-sickness	Tabacum; Cocculus.
Shingles (Herpes zoster)	Variolinum 200 t.d.s. in one day, repeat at lengthening intervals.
Small-pox	Malandrinum 10M, 3 doses in a week, or Variolin 200, 1M or 10M at 24 hours interval.
Sore-throat : recurrent (Allen)	Bar. C.C.M. or Psorinum M.
Stage fright	Ignatia 200, a few doses on the day of performance, and one dose just before.
Staphyloma : Protrusion of cornea on sclera	Nitric-ac. (Hrg.)
Styes, recurrent	Sulph. 10M (Kent).
Sun stroke	Nat-c., Gels., Glon.
Tetanus	Ledum; Hypericum 1M, 10M repeated doses.
Tubercular inheritance	Bacill. 10M - 50M - CM. (two doses of each on a day, successively at 6 to 8 weeks interval).
Vaccination — Septicemia, following : Acute effects	Malandrinum
Chronic effects	Thuja.
Whitlow	Sil., Nat-s., Dioscorea.
Yellow fever	Ars.-alb., Cimic. 1M Crotalus-horr. 1M.
Whooping cough	Pertussin 30 t.d.s in one day — Repeat at intervals of 3, 6 and 12 months upto age 6.

Appendix "D"

Causations

Complaint (or effect)	Caused by (Preceded by)	Remedy
Asthma	Measles or Whooping cough.	Carbo-veg.
Asthma	Anger	Arsenicum, Chamomilla.
Brain affection — paralysis or convulsions.	Exanthema, sudden retrocession of.	Opium (Zinc.)
Bleeding, profuse, from wound	After an injury	Millef. (Arn., Ham.)
Blindness	Lightning stroke	Phosphorus
Convulsions	Concussion of brain.	Cicuta
Cough	Weeping	Arnica
Diarrhoea	Apprehension of anticipated events, going for interview etc.	Arg-nit.
Diarrhoea	Coffee	Natrum-mur.
Diarrhoea	Excitement	Arg-n., Gels., Phos-ac.
Diarrhoea	Fright	Aconite, Gels
Diarrhoea	Fruits	Ars., Bry., Colo., Ipec., Nat-s., Puls., Verat.

Appendix "D"

Complaint (or effect)	Caused by (Preceded by)	Remedy
Diarrhoea	Milk, boiled	Sep., Nat-m.
Diarrhoea	Milk	Aeth., Calc., Mag-m., Nat-c., Sulph.
Diarrhoea	Sugar	Arg-nit.
Diarrhoea and vomiting	Bad food, food-poisoning, Ice-cream.	Arsenicum-alb. 30 to 10M.
Epilepsy	Blow on head	Melilotus
Facial paralysis	Wetting	Caust., Rhus-t.
Headache	Loss of sleep	Cimic., Coccul., Nux-v.
	Bathing	Ant-cr.
	Coffee	Nux-vom.
Indigestion	Anger	Colocynth.
	Night watching	Nux-vom.
	Pastry, fats, etc.	Puls.
	Vegetables	Arsenicum alb.
	Decayed vegetables	Ars-alb., Carb-an.
	Vexation	Cham.
Involuntary stool and urine.	Injuries	Arnica.
Nausea and vomiting	Odours of cooking food.	Colch., Cocculus, Ipec., Ars., Sep.
	Car sickness	Nux-v., Petrol.

Complaint (or effect)	Caused by (Preceded by)	Remedy
Nausea and vomiting	Sea sickness	Bry., Tabac.
	Air sickness	Cocculus, Borax
Respiratory troubles (bronchitis, emphysema, choking breathing).	Air pollution	Sulphurous acid.
Sleeplessness	Grief	Ignatia, Natrum-mur.
	Excitement	Coff. Hyos., Nux-v. Sep.
	Mental strain	Nux-v.
Surgical shock	Surgical operation	Stront-c.
Sciatica	Wet weather	Rhus-t.
Stiffness of limbs	Physical exertion, overlifting	Rhus-t.
Stool, urging to	Exciting news	Gelsemium, Sulph.
Tetanus	Splinters in the flesh	Cicuta; Hypericum.
Trembling of limbs	Fright	Opium
	Anger	Ran-b., Staph.
	Music	Ambra
Urine, retention of	After operation	Caust.

"Never well since .... " (Ailments or Bad effects from —)
Indications (Causation) *Remedies*
Air, hot, inhaled from fire (blacksmith or while cooking)   Carb-v.
Anger, suppressed; reserved displeasure : Aurum., Ipec., Staph.

Chagrin (mortification), Anger : Staph., Bry., Colo.

Appendix "D" 285

Indications (causation)	Remedies
Chilling, when overheated	Bryonia
Chloromycetin	Carb-v., Chloromycetin in potency (200th).
Cold drinks when overheated	Bellis, Nat-c.
Diphtheria anti-toxin (esp. laryngeal cases).	Antidote : Cal-c., Sulph. 10 M.
Drenching rains, exposure to	Phos., Sep., Rhus-t.
Eggs, bad	Carb-v.
Electric shock	Morphinum.
Exertion, slight — easy sprains; joint swell.	Ledum.
Exertion, unusual mental	Arg-nit.
Exhausting diseases	Carb-v., Chin., Phos., Psor., Selen.
Fire, heat of	Glon.
Grief, from death of loved ones.	Ign., Nat-m.
Head, getting it wet	Bellis, Rhus-t.
Injuries to bones	Heckla, Ruta, Symphytum, Calc.-p., Sil.
Injuries to eyes	Symphytum; Hamam (inflamed).
Injuries to head	Arn., Hyper, Nat-s., Cicuta.
Injuries to nerves	Hyper., Menyanth (teeth).
Injuries to periosteum	Symphytum, Ruta.

Indications (causation)	Remedies
Lifting, overlifting; sprains easily.	Carb-an., Calc., Rhus-t.
Measles (Asthma)	Carbo-veg.
Melon	Zingiber.
Odours, strong	Phosphorus
Overexertion of eyes	Onosmodium, Ruta, Sulph.
Overheating	Carb-v., Ant-c.
Overexertion of mind (loss of sleep).	Cuprum met.
Overstudy	Calc-ph., Nat-c., Phos-ac.
Pneumonia	Kali-c.
Poisoning from bad food	Ars. alb., Pyrogen.
Sunstroke, chronic effects (headache in hot weather).	Nat-c.
Sleep, loss of — from night watching.	Cocculus.
Serum therapy, suppressions from.	Phos., Puls, Sulph., Psor., Thuj.
Sprain, chronic effects :	Stront. c.
Sweat of feet, suppressed	Bar. carb., Silicea.
Tobacco — boy's complaints after using.	Arg-n., Ars., Verat.
Vaccination	Ant-t, (when Thuja fails, and Sil. is not indicated)

Indications (causation)	Remedies
Burns	Caust.
Climacteric	Lach.
Typhoid	Psor., Carb-v.
Wounds, clean cut (Surgical)	Staph.
Wounds poisoned	Lach.
Wounds, punctured (stings, bites, etc.)	Lach. Led.

SUPPRESSIONS — BAD EFFECTS OF

Complaint	Caused by suppression of	Remedy
Ailments from	Suppressed grief	Ign., Nat-mur.
Asthma	Urticaria	Apis
	Rash, in children	Puls.
	Itch or eruptions in general.	Ars.
	Measles, eruptions in general or miliary rash.	Ipec.
	Eruptions	Calc., Borax.
Brain affections	Repercussed eruptions.	Cuprum met.
Brain affections	Non-developed eruptions.	Zincum.
Brain congestion (rolls head from side to side; strabismus)	Suppressed diarrhoea	Podophyllum

Complaint	Caused by suppression of	Remedy
Convulsions	Suppressed eruptions.	Camph., stram., Zinc.
Chorea	Suppressed measles	Rhus-t.
Cerebral troubles	Suppressed eruptions	Cicuta
Deafness	After measles	Puls.
Deafness (tympanum thickens)	Suppressed head eruptions	Mezereum
Deafness (tympanum thickens)	After Otitis media or Scarlatina	Hydrastis
Deafness (tympanum thickens)	Measles, suppressed	Bryonia
Diarrhoea	Suppressed eruptions	Bryonia
Epilepsy	Suppressed eruptions	Agaricus, Psor., Sulph.
Epistaxis	Suppressed menses	Bryonia
Meningitis	Suppressed eruptions	Bryonia, Zinc.
Nervous paroxysms	Milk-crust, suppression of	Viola tricolor
Otorrhoea	Menses	Puls.
Typhoid	After suppressed measles	Puls.
Typhoid symptoms	After suppressed measles	Carb-v.

Appendix "E"

Organopathic Remedies

The elective action of drugs on particular organs, tissues, locations and systems in a peculiar pathological way depicts their inexorable tendency towards some distinct pathological ultimates.

The more the drugs are selected on the basis of their pathological sphere and are organopathic in nature (and the more the Characteristic symptoms are lacking in drug and disease), the greater the confidence with which the lower potencies and crude doses may be used. But these potencies may cause aggravation when the characteristic of drug and disease match in well-proved remedies.

Boger's Synoptic Key gives the region covered by each remedy. For a more detailed list of remedies covering various organs and their disorders, reference may be made to J.H. Clarke's "Clinical Repertory to the Dictonary of Materia Medica."

Sphere of Action	Remedies
Anus, Rectum	Aesc., Graph., Mur-ac., Nit-ac, Paeon., Ratan., Ruta.
Arteries	Cact., Calc-hypo., Crataegus, Lith-c., Lycopus-v, Polygon, Stront-c. etc.
Blood (Bleeding, haemorrhage)	Arnica, Bell., China, Cort-h., Kreos., Phos., Millif., Secale-c., Trillium, Ipecac., Sabina, etc.
Bones	Asaf., Calc, Calc-ph., Flour-ac., Hecla-lava, Mezer., Phos-ac., Ruta., Silic., Symphyt., etc.
Brain	Arnica, Baryt-c., Bell., Cicuta., Cocculus, Helleb., Kali-br., Nux-v., Passif., Pic-ac., Stram., Zinc-pic., etc.

Sphere of Action	Remedies
Female Sex	Alertris far., Aur-m-nat., Caulo., Hamam., Helon., Hydr., Jonosia asoka, Origanum, Ova testa, Puls., Secale cor., Senecio, Thlasp, Trill., Viburn., etc.
Glands	Baryta-carb., Calc-fl., Carb-an., Calc-iod., Clematis, Con., Iod., Lyc., Phyt., Sil., Thu. etc.
Hair	Graph., Mezer., Nat-mur., Petr., Pho., Flour-ac., Pho-ac., Thu., Vinc-m., Thall., etc.
Heart Remedies	Amyl-nit., Adonis-v., Apocyn., Cactus., Convall., Crataegus, Digit, Latrodectus. Lycopus-v., Moschus, Spartium., Spigelia, etc.
Joints	Calc-fl., Led., Phyt., Rhus-tox., Sanguin, Bry., Lyc., etc.
Kidneys	Berb-v., chimaph., Copaiva, Equis., Pareira-br., Petros., Rhus arom., Sabal-ser., Sarsap., Eel's Serum., Solidago, Verb., etc.
Liver and Gall Bladder	Berb-v., Carduus-mar., Chelidonium, Chionanth., Cholest., Chin., Myrica., Cerifera, Ptelia, etc.
Lungs	Aco., Ant.,t., Ars-iod., Ipecac., Lyc., Phos., Myrtus-com., Pix-liq., Illicium., Antars etc.
Lymph Glands	Phyt., Cistus, Rhus-t., Baryt-iod., etc.
Membranes, Mucous	Borax, Merc-sol., Sabad., Samb., etc.
Membranes Mucous, Serous	Apis, Bry., Canth, Scill, etc.

Appendix "E"

Sphere of Action	Remedies
Muco-Cutaneous Junction	Cundurango., Nitric-ac., etc.
Mammae (Female)	Bry., Corb-an., Con., Grap., Phyt., Phell, Castor eq., Sil., Lyc., Calc., Phos., etc.
Male Sex	Agnus cast., Calad., Damiana, Kali-br., Phos., Selen., Titanium., Yohimb., Zinc-ph., etc.
Nervous System	Alfalfa, Avena-sat., Hyper., Kali-ph., Lecithin, Picric-ac., Scutell., Zinc-ph., Zinc-pic., etc.
Parotid Glands	Jabor., Phyt., Cham., Bell., Rhus-t., Merc-sol, etc. Parotid.
Prostate Glands	Sabal-ser., Selen., Puls., Sil., Thuj., Con., etc.
Salivary Glands	Jabor., Pilocar., Phyt., Merc., Puls., Nit-ac., etc.
Spleen	Calc-ars., Ceonathus, Chin-sulph., Helianthus, Quercus, etc.
Skin	Apis, Ars. alb., Calc-c., Clematis, Caust., Graph., Hep-s., Kali-ars., Lach., Lyco., Merc., Sep, Sil, Sulph.; Hydrocot asiatica, Mez.,
Veins	Adonis, Bellis-p., Arnica, Digi, Hamam, Paeonia, Polygon, Vipera, Puls.

Appendix "F"

Some Important Differentiating Characteristics of Miasms

Psora	Syphilis	Sycosis
(A) Functional disturbances.	Ulcerative disturbances., ulceration of cornea, lids; ulceration of mouth.	Overgrowth, infiltration and deposits, more of overgrowth than destruction of tissue-warts, moles, papillomata, Gouty concretions.
Psora alone never causes structural changes.	Bones of nose destroyed only in this stigma.	Nasal stoppage from thickening of membranes and enlargement of turbinated bones.
Pathological developments very rare.	Structural changes in the dental arch; teeth come out deformed, irregular in shape and irregular in order of eruption.	Affects soft tissues, not bones.
Psora has no glandular involvement.	Teeth decay before they come out.	
(B) Psoric conditions are always itching; skin dry unwashed, unclean.	Eruptions do *not* itch, and there is very little soreness; there is little repair of tissues.	Worst forms of inflammations, infiltration of tissue, causing abscesses hypertrophies, cystic degeneration.

Appendix "F" 293

Psora	Syphilis	Sycosis
Eruptions do not suppurate, but dry down and become dead scales.	Psoriasis — Skin affections with glandular involvement.	Hair falls out in circular spots. Psoriasis (gouty element).
(C) Spends its action largely on nervous system, nerve centres, producing functional disturbances.	Spends itself on meninges of brain, affects larynx and throat in general, the eyes, bones and periosteum, principal sites of action.	Attacks internal organs, especially the pelvic and sexual organs.
Marked nervous reflexes, oversensitive to sound and strong odours.	Sense of smell lost. Nose bleeds very readily.	
(D) Restlessness esp. at new moon or at approach of menses.	Fixed ideas — Self-condemnation.	Fixed ideas — Self-condemnation.
Intelligent, alert, overactive and quick.	Idiotic; dull; stubborn. Imbecile. Slow and underactive mind; usually suspicious.	So suspicious that he does not trust himself, goes back to repeat what he has done.
Easily fatigued, mentally and physically.	Fixed moods. Keeps his depression to himself; close mouthed.	Mischievous; mal-active mind.
Source of all subjective symptoms and "sensations as if;" has valuable concomitants and modalities.	Desire to escape get away from self and so, without forewarning one hears "he has committed suicide."	Marks secret of everything, and suspects others of doing so.

Psora	Syphilis	Sycosis
	Wanting in attention and comprehension; mind slow, as if paralysed.	Worst form of degeneracy. Suspicious, quarrelsome, tending to harm others, even animals. Cruelty, cunning deceit. Bereft of all sense of righteousness. Liars, vicious scoundrels, mean, selfish; Sycosis makes a beast out of man.
(E) Has dropsical conditions more than in Sycosis.	Succumbs before dropsical condition becomes marked.	
(F) Always hungry; desires and longings for various things; craves sweets, sour things. Desires hot foods; Meat. Most aggravations occur after eating. Lack of power of assimilation.	Prefers cold food; aggr. from milk. Aversion to meat.	Wants food either hot or cold. Meat aggravates.
(G) Heart : functional disturbances; violent rushes of blood to chest, with anxiety and fear.	The syphilitic and sycotic patients deny they have any cardiac troubles; they are usually unaware of them. They have very little mental disturbance even in critical periods. They die suddenly without warning.	

Psora	Syphilis	Sycosis
Fear of dying from heart trouble, but lives long. Heart affections from fear, disappointment, loss of friends or overjoy.		The sycotic heart patient has better motion as walking, riding or gentle exercise.
(H) Ameliorated by natural eliminations like urine, sweat, stool.	Amel. by unusual discharges (leucorrhoea, catarrh, ulcer). No Amel. from sweating, urination.	Amelioration from unusual eliminations through mucous surfaces, such as leucorrhoea, free nasal discharges. Menses Amel.
(I) Time : Agg. daytime, from 9 or 10 a.m. to evening.	Agg. from evening up to 2 or 3 a.m. — Dreads the night, restlessness drives him out of bed.	Agg. from 2 or 3 a.m. upto 9 or 10 p.m. Aggr. day time.
(J) Diseases of blood vessels, liver, deposits beneath the skin.	Rheumatism. Bright's Disease, Phthisis.	Red nose with prominent capillaries.
Fears, anxieties and delusions of all kinds.	Neuralgias agg. at night and from heat.	Carcinoma of breast or Uterus.
Vertigo of various types. Constipation diarrhoea, worms.	Skin affections with glandular involvement.	Bright's disease, Diabetes.
	Ptosis of lids.	Rheumatic troubles in heat.
	Seldom attacks Ovaries or Uterus.	Slow recovery, slipping back on progress.

Psora	Syphilis	Sycosis
	Rickets — Varicose Ulcers	Tumours, Piles.
	Sense organs (eye, ear, nose, lips).	Uterine and ovarian troubles.
	Ulceration of Muc. membranes : Nose throat, caries of Bones.	Appendicitis.
		Sterility in women.

Appendix 'G'

Pseudo-Psora or Tubercular Miasm

Structural changes in Arteries. Blood Pressure.
Lupus of nose, allied to Tuberculosis.
Ravenous hunger, craving for undigestible things; craving for salt especially, for unnatural things; for potatoes.
Nose bleed, haemorrhage at slightest provocation.
Widely dilated pupils in children and young people.
Averse to meat.
Tubercular diathesis is soil in which Impetigo flourishes.
Skin affections with glandular involvement.
Wounds do not heal.
Stitch abscess after surgery.
Tubercular diathesis produces drunkards.
A picture of "Problem Child" — slow in comprehension, dull, unable to keep a line of thought.
Unsocial — keeps to himself and becomes sullen and morose.
In children, ulceration of umbilicus with yellowish discharge, which smells offensive, carrion like.
Tubercular children suffering from bowel troubles, develop a sudden brain stasis, or brain metastasis. Manifestations in brain alternate with bowel difficulty. Characteristic diarrhoeas Verat-alb., Ars., Camph and Cup-m. Die within 48 hours after sudden attack.
Tubercular child cannot use cow's milk in any shape.
Least exposure brings on diarrhoea.
Inability to assimilate much starch.
Chest wall narrow — breathing difficult, reduced oxygenation of blood.
Cough, deep, hoarse, on least exposure to cold.
Expectoration, purulent, greenish yellow, offensive, sweetish or salty.
Hysteria and lungs conditions alternate.
Haemorrhage from rectum (also Sycotic Piles).
Suppressed piles cause Asthma or Heart troubles.
Nocturnal enuresis. Prostatic troubles. Nightly emissions.

Appendix 'H'

Miasms and the Children

Psora :
Epistaxis more or less profuse, more or less frequently.
Nostrils stuffed up.
Fears death; fear of strangers.
Timid about going to school.

PSEUDO-PSORA (TUBERCULAR)

"Problem Child" — See under Pseudo-Psora.
Ulceration of Umbilicus — under Pseudo-Psora.
Weak wrist and ankle joints — drops things, or stumbles easily.

Syphilis :
Head large, bulging, often open sutures, bones soft, cartilaginous (also Tubercular).
Makes serious inroads upon the structures of the eye, or on lachrymal apparatus.
Snuffles in children.
Dental arch imperfect, etc. — See above.
Painful dentition, with diarrhoea, dysentery, spasms, convulsions, middle ear abcesses, meningeal congestions. These children cannot endure extremes of heat or cold.

Sycosis
Child smells sour.
Chronic corneal ulcers in children where there is no trace of syphilis, but based on tubercular diathesis.
Sycotic babies (born of sycotic parents) sometimes have Ophthalmia Neonatorum.
Gouty concretions in ears of sycotic babies.
Snuffles in children, usualy moist, no ulceration and no crust; if purulent, is very scanty and has odour of fish brine or stale fish. In new sycotic babies (of Sycotic parents).
Snuffles : Nose dry, stuffed up. Child will scream, usually followed by something more serious, especially if local measures are applied to "relieve".
Sycotic children, complicated with gout take cold easily, on

Appendix "H"   299

slightest exposure.

Gouty concretions in the mouth of young sycotic babies.

Patient, especially child, is worse by eating any kind of food whatever, and is better lying on stomach or by pressure over the region of stomach.

Sycotic children often suffer from colic almost from the moment of birth; the suffering is indescribable, better by pressure or by lying on stomach, or by being carried about, or rocking gently. (Lyc., Arg-nit.)

Colicky pains in bowel troubles of children, better doubling up, by motion or hard pressure. Simplest food produces colic.

Ulceration of Umbilicus, pus yellowish green, then excoriating often of fishy odour.

Stool like *Rheum.*, *Chamomilla* and *Magnesia-carb.*, gripping colic and tenesmus. Stools forcibly ejected, like *Crot-tig.*, *Cham.*, *Lauro.*, *Colocy.*

Sour smelling babies, with cutting colic; stools sour.

Sycotic colic (Dulcamara). Grass green stools of *Ipec.*, *Mag.c.*, *Cort-t.*, *Gratiol, Argenium-nit.*

Child screams when urinating (*Lycopodium, Sarsaparilla*) Gouty concretions of urethra of young (Sycotic) babies.

Appendix "I"

Exercises for Repertorisation

(It is only through practical application of the rules that one acquires mastery. Do your best to work out these exercises before referring to the solutions. Use the eliminative method.)

Case No. 1 : Mrs. Kusum aged 40 suffered from pain in the coccyx since a couple of years. Sitting on the painful part was very painful and sore, and any pressure, or a ride in the rikshaw aggravated the pain. Her hands became numb at night; stools were difficult with a feeling of constriction of the rectum during stool. She was worse from cold weather and could not stand draft of air even during fairly warm days.

Case No. 2 : A gentleman aged 37 had cramping pain in the abdomen every night between 2 and 4 a.m. only. The pain increased gradually to a pitch and subsided equally gradually. He was relieved by hard pressure on the abdomen or by bending forward. He had a sense of fullness in the stomach after eating.

Case No. 3 : Vertigo as if he is turning in a circle, for the last several months. Worse from moving his head, and relieved only when he closes his eyes. His wife has gone to her parent's house after a quarrel since the last three years.

Case No. 4 : Child aged 2 years, becomes stiff and blue in the face from suffocative, choking, croup cough. The cough is exhausting and is ameliorated somewhat following expectoration which is thick and yellow, difficult to raise. With the cough there is nausea and aversion to food.

Case No. 5 : A male patient Mr. G. came with the complaint of noises, like the sound of crickets in monsoon, in the ears, which started after an accident, in whcih he hurt his head badly. Now unable to stand music. Even lively music saddens him. Disgusted with life, he had suicidal inclinations and had to restrain himself from doing so. I also observed multiple small warts on the patient's face. (Dr. Parinaz Humranwala).

Appendix "I"

Case No. 6 : A girl 21 years, with greasy, oily complexion came with complaint of recurrent headache since 3 years. Worse on touch. She felt as if a thousand hammers were pounding on her head. On probing the history, it was found that she was disappointed in love-life and eversince had progressively worsened. When she is depressed, she wants to weep but is unable to do so. At such times she hates to be consoled.

Her first menses set in at the age of 18 years, after which they have been quite regular. (Dr. Parinaz Humranwala)

Case No. 7 : Mr. S, a pilot by profession, aged 29 years came to me looking very tensed and nervous. Just as he started to narrate his difficulty, he asked me to excuse him for a few minutes, as he wanted to visit the toilet. On returning I reassured him not to worry but to explain his trouble.

He had joined the Airlines 4 years ago and travelled all over the world but suddenly since a month he has developed some fear that something will happen. Being a pilot, he never feared heights but now he dreads to look out of the window. The sight of high houses makes him feel dizzy. Someone had suggested to him that he should go for long brisk walks in the evening and relax himself. But on doing so, he found that the faster he walks, the faster he thinks he must walk and he walks till he gets extremely tired.

Just before he was to meet me, he became anxious and apprehensive. The other day when he had been to his friend's wedding, he had anxiety, followed by diarrhoea.

Now he has a constant fear that his aircraft is going to crash and that he is going to die.

Memory has also been impaired. While giving the history he paused for a moment, was lost in deep thought and started again. He said, "Sorry doc, but I just forgot what I was about to say".

A few doses of the similimum removed all the fear complex from this man, and he continues to be a successful pilot to this date. (Dr. Parinaz humranwala).

Case No. 8 : Mrs. G. 30 years. 1st child 2 months old. Lactating. Hard, very painful lump in left breast. Walked with hand on breast. Able to feed. High fever. Sweating ++. Thirst +++. Lethargy. No redness. (Dr. Prabha Patwardhan, M.D.)

Case No. 9 : Mr. D.Z., 46 years. Frequent attacks of sore throat with fever since one year. Pain throat, left to right and again to left. Cold drinks amel. Agg. empty swallowing. Concom : Salivation, loose stools. Gen : Rundown, weak. App. Extra salt. Thirsty. Mentals : Fear being alone. Claustrophobia. P.H. — Jaundice, typhoid, kidney stone passed. (Dr. Prabha Patwardhan).

Case No. 10 : Miss K. 12 years. C/o. Intense pain, both lower limbs since 3 days. Pain agg. walking; touch. Would wince if touched Stiffness++. Could not flex legs. Jerks normal. Routine Tests : NAD. Gen. Exam. : NAD. Then, noticed that when engaged in talking of films, she relaxed; not so stiff. No wincing with pain, was asked to wait outside Consulting Room to take the full history from mother.

Mentals : Obstinate, wanted her way all the time. Joint family. Very selfish. Wanted to listen to music all the time. Saw one particular movie ten times. Complaints about other people, to get her way.

When called back to Consulting Room., got up suddenly and walked a few steps normally. Then went back to original stiff gait. Obvious; Feigning.

Cause : Did not want to do examinations. Had done this kind of thing earlier. (Dr. Prabha Patwardhan)

Case No. 11 : Miss A.G age 2 years & 3 months, had recurrent episodes of fever associated with cold and cough. She had three such attacks in the last 1 1/2 months. The mother brought the child with fever 103'F since last night. She is very dull and listless with fever and even more sleepy than normal. Demands a lot of attention during fever. The child generally liked sour foods, even pickles, and is prone to frequent stomach upsets with undigested stools. Normally she feels the heat a lot and avoids going out when it is hot. In the mother's lap child was quiet and looking suspiciously at me, as she is wary of adults and strangers. Today she was lying perfectly still, but when I approached to examine her physically, she started howling the moment I looked at her, and even more when I touched her. Cracked corners of mouth and slight white coating of tongue. The child was all right with three doses of the indicated medicine. (Dr. Sunil Anand)

Case No. 12 : Miss A.S., age 2 years presented with acute diarrhoea and vomiting along with high fever.

The history given by the mother was as follows. On the night prior to all these symptoms appearing, the child was constipated and had passed a very hard black stool with a lot of straining. She was listless all day. From the next day severe purging along with vomiting started. She had been having lot of mangoes prior to this illness. When I touched her body it was very cold to touch inspite of the fever. There was cold sweat on the forehead. Also while I was examining the child the mother anxiously warned me not to change the position of the child as she was afraid that with too much movement the child may start vomiting or purging as that had happened earlier. The child was asking for juices and cold things, but the mother was afraid to give them. Inspite of not being able to retain anything (the moment she took anything she would vomit or pass a stool), she wanted to eat or drink something and kept demanding, and the mother was perplexed as to what to do. The child's urine output had fallen drastically and her abdominal skin was very lax indicating moderate dehydration. The child improved rapidly from the first dose of the medicine. (Dr. Sunil Anand).

Case No. 13 : Mr. G., 54 years, railway guard, was suffering from diabetis and high blood pressure. He was feeling very weak. He also had pain in the right knee without any modality. He was passing frequent urination at night. He had constipation. Had very poor sleep; full of dreams which he could not remember. Had craving for sweets, fatty food, poor thirst. Scanty perspiration. He had suffered from piles and fissure. Mind : Very sensitive. Likes to be alone. Tremendous anxiety for his health. His family doctor said he had a slight high blood pressure. He came to confirm this, after consulting four more doctors (who had confirmed his high B.P.). Patient was repeatedly asking me whether "I have high B.P. or not." A fortnight after the medicine was given, he reported that his sleep had improved a lot, his B.P. was normal and he was feeling energetic. Since he did come to me again, the question is whether his mistrustful nature has also changed ! (Dr. Sujit K. Chatterjee).

Case No. 14 : Mrs. Z. was suffering from left sided otorrhoea with intense itching for the last 12 years. Had yellowish-green offensive discharge from the left ear. Agg. from draft. Hears ringing noises in the ear, which is agg. stooping. Craving for spices, sweets and aversion to milk. Thirst not marked. Poor perspiration. Salivation at night. Husband reported offensive odour of mouth. She was a hot patient; could not tolerate hunger and used to have severe giddiness while fasting. Mental symptoms not marked. Complaint cured in a few days. *(Dr. Sujit K. Chatterjee)*

Case No. 15 : An acute emergency was called for a visit on a Sunday night to see Mr. N.M., 45. He had massive eruptions on the left leg with severe oedema, with watery, sticky discharge and itching with severe burning pain. He had 104'F fever. When asked what foods he liked or disliked, he said he had great liking for sour things, and he hated sweets. He was a chilly patient. The attacks of fever and restlessness came at 11 a.m. and about midnight. No sleep. Tongue very thickly coated. Thirst for small quantities of water every half an hour. The burning sensation in the leg was severe. The patient was very restless with great fear of death. He was surrounded by many relatives. The indicated remedy was given, three doses, four hourly, with instructions to let me know after 15 hours, so that if required he could be admitted to hospital. Next morning (less than 12 hours after), the pleasant report was that in three hours the patient had good sweat, fever came down, had good sleep and appetite, the pain and burning was much relieved, and so was his anxious state. Thanks to Hahnemann and other masters, homoeopaths are capable of tackling emergencies. *(Dr. Sujit K. Chatterjee)*

Case No. 16 : Drug addiction : A 25 years old boy was taking drugs (brown sugar) since the last four years. His chief complaints were insomnia; he could not apply his mind to any work. Just before this addiction, his father had a loss in business. He had borrowed a large amount from the patient's elder brother's father-in-law. His father could not return the money in time due to his losses. The daughter-in-law was insulting everyone in the family. The family was very sensitive about it. He was worse from heat. Desires sweets. Always sleeps on abdomen. Is generally worse when away from Bombay (seashore). Washes his hands frequently. Warts on the nose. His relative complained that he steals wrist watch, transistor, etc. from home every day. After the well-selected remedy, (1M four doses 12 hourly), he started improving fast, getting sound sleep: Within a year his confused state of mind vanished. One dose was repeated after three months on a complaint of severe constipation. This was also cured in a day. *(Dr. Sujit K. Chatterjee)*

Case No. 17 : A lady, 46, suffering with a congestive headache requested to bring my "hypodermic syringe or chloroform". Of course, I didn't take them. She had dark complexion, black hair and eyes, and usually enjoyed good health except an occasional headache. Menses NAD. The present attack of headache followed some mental excitement. The pain began in the evening, and the violence of the attack soon compelled her to leave the bed, to seek relief by walking as rapidly as possible from end to end of a three room suite, while pressing the head with both the hands. A few pellets of the remedy, 200th, prepared in water were given, a teaspoonful every ten minutes until relieved. Before the time for the third dose had arrived, she went into sleep. the next day she was as well as usual. Could the "hypodermic" do the work as quickly? *(Dr. H.C. Allen)*

Case No. 18 : A farmer 55, since 3 years had a morbid growth from the inner angle of the eye, thick, opaque and rich with blood vessels, looking like a muscle extended over the sclerotic. It covered more than one half of the pupil, rendering the patient nearly blind. The conjunctiva of the remaining portion was deeply injected. There was much purulent discharge from the inner canthi. Patient was unable to endure light and was compelled to protect his eyes during daytime. Reading was out of the question. There was sore pricking pain in the inner angle of the eye, worse in the evening and night. Also severe pressing pain at the root of the nose with considerable lachrymation. The remedy, four doses in 200th, started giving relief from the third day. It had to be repeated thrice at long intervals. Growth diminished very much; sight fully restored. *(Dr. Carroll Dunham)*.

Case No. 19 : Mrs. V. aged 40, timid and of quiet disposition, who was frightened easily, had a number of disappointments in life such as late marriage and the death of her first child. She became a subject of peculiar fears. She began to feel that she was being pursued by enemies, and that they are planning to kill her.

She was so afraid of being alone that, when her husband had gone to office, she called in her neighbour to be with her. She passed sleepless nights with fearful thoughts passing through her mind. As a result her face was flushed, and she looked confused.

Case No. 20 : A boy aged 7 from a good family was brought by his mother with the complaint that he had recurrent fever with tendency to colds, and inflammation of tonsils. He was also a problem in the family, as he was very rude with other childern, abusing, kicking, pinching and pulling their hair. He had excessive hunger, and craving for sweets. The well-selected remedy, given as need arose, reformed him mentally and physically. (Dr. Asif Chunawala)

Appendix "J"

The writer is fully conscious that presenting this feature of "minimum syndrome of the maximum value" is no child's play, as it involves the identification and bringing up from depths of the ocean of Materia Medica only those Gems of proved value. Yet he is making a bold attempt to present such a minimum group for a few remedies, in the hope that it will spur others to contribute more and better drug pictures highlighting the few indispensable characteristics that help us to straightaway "think of the remedy".

Thereafter, we have to examine if the remaining symptoms of the case fit into it. Let it be emphasised that it is not any single symptom, however characteristic, that decides the remedy, but the three or five-legged stool, the tout ensemble, that does it.

Bryonia

A remedy notable for : (1) Agg. from Slightest Motion; (2) Amel. from Pressure; (3) Dryness of Mucuous membranes; Exudation of Serous Membranes ; (4) Great thirst; (5) Stitching pains; (6) Slow and insiduous development of complaints; (7) Irritable, angry disposition; talks and dreams of business only; eccentric desires; (8) Ailments from Suppressions; (9) Right-sidedness; (10) Agg. from warm weather; Summer.

1. Worse from or even dread of slightest any motion (even diarrhoea); Amel. by absolute rest, mental and physical. Dizziness, nausea or fainting on sitting up (motion).

2. Amel. by lying on the Painful Side (pressure amel. Except abdomen);- (rev. *Bell. Kali.c.*)

3. Dryness ("Bryonia") — Excessive, of mucous membranes- from lips to anus. Stool dry as if burnt; cough dry, hard racking, with scanty expectoration; urine dark and scanty and (because of dryness great thirst).

4. Inflammation and Exudation of Serous membranes (synovitis). Inflammation red (*Bell* : vermilion; *Apis* : rose red).

5. Irritable, inclined to be vehement and angry (only a shade of Nux-v). A ragged businessman, forever planning and watching for opportunity for profit in business (even dreams of business). Wants to go home (in delirium). Eccentricity : Hard to please, as he does not know what he wants. Anxiety about future (monetary).

6. Agg. at 9 p.m., evening. Worse, becoming overheated; in hot weather, change from cold to warm. Child kicks the covers.

7. Great thirst for large quantities.

8. Stiching pains (pleurisy, Synovitis)

9. Attacks are insiduous, develop slowly (rapid, violent : Ap., Bell.

10. A.F. Suppressions : of discharges (menses, lochia, milk), of eruptions (or tardy appearance of eruptions) in measles. (cf. Ap. Bell.) Cup, Hell, Sulph., Zinc. Suppressions cause vicarious discharges : Epistaxis, milk in breasts, running ear.

11. Right sided complaints.

Case : A young man complained early morning of severe pain in the whole of right arm. Any motion, was very painful. He had passed sleepless night because of the pain. Was asked to lie down on the right side and tell after ten minutes whether he felt better or worse. He reported he was better lying on the painful side. *Bry.* 1M 2 doses four hourly cured him by evening.

To sum up : A patient with severe stitching pains, worse from the slightest movement, worse for sitting up; better for pressure ; very thirsty for large drinks of cold water; very irritable; angry and not only angry, but with sufferings increased by being disturbed mentally or physically; white tongue; in delirium "wants to go home". (even when at home); busy in his dreams and in delirium with his everyday business — with these you can administer *Bry.* and bet on the result ! Margaret Tyler.

BELLADONNA

A remedy of (1) Violence, (2) Congestions Inflammations hot bleeding Skin scarlet red, (3) Suddenness, (4) Photophobia,

Appendix "J" 309

(5) Great sensitiveness (6) Craves Lemonade, (7) Spasms, (8) right-sided complaints, (9) Delusions, wild, ferocious.

1. **Violence** : Of Headache, dysmenorrhoea, labour pains, bearing down; grinding of teeth; convulsions, tenesmus; gall-stone colic; neuralgia.

2. **Congestions** : Rush of blood to head, face, eyes congested. Face flushed. Throbbing brain and carotids. Inflammatory conditions. Hence, sleepy but cannot sleep. Hence pupils dilated and photophobia. Hot head with cold limbs.

EFFECTS OF CONGESTION

Inflammations : In all inflammations there is extreme heat, shining redness, burning, throbbing carotids; sensitiveness to pain. In mastitis red streaks radiate from the centre.

Bleeding : Blood feels hot as it passes (nose-bleed, uterine haemorrhage; profuse, bright red blood).

Position : Lying down is the worst position; better by standing or sitting erect. (Glon. better lying down).

Skin : very red, scarlet red and hot; seems to radiate heat; shining, smooth; dry and hot; intense dermatitis. Sweat on covered parts.

3. **Photophobia** : With intense, burning fever.

4. **Suddenness of all complaints** : Pains come suddenly, last a short time and disappear suddenly. Colics; swellings; convulsions; hoarseness, etc. Children moan or cry during sleep (earache). Start as in fright during sleep.

5. Sensitiveness to pain: Agg. from noise, slightest motion or jar; slightest touch; light. Sensitive to cold; washing head.

6. **Craves** : Lemonade, (or lemon water) which agrees. Aversion to meat, acids, coffee, milk, beer.

7. **Spasms** : Spasmodic hiccough; Twitching of face; jerkings; Convulsions in children with fever, hot head, red face, violent distortion of body. Sudden jerkings when falling asleep. Chorea.

8. Right-sided remedy, predominantly (right eye, right ear, right leg, right hand, right chest, but left side of mouth and throat). Paralysis right side of face. Paralysis of one side, spasm of the other.

9. **Delusions** : Delirium wild, ferocious; wants to bite, strike, spit; wants to escape. (Hyos. Stram., Hell.). An angel when well, a devil when sick.

Case 1 : Dr. Miller had a severe attack of angina pectoris. He could not lie down for several days and nights. After slight improvement for a few days, his left arm suddenly became numb, during a quiet sleep about midnight. He found that the right half of his person was completely paralysed. At first he was speechless, but after considerable effort, he said "spasms of left side and paralysis of the right" — "Raue". In ten to fifteen minutes after administering a dose of *Bell* Dr. M. could speak distinctly and use the paralysed limbs. So prompt a cure of hemiplegia was entirely unexpected to all. (L.B. Wells HH 8/82)

Case 2 : The mother of a boy complained that he had suddenly developed high fever, 103 degree. In answer to each question she answered that the fever was burning hot to touch. The face and eyes were red and congested. The boy turned his face from light. He had throbbing pain in the temples. He was asking his mother to sit gently on his cot. He was muttering in sleep about his school. He asked for lemon-water frequently. One dose of *Bell.* 200 brought down his temperature, with profuse perspiration in three hours. (Dr. Sujit K. Chatterjee)

Rhus-tox

1. A.F. (Ailments from) getting wet, especially after being overheated; or swimming too long in a lake; or overlifting and spraining muscles and tendons. Getting wet while perspiring.

   A.F. Overexertion — even dreams of great exertion of body.

Appendix "J" 311

2. Great restlessness — anxious driving out of bed. Cannot remain in bed long in one position. Must change position often to obtain relief. Agg. when at rest.

3. Lameness, stiffness, pain from first motion, after rest or sleep. Amel. by continued motion. (Rheumatic complaints).

4. Sensitiveness, highly, to open air, to cold wet rainy weather. Even putting the hand out from under the bed cover brings on cough (Bar. C., Hep.) Amel. by warm covering.

5. Mentally restless. Fear that he will die. Delirium with fear of being poisoned. Sensorium cloudy. Anxiety with fear; anxiety about the future.

6. Agg. after midnight.

7. Sore painfulness of affected parts; of whole body before and during fever. Sore to touch.

8. Paretic — paralytic : "The great anti-paralyticum" (Lilienthal). Paralysis following parturition; sexual excesses; after malaria; after typhoid. Infantile paralysis from exposure to damp, wet, foggy weather (Kent). Facial paralysis from left to right.

9. Freakish : Hunger without appetite ; chilliness even when near the fire ; craves cold water, which is vomited immediately. Cough during chill, urticaria during heat.

10. Yawning - constant and irresistible desire to yawn.

11. Skin : Vesicular eruptions with oedema, burning and itching (not amel. by scratching), and tingling. Dusky redness of affected part.

12. Side : left side of body, arm, chest, lower extremeties — Right abdominal ring. Aching left arm with heart disease.

Case : Was asked to see a moribund lady with congestive heart failure due to mitral stenosis with regurgitation, rejected by top Cardiologists. Aged 34, mother of 3 children. Was lying in semi-orthopnoeic position with back rest, general anasarca, moderate cyanosis. Was warned by cardiologists against any movement, but rest actually aggravated her breathing distress. This forced rest was a cause of agony, as rest increased the body-ache she was having all along. She was an out and out Rhus tox case from the beginning of her whole illness. Even for dyspnoea she could not stand fanning, body remaining covered by sheet; was so chilly. Dominated by *Rhus tox* type of anxiety. Under Rhus tox 200, 2 doses, she responded dramatically, in a week became ambulatory. Relapses at longer and longer intervals were helped by Rhus tox higher potencies. End of one year. Cardiologists could not detect any organic defect in her heart. (Dr. J.N. Kanjilal — *HH* 5/86).

CALCAREA CARB

1. Defective power of assimilation of calcium, and imperfect ossification (bony growth). Consequently patients either grow fat and flabby or run into a marasmic state. (Children : Open fontanelles; delayed dentition; difficult learning to walk or stand; will not even try to stand).

2. Irregular development : Curvature of spine and long bones; Large abdomen, looking like an inverted saucer, while the rest of the body is emaciated. Perspiration on head during sleep, wetting the pillow; feet habitually cold and damp. Fair, fat (unwieldy), flabby. Fat without fitness. Sweat of single parts.

3. Easy sweat; easy taking cold. Worse cold air, wet weather; from washing. Takes cold at every change of weather.

4. Craving for eggs; undigestible things like chalk. Aversion for meat, coffee. Disagree : milk, cannot digest it. Child vomits sour curds; eggs.

5. Lack of stamina : Pale, weak, easily tired. Worse from mental or physical exertion. Dyspnoea from ascending steps or walking fast; from slight exertion. Hence indolent, sluggish, slow.

6. Weakness of mind : Children, dull lethargic, do not want to play; obstinate and inclined to grow fat. Worse from

mental exertion. Sensitiveness (fear) to horrible things, sad stories; reports of cruelties, bad news. Fears of various kinds : of death, of insanity. Fear of being observed. Mind prostrated, confused, restless, nervous. Timidity. Easily frightened. Finally, despair of recovery.

Case : Vertigo (Dr. Swan) : A lady was afflicted with vertigo in the back of the head, accompanied with a feeling as if the head was enlarged; while at the table she would lose her consciousness in consequence of it, and thought that those about her would observe it ; she had it at night while in bed, as well as during the day. Dr. Piersons suggested *Calc. carb.* Dr. Caroll Dunham said that Petrol had the vertigo in the back of the head, accompanied by the sensation as if falling. Phos. was also suggested to his mind, as well as *Silicea. Calc. carb.* helped the lady. (*H.H.* 3/82 (89)).

NUX VOMICA

1. For very careful zealous persons; irritable and impatient; fault-finding; Easily offended. Uncontrolled fiery temper (like one intoxicated), may lead to violence. Dread of mental exertion.

2. Chilly : Repugnance to cold air, chilly on least movement; from being uncovered; must be covered in every stage of fever (chill, heat and sweat). Burning heat, yet cannot move or uncover in the least, without feeling chilly.

3. A. F. Sedentary habits; lack of physical exercise with over-exertion of mind. Over-eating, excess of coffee, highly spiced food, tobacco, alcoholic stimulants. Over-use of drugs. Gastric complaints with costiveness, loss of sleep and irritability.

4. Ineffectual urgings : Frequent and unsuccessful desire for stool (passes, small quantity at a time). Ineffectual labour pains which extend to rectum with desire for stool or urination. Ineffectual, painful urging to urinate. Ineffectual desire to vomit; says "if only I could vomit."

5. Cravings : Fats, alcohol, pungent, bitter things. Aversions : Meat (makes him sick); tobacco.

6. Sleep : Sleepy, hours before bedtime, awakes at 3 or 4 a.m., lies awake for an hour or two, then falls into heavy sleep; awakens late in the morning feeling tired and unrefreshed.

7. Oversensitive to least pain, to least noise, to least even suitable medicine; faints from odours. Trifling ailments unbearable.

8. Agg. morning : Feels worse in the morning soon after awaking (Lach., Nat-m.), awakes tired and weak with many complaints.

9. Spasms, sensitiveness and chilliness — three general characteristics, convulsions with consciousness, brought on by anger, emotion. Spasms cease as soon as he is tightly grasped; and renewed by slightest touch.

10. Other indications : Backache, as if broken, must sit up to turn in bed. Menses : Too early, profuse, long lasting with cramps in abdomen, with nausea. Diarrhoea or dysentery : Pain much relieved after every stool (rev. Merc. cor.)

Case : Male aged 55. Ill on and off for 6 months. Digestion all wrong. Feels chilly; he never used to feel the cold. Very fond of fat. Is a worrier. Is sensitive and frightfully irritable. Wants to be left alone. Miserable, wept telling his symptoms. Lost two relations in the blitz. *Ignatia* given with no result.

Case now reconsidered and *Nux-vom.* 30 prescribed. Returned a different man; brighter; can walk upright. Digestion much better. It is often difficult to choose between Ignatia and *Nux-vom.* Both contain strychnine, which explains the resemblances. Both are over-sensitive. This over-excitability is manifested in *Ignatia* by brooding, melancholy and tears, which the patient conceals as far as possible, whereas *Nux-vom.* exhibits gross irritability — H.H. Feb. 1987.

PULSATILLA

1. Agg. by heat in any form — warm, stuffy closed rooms; warm applications. On the contrary, cool open air, cold drinks, cold applications are comforting.

Appendix "J"

2. Erratic : Chilly with pain; chilly, yet averse to heat. Menses scanty or protracted and intermittent. Easily moved to laughter or tears. Mouth dry, but no thirst.

3. Mild, gentle, yielding (timid), disposition. Sad and depressed. Weeps easily when telling her symptoms. Affectionate. Slow and irresolute. Likes sympathy.

4. Thirstlessness with nearly all complaints, though mouth is dry. Thirstless even during height of fever. But great thirst when she sweats.

5. Wandering pains : they travel from one part to another (*Kali-bi., Lac.c.*)

6. Changeability : Now irritable and in a moment Mild and pleasant. Haemorrhages flow, stop, and flow again. No two stools alike. No head or tail to the case. (Erratic).

7. Food and Drinks : Craves : indistinct (knows not what erratic), sweat, sour. Aversion to : Fat foods, milk, meat, bread (Nat-m.), butter, Onions (Thu.)
Don't agree : Cakes, rich fat food, pork, eggs, frozen food.

8. Menses : Too late, too scanty or suppressed. Flow more during day (on lying down ; Kreos.; more during night; *Mag-c.*). Pains begin with the flow (*Lach.* pains subside when flow begins).

9. Digestion, disorders of : From fat foods; bad taste in the mouth, especially, early morning.

10. Hanging down of limbs, aggravates complaints. (*Amel., Con.*).

11. Metastasis : Of mumps to mammae or testicles.

12. Pains : Appear suddenly and leave gradually, or let up with a snap.

13. Complaints Agg. : Evening; when at rest (amel. by gentle motion); lying on the painless side (erratic); lying on the left side.

14. One-sided complaints : headache, sweat, one-sided pains.

15. Others : Ophthalmia neonatorum (Asphyzxia neonatorum : Ant-t.); Orchitis (right); Corrects malposition of foetus in the womb; milk in breasts of young virgins.

"In any of the local affections, we should expect to find the Mind and Modality of the remedy present, or not be very confident of a brilliant cure". — E.B. Nash.

Any three or four of these symptoms can make you think of Sepia.

SEPIA

1. Averse to company, yet dreads being alone. Great sadness, weeping. Indifferent to one's family, averse to loved ones, to one's occupation. An exertion to think. Greedy, miserly. Averse to coition. Fond of dancing, which amel. (dyspnoea).

2. Complaints amel. by exertion, occupation. Symptoms due to congestion of veins (sluggish circulation), amel. by exercise or brisk walking.

3. Aversion to milk; diarrhoea from boiled milk.

4. Women's remedy : Menses : Irregularity of every form Leucorrhoea. Morning sickness of pregnancy. Prolapse of uterus or vagina, with bearing down pains as if everything would protrude from pelvis — must cross limbs tightly.

   Climacteric : Flushes of heat with anxiety, sweat, throbbing in veins; flushes ascend from pelvis. Abortion in fifth month. Complaints at puberty, childbed or lactation.

5. Cold agg. Chills so easily; dreads to bathe; feels cold even in warm room. Agg. from dampness; Washerwomen's remedy (worse washing, getting wet). Worse at rest; before thunderstorm. Amel. heat of bed or applied heat. Exercise.

Appendix "J"

6. Ascending (upward direction). Complaints : From rectum or vagina; Uterus to umbilicus.

7. Yellowness : Of face, conjunctiva, spots on chest. Yellow saddle across upper part of cheek and nose.

8. Pot-bellied mothers (child: Calc.), exhausted by frequent child-bearing, or nursing a vigorous child.

9. Sensation of Ball or Plug : In inner parts, in throat, rectum with constipation, diarrhoea or piles; in uterus (during menses); in anus not amel. by stool.

10. Nausea : At the sight, thought or smell of cooking food. Nausea while riding in a carriage.

Case : See Case No. 17 in the Exercises for Repertorisation.

A Remedy of imperfect nutrition (assimilation), and its consequences.

1. Lack of self-confidence : Dreads failure; undertakes nothing lest he fail. Lack of grit — Concentration difficult. Agg. from mental exertion. Mind prostrated from reading. Sensitive to slightest noise. Timidity for appearing in public, or talking to children, cry when spoken kindly to. Dreads any work, but improves on being warmed up to it.

2. Lacks vital heat : Always chilly. Can sweat all over only after a good deal of exercise, but sweats as soon as he falls asleep. Worse from cold air, becoming cold, from draft. Better when warmly wrapped, or hot bathing. Body, especially limbs cold to touch.

3. Offensive sweat of hands, feet, toes, axilla.

4. Constipation from inactivity of rectum. Shy stool — stool partly expelled recedes again (just as shyness in public).

5. Ailments from bad effects of vaccination (especially abscesses and convulsions.

6. Has wonderful control over the suppurative process : even suppuration of glands, soft tissue, periosteum or bones (Calendula and Hep. act chiefly on soft tissue.) Promotes expulsion of foreign bodies from tissues (fish bones, needles, bone splinters).

7. Emaciation : Whole body is emaciated, wasted while the abdomen is distended and head is large. (Calc. is fat and flabby.)

8. Craving : Indigestible things. Aversions : Meat, mother's milk. Agg. from : Potatoes; sight or smell of food; wine.

9. Modalities : Agg. cold, damp weather; draft; cold changes in weather. During new full moon; when uncovering, especially the head.

10. Skin : Unhealthy; every injury tends to ulceration with discharge of pus, and with no tendency to heal. Sil. has inflammation, swelling, ulceration and necrosis (sensitive and tender to touch).

Case : (Dr. A.K. Boman Behram - (H.H. 1/87) : A maid was suffering from profuse leucorrhoea which went down to the heels and prostration from least physical exertion. On examination she has extensive erosion with multiple deep ulcers on the cervix, and the uterus was fixed to the sacrum. She was very chilly and was always clammy and cold to touch. Repeated doses of *Silica* stopped her leucorrhoea and greatly improved her general condition. On re-examination, the cervical erosion and ulcers had healed but the uterus was still fixed posteriorly. There was no recurrence of the leucorrhoea during follow-up period of more than 4 years. (A good lesson from this case : One should not always base one's prescription on the mental symptoms alone nor give a high priority to them. Actually there should not be any distinction made between a physical and a mental symptom because both are the expression of one and the same individual (who is indivisible) and both can be peculiar to a given individual. In this case (and others given in his article), the prescription was based on the peculiarities of the physical symptoms and modalities. Where the physical symptoms were more characteristic in the individual, the mentals were ignored).

Appendix "J"

LACHESIS

1. Intolerance of heat : Agg. in summer cannot stand the sun, heat of the sun, yet occasionally cannot stand draft of air. Warm food and drinks agg.

2. Sleep — Complaints agg. during sleep, wake him up. Worse after sleep; agg. in morning after waking.

3. Touch and pressure : Aggravation from. Feels uneasy by slight touch. Intolerance of tight clothes, or even weight of bed covers. About throat, waist, chest.

4. Swallowing (Peculiar) : Empty swallowing is agonising, liquids are swallowed with less pain, solids with the least pain.

5. Left-sidedness of all complaints (or left to right) : Sore throat, diphtheria, headache, tonsillitis, lung troubles. Ovarian pain. Left iliac region tender, agg. from slightest pressure.

6. Menses : Many complaints agg. before menses, and are amel. as soon as the menstrual flow is established. Feels better during the menstrual flow. Agg. from retarded discharges, better from discharges. Headache better from Coryza. Asthma relieved by expectoration.

7. Loquacious : Jumps from one to another subject. Jealous. Suspicious. Religious. Deranged time sense.

8. Climacteric Ailments : Flushes of heat, with profuse perspiration. Haemorrhages. Rush of blood to head.

9. Bluish or purplish swellings : Of boils, carbuncles, varicose veins, gums, cancer of breast; even gums bluish, swollen.

10. Upward extension of sensations and complaints.

11. Haemorrhagic tendency, but the blood is dark, decomposed, may be like charred straw. (*Phos.* is bright red).

Case : (Dr. A. J. Brewster — *H.H.* 11/86) : A young lady had a severe attack of diphtheria, located on the left side. The parotid was swollen and very sensitive to touch : the tonsil was also swollen, was of purplish red colour and extremely sore ; deglutition very difficult. The left side of the next swollen, very sore and dark purple or bluish in colour. Violent pains darting up the left side of the neck into the head . . . Great prostration . . . aggr. of all symptoms during sleep. On these symptoms *Lachesis* 200th potency given, which gave prompt relief. But in two days the case was getting worse. As symptoms had not changed, concluded that the severity of symptoms called for greater dynamic force. Hence, *Lachesis* CM, one dose dry on the tongue at night was given. Improved much in morning, but return of the same symptoms in evening necessitated repetition of dose morning and evening for a few days. Patient declared convalescent. Disease force yielded to the dynamic force.

NATRUM MUR.

This is an evolutionary analysis of the Natrum mur. mind based on a study of the mental symptoms given in Kent's Repertory. Correlation of the mental state with the physical symptoms leads to the similimum with certainty. Readers should try to make similar studies for other remedies.

Each remedy is a personality which develops according to its in-born tendencies, and in response to stresses and strains of life, exhibits personality traits peculiar to itself. Let us see how Natrum mur. personality evolves in response to the environmental stresses.

The main characteristics of Nat-mur. are that he is very emotional and sensitive, but his tendency to suppress his emotions leads to the manifestation of a variety of mental reactions and problems.

To begin with, he is mild, gentle, affectionate and sympathetic. The emotional nature makes the girl fall in love with a married man against her (intelligent) will. In consequence, she may have ailments from disappointment in love. Being emotional she will be tearful, weeping, and even laugh and weep alternately. She may even be remorseful. With her emotional nature, she is haunted by unpleasant subjects and persistent thoughts which she is incapable of getting rid of; dwells on disagreeable occurrences.

She is very sensitive by nature, and as such, she is easily frightened also easily offended. Startled by least noise. Her dominant nature is to suppress her emotions. Hence, she becomes reserved ; averse to company, averse even to being spoken to. She does not like to be pitied, and hence consolation aggravates her complaints. She cannot cry even in grief, and if at all she cries she will do so when alone, when no one can know her mental anguish. She is struggling to adjust herself, compensating for the difficulties she is facing.

A heightened phase of this compensation effort will be when she becomes irritable, angry and quarrelsome. Discontented with everything. Becomes censorious. Wants to do things in a hurry. Occasionally, her innate mildness prevails and she has irritability alternating with cheerfulness. All this strain causes mental exertion which she cannot stand. When this stage is passed without avail, she gives way — she becomes sad, depressed and hypochondriacal. Becomes weary of life, loathing of life. Develops fears of all sorts, of robbers, fear in a crowd, of evil, of insanity, fear that something will happen, fear of trifles. Frightened easily. Complaints from fright. Hatred of persons who had offended her. Heedless. Hysteria. Indifference, Apathy even to pleasures of life.

NAT MUR — PHYSICAL GENERALS

1. Great emaciation : Losing flesh while living well. Emaciation of throat and neck. Face oily, shiny, as if greased.

2. Tongue, mapped, with red insular patches : Geographical tongue, speech heavy, difficult. Children slow in learning to walk, and talk.

3. Craving for salt and salty things. Bad effects from excessive use of salt. Averse to bread, meat, coffee. Thirsty, drinks large quantity of water.

4. Worse : Exact periodicity 9 to 11 a.m.; Worse with the sun, heat of sun, summer. Worse at sea shore or from sea air. Full moon.
Better : Open air; cool bathing. Going without regular meals.; feels better on an empty stomach.

5. Constipation on alternate days, or skips 2 or 3 days. Stools dry, hard, crumbling.
6. Urine, involuntary on coughing, laughing, sneezing.
7. Skin : Dry eruptions on the margin of hair.

Appendix "K"

Solutions of Repertorial Exercises

Case No. 1 :
Page 1344 - Draft aggr.
Page 912 - Pain Coccyx after a carriage ride
Page 912 - Pain Coccyx aggr. pressure.
Page 934 - Pain sore, coccyx, sitting when
Page 658 - Urine frequent, at night
Page 1038 - Numbness hand at night, during sleep
Page 609 - Stool difficult with a feeling of constriction of rectum during stool.

Silicea 200 b.d. for 3 days and once a week thereafter; to be stopped when better and resumed for 3 days on recurrence.

She was completely relieved of the pain after a few months of this long standing complaint.

Case No. 2 :
Page 1377 - Pain appears and disappears gradually.
Page 1390 - Periodicity
Page 575 - Abdomen, cramping pain amel. by bending forward.
Page 575 - Abdomen pain, pressure amel.
Page 498 - Stomach, fullness after eating.

Stannum 200 b.d. for 3 days relieved him completely. He reported recurrence after seven months, and a repetition of the dose cured him fully. Nearly two years have elapsed since then.

Case No. 3 :

			con.
1.	Sexual desire, suppression of	1399	3
2.	Vertigo amel. on closing eyes	98	2
3.	Vertigo agg. moving the head	101	3
4.	Vertigo, as if turning in a circle	105	3

Conium.

Case No. 4 :

		Bell.	Caust.	Ipec
1.	Face discoloured bluish, cough during 358	1	1	1

			Bell.	Caust.	Ipec
2.	Extremities stiff, cough during	1191	1	1	1
3.	Cough, choking	783	-	-	3
4.	Cough, Croupy	785	2	-	2
5.	Cough, suffocative	806	1	2	3
6.	Cough, exhausting	790	1	1	2
7.	Cough, amel. by expectoration	790	1	1	2
8.	Expectoration thick	819	-	2	1
9.	Expectoration yellow	821	1	1	1
10.	Expectoration difficult	815	-	3	3
11.	Nausea during cough	506	-	-	3
12.	Aversion to food	481	2	1	1

Note : See how Ipecac. covers this wide range of symptoms in an acute case.

Case No. 5 :
K - 295 (1) Ear - noises - chirping
K - 128 (2) Injuries of the head, after
K - 56 (3) Mind - Injury - must use self-control to prevent shooting himself.
K - 28 (4) Sadness from music.

Nat. Sulph. 1M, 3 doses for two days followed by S.L. for 2 weeks. Nat. Sulph. repeated twice in the same potency.

Case No. 6 :
K -   63 (1) Mind - love ailments from
K -   78 (2) Sadness - can't weep
K -   16 (3) Consolation agg.
K - 140 (4) Head pain hammering
K - 1407 (5) Generalities - touch agg.
K - 726 (6) Menses delayed in girls — first menses.

Nat-mur. 200, 3 doses everyday for seven days followed by S.L. for three weeks. Nat Mur 1M 3 doses for 3 days followed by S.L. for three weeks. No more headaches.

Case No. 7 :
K - 45 (1) Mind - fear, high places
K - 4 (2) Anticipation.
K - 43 (3) Fear - accident
K - 45 (4) Fear - something will happen.
K - 65 (5) Memory - weakness for what he was about to say.

Appendix "K" 325

K - 44 (6) Fear - death
K - 92 (7) Walking rapidly from anxiety
K - 613 (8) Rectum - Diarrhoea - fright, after.

Argentum nitricum 200, 3 doses everyday for seven days. Followed by S. L. for three weeks. Argentum nitricum repeated only once more in the same potency. All the fear complexes disappeared and he still works in Airlines as a successful pilot.

Case No. 8 : Bryonia
K - 835 - Induration, mammae 2
K - 1369 - Jar agg. 3
K - 529 - Thirsty during fever 3
K - 1280 - Burning fever at night
    with sweat 1
K - 1411 - Walking agg. 3

Case No. 9 : Lac.-Can.
K - 1400 - Sides, alternating 3
K - 458 - Throat pain, amel. 1
K - 458 - Throat pain, agg. empty
    swallowing 2
K - 417 - Salivation 2
K - 486 - Desires salt 3
K - 43 - Fear being alone 2
K - 643 - Stools loose, watery 2
K - 1413 - Weakness 2

Case No. 10 : Tarentula Cub.
K - 69 - Obstinate 3
K - 79 - Music amel. 3
K - 48 - Feigning 2
K - 12 - Complaining 1

Case No. 11 : Ant. Crud.
K - 62 - Looked at cannot bear to be 2
K - 89 - Touched, aversion to being 3
K - 486 - Stomach disordered 3
K - 486 - Desires sour 2
K - 485 - Desires pickles 2
K - 402 - Discolouration, tongue, white 3
K - 1250 - Sleepiness during heat 2
K - 1412 - Warm air agg. 2
K - 357 - Mouth, cracked corners of 2

Case No. 12 :   Verat. Alb.
K - 478 - Appetite ravenous with diarrhoea   2
K - 532 - Diarrhoea during vomiting   3
K - 222 - Perspiration, forehead   3
K - 484 - Desire, cold drinks   3
K - 688 - Urine scanty   2

Case No. 13 : Here is a patient who is distrustful. He does not believe any doctor. He is tremendously anxious about his health.   Nit - ac.
K - 86 - Suspicious, mistrustful   2
K - 7 - Anxiety about health   3
K - 485 - Desires fat   3

Phatak's Materia Medica — Sleep, Rx=Nit-ac. unrefreshing with frightful dreams — Nitric Acid.

Case No. 14 :   Sulphur
K - 1367 - Agg. hunger   3
K - 1412 - Agg. warm   2
K - 1344 - Agg. draft of air   2
K - 486 - Desires sweets   3
K - SR- 272 - Desires spices   3
K - 481 - Aversion to milk   2
K - 409 - Mouth odour, offensive   3
K - 286 - Ear discharge, fetid   3

Case No. 15 :
Agg. mid-day and mid-night (K-1341 & 1343)
Thirst for small quantities, often (K-529);
Chilly patient — worse from cold (1348);
Restlessness during the heat (74); — Fear of death (44)
Eruptions burning (1309) — All these characteristic symptoms clearly pointed to Arsenicum Alb.

Case No. 16 : (1) SR-I-1061 — Washing her hands; (2) K-1344 — Air seashore, amel. (3) Desires sweets; (4) (SR —) Lies on abdomen; (5) SR-I-898 — Sensitive; (6) K - 13 — Confusion of mind; (7) K-1251 — Sleeplessness. All these pointed to Medorrhinum.

Case No. 17 — Allen comments : "The character of the pain, the intense congestion of head, face, eyes and throbbing carotids certainly pointed to Belladonna. but the manner of obtaining

relief from rapid motion, promptly excluded that remedy. Any remedy that would cure this case must contain among its totality, this peculiar symptom, which is a characteristic of Sepia."
However, we are showing the repertorial working :   Sepia

K - 1358 - Exertion (walking rapidly) amel.   3
K - 178 - Headache bursting   2
K - 179 - Continued hard motion head (Head)   1
K - 179 - Head, pain, sleep amel.   1
K - 1392 - Pressure amel.   2
K - 110 - Head, congestion   2

Case No. 18 :
(1) K-258 — Eyes pain sore, inner canthi; (2) K-248 — Eyes pain, agg. evening; (3) K-249 — Eyes pain, agg. night; (4) K-245 — Lachrymation; agg. evening; (5) K-245 - Lachrymation, agg. night; (6) K-346 — Pain, pressing, root of nose ; (7) K-238 — Discharge muco-pus from inner canthi; (8) K - 262 — Photophobia, daylight; (9) K - 262 — Pterygium.

Case No. 19 :
(1) K - 49 — Frightened easily ; (2) K - 43 — Fear, being alone ;
(2) K - 30 - Delusion, being pursued by enemies;
(3) K - 29 - Delusion, that she would be murdered;
(4) K - 1254 - Sleeplessness, from activity of mind;
(5) K - 361 - Face red (flushed); (7) K - 374 - Expression confused.

Rx=Hyoscyamus

Case No. 20 :   Lycopodium
K - 75 - Rudeness   3
K - 486 - Desires sweets   3
K - 478 - Excessive, ravenous, hunger   3
K - 1349 - Colds, tendency to take   3   Rx=Lyco.
SR - 605 - Impolite children   1

Appendix "L"

Depth of Action of Remedies

Shallow Remedies:
Acon., All-c., Arnica, Arum-t., Bapt., Bell, Bry., Cact., Camph., Cann-i., Caps., Chel., Coffea, Coloc., Croc., Dios., Eupper., Euphr., Gamb., Glon., Ham., Hyper., Ign., Ipec. Kalm., Laur., Meph., Mill., Mosch., Nux-v., Par., Rheum., Rhus-t., Samb., Stram., Viol-o., etc.

Remedies of Medium Depth:
Acet-ac., Aesc., Aeth., Agn., Ang., Ant-t., Apis, Asar., Berb., Bov., Bry., Cham., Cimic., Chin., Cina., Clem., Colch., Cycl., Dulc., Gels., Hell., Hyos., Kreos., Led., Lil-t., Meny., Podo., Puls., Rhus-t., Ruta., Sars., Seneg., Spong., Spig., Teucr., Verb., Verat., Viol-t., etc.

Deep Acting Remedies:
Agar., Aloe., Ambr., Am-c., Am-m., Anac., Ant-c., Arg-m., Arg-n., Ars., Asaf., Asc-t., Bism., Bor., Brom., Calad., Carb-an., Carb-v., Cic., Cocc., Con., Dig., Dros., Dulc., Euph., Ferr-m., Fl. ac., Gels., Guaic., Hell., Hep., Iod., Kali-bi., Kali-i., Kali-n., Lach., Mang., Merc-s., Mez., Mur-ac., Nat-m., Nit-ac., Nux-m., Petr., Phos., Plat., Plb., Podo., Psor., Puls., Ran-b., Ran-s., Rhod., Ruta., Sars., Seneg., Sep., Stann., Sul-ac., Tell., Zinc., etc.

Very Deep-acting Remedies:
Alum., Asc-t., Aur-met., Bar-c., Calc., Calc-p., Caust., Cupr., Graph., Kali-c., Lyc., Merc., Mez., Nit-ac., Sep., Sil. Sulph., Thuja, etc.

(Hahnemannian Gleanings, May, 1978)

Appendix "M"

Anti-Psoric Remedies

Abort., Acet-ac., Agar-musc., Aloe., *Alum.*, Ambr., Amm-c., Amm-m., *Anac.*, Ant-c., Apis., Arg-m., Arg-n., Ars., *Ars-iod.*, Ars-s-r., Arum-t., Aur., Aur-m., *Bar-c.*, Bell., Benz-ac., Berb., Bor.-ac., Bor., Bov., Bufo., *Calc-ar.*, *Calc.*, *Calc-p.*, *Calc-s.*, Carb-an., *Carb-v.*, *Caps.*, Caust., Chin., Cist., Clem., Coc-c., Coff., Coloc., *Con.*, *Crot-h.*, Crot-t., Cupr., Dig., Dulc., Euph., Ferr-p., *Fl-ac.*, *Graph.*, Guaj., HEP., Hydr., Hyos., Ign., IOD., *Kali-bi.*, Kali-c., *Kali-i.*, Kali-n., Kali-p., Kali-s., Lac-c., LACH., *Led.*, Lob., Lyc., Mag-c., Mag-m., Mang., Mez., Mosch., Mur-ac., Nat-a., *Nat-c.*, NAT-M., *Nat-s.*, *Nit-ac.*, Nux-v., Orig., Petr., Podo., *Phos.*, Pho-ac., Plat., Plb., PSOR., *Pyrog.*, Rhodo., Ruta., Sars., Sec., *Sel.*, Seneg., SEP., SIL, Stann., *Staph.*, Stront., SULPH., Sul-ac., Tell., *Tarent.*, Ther., TUB., Vip., Zinc.

Full names of remedies corresponding to the above abbreviations will be found in Kent's Repertory.

Appendix "N"

Anti-Sycotic Remedies

Agar., *Alumn.*, *Alum.*, Amm-m., Anac., Ant-c., Ant-t., *Apis.*, Aran., *Arg.-m.*, *Arg-n.*, ARS., ARS-I., *Aster.*, Aur., *Aur-m.*, Aur-m-n., Bacill., Bar-c., Bar-m., Benz-ac., Berb., Bism., Bor., Brom., *Bry.*, Bufo., CALC-AR., CALC., Calc-p., Canth., Carb-an., Carb-s., Carb-v., Cast., *Caust.*, Cedr., Cham., Chrys., Cimic., Cinnb., Clem., Cocc., Colch., Cop., *Dulc.*, Euphr., *Ferr.*, *Fl-ac.*, Gels., *Graph.*, Hep., IOD., *Kali-bi.*, *Kali-c.*, *Kali-i.*, KALI-S., *Lach.*, Lith-c., *Lyc.*, Mag-c., Mag-m., Mag-p., *Mang.*, MEDOR., Merc., *Mez.*, MUR-AC., Nat-ar., Nat-c., NAT-M., NAT-S., NIT-AC., Petr., Pertus., Phyt., PHOS., PH-AC., Plan., *Plat.*, *Psor.*, Puls., PYROG., Sabin., *Sars.*, *Sec.*, *Selen.*, SEP., SIL., *Staph.*, Stront., Sul-i., *Sulph.*, Tell., THUJ., TUB.

Appendix "O"

Anti-Syphilitic Remedies

Aethiops., Anac., Ant-c., Arg-m., Arg-n., *Ars.*, ARS-I., *Ars-s-f.*, Asaf., Aur-i., AUR., AUR-M., AUR-M-n., Bad., Bapt., Benz-ac., Berb-acq., *Calc.-ar.*, Calc-f., *Calc-i., Calc-s.*, *Carb-an.*, Carb-s., Carb-v., Cinnb., Clem., *Con., Cor-r.*, Coryd., Crot-h., Echin., Fl-ac., Gels., Guaj., Guaco., Hecla., *Hep., Iod.*, Jac., *Kali-ar., Kali-bi., Kali-c.,* KALI-I., *Kali-m.*, KALI-S., Kreos., LACH., LYC., MERC-AUR., MERC-C., MERC-D., MERC-I.F., MERC-I-R., MERC., Mez., Mur-ac., *Nit-ac., Petr., Phos., Ph-ac., Phyt.*, Plat., Psor., Rhus-g., *Sars.*, Sec., *Sil., Staph.*, Still., *Sulph.*, Sul-ac., *Sul-i., Syph., Thu., Tub.*

Appendix "P"

Anti-Pseudo-Psora (Tubercular)

Acet-ac., Aesc., Agar., Ambr., Amm-c., Amm-m., *Ang.*, Apis., *Arg-m.*, Ars., *Ars-i.*, Asaf., Aur-ars., BACILL., Bell., Berb., Bor., Brom., *Bry.*, CALC-AR., CALC., Calc-f., *Cal-hypop.*, Calc-i., Calc-p., Carb-s., *Carb-v.*, Caust., Chel., *Chin.*, Chin-ar., Coca., Cocc., Con., Cupr., *Dros.*, Ferr-ar., *Ferr.*, Graph., Guaj., Ham., Helon., Hep., *Iod.*, Ip., Kali-bi., KALI-C., Kali-i., Kali-n., *Kreos.*, Lac-d., Lach., Lachn., *Led.*, Lil-t., *Lyc., Mang.*, Merc., Mez., Mill., Mur-ac., Myos., Myrt-c., Nat-ar., Nat-c., Nat-m., Nux-v., Oleum-j., Petr., *Phos-ac.*, PHOS., Pineal-gland., Podo., Polyg., PULS., Ran-b., Sarrac., Salen., Seneg., Sep., *Sil.., Spong.,* Stann., *Sulph.*, Ther., Thyroid., TUB., Urea., Vanad., Yerba., Zinc.

References

Homoeopathic Pamphlet Series — Jain Publishing Co., Five in One — B. Jain Publishing Co.

Brief Study Course in Homoeopathy — Dr. Elizabeth Hubbard — B. Jain Publishing Co.

On the Comparative Value of Symptoms — R.G. Miller — B. Jain Publishing Co.

How to Use the Repertory — G.I. Bidwell — B. Jain Pub. Co.

Different Ways of Finding the Remedy — Tyler.

Pneumonias — Douglas M. Borland — B. Jain Pub.

A Comparison of the Chronic Miasms — Phylllis Speight.

Chronic Diseases — Its Cause and Cure — P.N. Banerjee — B. Jain Pub.

Accoucher's Emergency Manual — W.A. Yingling — B. Jain Publishers (P) Ltd.

Beginners Guide to Homoeopathy — T.S. Iyer — B. Jain Pub.

The Lesser Writings of Von Boenninghausen — B. Jain Pub.

New Remedies, Lesser Writings, etc. — J.T. Kent — B. Jain Pub.

The Principles and Art of Cure by Homoeopathy — H.A. Roberts — B. Jain Pub.

Chronic Miasms — J.H. Allen — B. Jain Pub.

Lectures on Homoeopathic Philosophy — J.T. Kent — B. Jain Pub. Co.

Organon of Medicine — Hahnemann-Commentary by B.K. Sarkar — M. Bhattacharya & Co.

Principles of Prescribing — K.N. Mathur — B. Jain Pub.

Fifty Reasons for being a Homoeopath — J.C. Burnett — B. Jain Pub.

Homoeopathy — An Explanation of its Principles by Sir John Weir — Roy & Co.

A Study of Kent's Repertory by M.L. Tyler — Roy & Co.

How Not to Do It M.L. Tyler — Roy & Co.

Different Approaches to Finding the Simillimum — J.N. Kanjilal — *Hahn. Gleanings*, March 1971.

Second Prescription — J.N. Kanjilal — Hahn. Gleanings, Feb. 1971.

Presidential Address, 18th All India Hom. Med. Cong. — Jugal Kishore — *Hahn., Gleanings*, Jan., 71.

The Potency Problem — P. Sankaran — Homoeopathic Medical Publishers, Santacruz, Bombay, 54.

Homoeopathy, a Science of Drug Therapy by Sir John Weir — *Homoeopathic Heritage*, July 1977.

The Influence of Drs. Hughes, Cooper and Burnett on Presentday Homoeopathy by John H. Clarke — *Homoeopathic Heritage*, July 1977.

The Finding of the Homoeopathic Remedy in Heart Conditions by H.A. Roberts — *Homoeopathic Heritage*, Oct. 1977.

The Chronic Miasms by Edward Whitmont — *Hom. Heritage*, Nov. 1977.

Law of Similia not only concerns Loncation, Sensation and Modalities, but also depth, pace and duration of Symptoms — J.N. Kanjilal; Editorial, *Hahn. Gleanings*, May 1978.

Management of Chronic Disease — J.N. Kanjilal, *Hahn. Gleanings*, Dec. 1971.

Homoeopathy in Acute Cases — Some Hints — A.R.A. Acharya; *Hahnemannian Gleanings* Dec. 1974.

References

Diet and Other Restrictions in Homoeopathy — V. Krishnamurthy Iyer — *Hahnemann Gleanings*, March, 1976.

Second Prescription, Syed Anwar Hossain — *Hahnemann Gleanings*, June, 1977.

Repetition of the Remedy — R. Gibson Miller — *Hahnemannian Gleanings*, Sept. 1974.

The Homoeopathic Aggravation — Dewan Harish Chand, *Hahnemannian Gleanings*, Jan. 1980.

Follow up of the Case — Dewan Harish Chand, (29th International Congress of Hom.) — *Hahnemann Gleanings*, April 1975.

Management of the Case — P. Sankaran — *Hahnemannian Gleanings*, April 1976.

The Science and Art of Prescribing — A. Pulford — *Hom. Heritage*, July 1979.

Nosodes — Guy Bukley Stearns — *Homoeopathic Heritage*, July, 1979

Homoeopathic Regimen — J.N. Kanjilal — *Hahnemannian Gleanings*, Feb. 1976.

Hahnemann's Doctrine of Psora in the Treatment of Diseases in Children — Wm. Boericke — *Hom. Heritage*, Oct. 1979.

Editorial reply to Readers on "Etiology, its importance" — S.P. Koppikar — *Hom. Heritage*, Oct. 1979.

Hahnemann's Conception of Psora, M.L. Tyler — *Hom. Heritage*, July 1980.

Hahnemann's Conception of Chronic Diseases — M.L. Tyler — *Hom. Heritage*, Aug. 1980.

Pyrogen — P.C. Majumdar — *Hom. Heritage*, Aug. 1980.

Modern Concept of Psora and its Implications in Medicine — S.P.Koppikar — (International Hom. Congress, 1980)

Carrying Hahnemann's Great Work Forward — M.L. Tyler — Hom. Heritage, Dec. 1980.

Chronic Expressions of Venereal Diseases and their Homoeopathic Treatment — Allen C. Neiswander — Hahn. Gleanings, July 1975.

Relationship of Remedies — S.P. Koppikar — Journal of Hom. Med. Apl.-June. 1962; Oct.-Dec. 1962; January, Mar., 1963.

The Administration of the Remedy — J.T. Kent — Indian Journal of Hom. — Nov. 1953.

Importance of Diagnosis in Hom. Practice — P. Sankaran — Ind. J. of Hom. — Nov., 1953.

The Unrecognised Use of Homoeopathy in Conventional Medicine — R.H. Savage, British Hom. Journal — April, 1980.

Experiences with Some Nosodes and Antidotes — N. P. Sukerkar — Journal of Hom. Medicine — July-Sept. 1963.

Poisons — Samuel Swan, — Hom. Heritage, 1980.

Clinical Verifications and Reflections — S.P. Koppikar — Harjeet & Co.

Repetition of Fifty Millesimal Potency — Brahmanand Prasad — Hahn. Gleanings, Feb. 1977.

Homoeopathic Philosophy in Chronic Diseases — Dwight Smith — B. Jain Pub.

Homoeotherapeutics and the Current Medical Scene — H.N. Williams — Lecture: National Centre for Instruction in Homoeopathy — Hahnemann Gleanings, Dec. 1977.

The Art of Symptoms Evaluation — Dr. P.S. Krishnamurthy — Hahnemann Gleanings, April 1976.

The Causes of Rise and Fall of Homoeopathy in the U.S.A. — J.H. Kanjilal — Editorial, Hahnemannian Gleanings, Oct. 1974.

References

Experiences with Some Nosodes & Antidotes — N.P. Sukerkar — Journal of Hom. Medicine, July-Sept. 1963.

Iatrogenic Disease — Editorial, Journal of Hom. Med. — Oct.-Dec. 1966.

The People of the Materia Medica World — F.E. Gladwin — National Hom.. Pharmacy, New Delhi.

Genius of Homoeopathy — Dr Stuart Close.

Use of Repertory — J.T. Kent and M. Tyler.

A Study Course in Homoeopathy — Phyllis Speight.

The Value and Use of Repertory in Clinical, and Clinical Research Work — An Aspect — By Sarabhai Kapadia.

Homoeopathy in Paediatrics — International Homoeopathic Congress, 1977 — Sarabhai Kapadia.

Posology — Indian Journal of Homoeopathic Medicine — Sarabhai Kapadia.

Pneumonias — Dr. Douglass M. Borland.

BJAIN
serving Homeopathy since 1966

Another milestone in the history of BJAIN

BJAIN Pharmaceuticals (P) Ltd.

Base: Experience of working with Homeopathy for more than 40 years.
Aim: To provide high quality homeopathic medicines.

Key Features

- GMP certified, state of the art manufacturing unit
- Medicines prepared as per strict guidelines of Homeopathic Pharmacopeia
- As per International Standard names of quality and purity